Spatial Representation

Oxford Series in Developmental Cognitive Neuroscience

Series Editor
Mark H. Johnson, Centre for Brain and Cognitive Development,
Birkbeck College, University of London, UK

Attention, Genes, and Development
Kim Cornish and John Wilding

Neuroconstructivism, Volume One: How the Brain Constructs Cognition
Denis Mareschal, Mark H. Johnson, Sylvain Sirois, Michael W. Spratling,
Michael S.C. Thomas, and Gert Westermann

Neuroconstructivism, Volume Two: Perspectives and Prospects
Edited by Denis Mareschal, Sylvain Sirois, Gert Westermann, and
Mark H. Johnson

Toward a Unified Theory of Development: Connectionism and Dynamic Systems Theory Re-Considered
Edited by John P. Spencer, Michael S. C. Thomas, and
James L. McClelland

Spatial Representation: From Gene to Mind
Barbara Landau and James E. Hoffman

Spatial Representation

From Gene to Mind

BARBARA LANDAU
JAMES E. HOFFMAN

OXFORD
UNIVERSITY PRESS

OXFORD
UNIVERSITY PRESS

Oxford University Press is a department of the University of Oxford. It furthers the University's objective of excellence in research, scholarship, and education by publishing worldwide.

Oxford New York
Auckland Cape Town Dar es Salaam Hong Kong Karachi
Kuala Lumpur Madrid Melbourne Mexico City Nairobi
New Delhi Shanghai Taipei Toronto

With offices in
Argentina Austria Brazil Chile Czech Republic France Greece
Guatemala Hungary Italy Japan Poland Portugal Singapore
South Korea Switzerland Thailand Turkey Ukraine Vietnam

Published in the United States of America by
Oxford University Press
198 Madison Avenue, New York, NY 10016

Library of Congress Cataloging-in-Publication Data

Landau, Barbara, 1949-
Spatial representation: from gene to mind / Barbara Landau, James E. Hoffman.
p. cm.
Includes bibliographical references and index.
ISBN 978-0-19-538537-3 (pbk. : alk. paper)
1. Williams syndrome. 2. Cognition disorders. I. Hoffman, James E. II. Title.
RJ506.W44L36 2012
618.928—dc23
2012011723

9 8 7 6 5 4 3 2 1
Printed in the United States of America
on acid-free paper

To Robert, Matthew, and Simon
without whom, nothing

and

To Lou

Contents

Preface

This project began around 1993, with news from a colleague that Ursula Bellugi had just described a fascinating cognitive profile resulting from an unusual genetic deficit. People with Williams syndrome were described as highly verbal and fluent, but also severely impaired at even the simplest spatial tasks, suggesting a clean dissociation between space and language due to missing genes. The idea that a genetic syndrome might result in destruction of one cognitive system with no effect on the other was fascinating to the communities of cognitive scientists, neuroscientists, and linguists interested in the biological basis of cognition. As with other genetic deficits, such as FOXP2, Down syndrome, or autism, Williams syndrome seemed to be a perfect case to study the role of genes in human cognition. For us, Williams syndrome also offered a unique opportunity to gain special insight into the nature of spatial representation and how it might develop under genetic deficit, the nature of language under such deficit, and the relationship between the two systems: If people with WS had severely impaired spatial understanding, but unimpaired language, what would the result be for spatial language?

Several years after hearing about WS, we began to think in earnest about studying this population. The conversation began in the hallways and in our offices; Barbara had begun to collect data from a few young children with WS, and Jim was interested enough to listen and comment,

As time went on, experiments were proposed, data were gathered, conversations became deeper and broader, and the project grew. The collaboration was in many ways ideal, with each of us having complementary scientific interests and strengths—one of us a cognitive scientist specializing in space, language, and development, and the other a vision scientist specializing in spatial attention and its underlying mechanisms.

As often happens in science, the questions we thought we were pursuing were not necessarily the ones we ended up answering. Initially, we wanted to know why people with WS were so impaired at what seemed to be a very simple spatial task—the block construction task, in which people must assemble blocks to copy an existing design. Our goal at that point was just to understand this aspect of spatial cognition. It seemed like it would be quite tractable, especially given our sophisticated experimental techniques. One of us even claimed that we would have this "understood and wrapped up" after a few well-chosen experiments.

We decided to start by setting up a computerized version of the block construction task in which we could observe not only the final copy people made, but each step of their solution, by measuring both where people moved blocks and where they looked as they did so. This first study was an eye-opener. We observed children with Williams syndrome around age 11 and normally developing children of around age 5 or 6 purposively solving the copy tasks, using many of the same cognitive strategies—they looked at the model, picked up a block, placed it in the copy, repeated the cycle, and checked back and forth between their copy and model as they went along. But strikingly, the end copies were vastly different in the two groups. The children with WS made many mistakes, selecting the wrong blocks and placing them in the wrong locations. When they noted that they had made a mistake, they conscientiously removed an offending block—sometimes all offending blocks—and started over. Remarkably, they then proceeded to make the same kinds of errors as they had on the first round. Normally developing children, who were matched for mental age and were considerably younger, performed much better. Although they, too, made mistakes and restarted the process, the number of mistakes was much lower, and therefore fewer tries were required; and when there were new tries, they more often resulted in success. Thinking about what was going on in the block construction task—and especially understanding how complex this task really is—led us to recognize that understanding the spatial disorder in Williams syndrome would not be wrapped up in a few experiments, but, rather, would be a large and complex undertaking.

Ensuing phases of the project took us more broadly into many more aspects of spatial representation than either of us had anticipated. Although Bellugi had pointed to "peaks and valleys" in WS spatial cognition, we found, as we thought through the conceptual structure of the block construction task, that any investigation of spatial impairment would have to cover a broad range of spatial functions, each one with its own unique cognitive structure and function. Doing so would allow us to determine whether the impairment was restricted to certain spatial functions or was ubiquitous. We also realized that we would need to move beyond the typical model of research in developmental abnormalities, which relies on comparing abnormal populations with normally developing people who are matched for either chronological age and/or mental age—a roughly derived measure of intelligence for age. Rather, we recognized that no simple "control" group would really be the right match, and that examining the nature of spatial representation and language in people with WS would require using the developmental trajectory for normally developing children as the benchmark against which we could evaluate the WS deficit. Thus the studies grew by including more areas of spatial representation; but they also grew by including a wider normal age range—required to generate a fuller normal developmental timetable for different kinds of spatial representation. Our theoretical goals became clarified: Understanding Williams syndrome required understanding normal development, and vice versa. As with many "experiments of nature," the study of WS could also shed unique light on the nature of normal spatial development.

We decided to examine object representation, which clearly is a spatial function, but had never been observed to be impaired in WS. We studied biological motion perception, motion coherence, and form-from-motion—each of which requires the processing of individual elements forming a whole. We studied basic visual processes such as perception of illusions and the discrimination and integration of orientation elements. We examined multiple object tracking as a way to understand this special function of spatial attention. We looked at vision for action in simple tasks such as reaching and grasping. We studied subitizing and some basic numerical functions. We carried out studies of navigation, especially reorientation. We examined and reexamined the nature of copying. And we studied the use of spatial representation in a completely separate function—spatial language.

Across all of these studies, we began to see a pattern: It wasn't that space was impaired and language spared in people with WS. Rather, each different cognitive function—across space and language, and within each domain—had a unique normal developmental timetable. In normally developing children, some of these functions emerged early in development and by age 3 or 4, were at or close to maturity. Other functions underwent quite protracted normal developmental timetables, not reaching maturity until adolescence or beyond. The WS profile looked as if it grew with these same constraints, but at a much slower rate, ultimately undergoing arrest, with no further development.

Coming to this conclusion took a village—one that underwent considerable change over the roughly 15 years of the project. During this time, we were extremely fortunate to have many wonderful graduate students and postdoctoral fellows taking on pieces of the project; these young scientists worked on the project with enthusiasm, intelligence, and a passion for understanding not only Williams syndrome, but the nature of normal development. Included in this group are Banchi Dessalegn (JHU), Danny Dilks (UD/JHU), Matt Doran (UD), Katrina Ferrara (JHU), Emma Gregory (JHU), Heather Jordan (UD), Laura Lakusta (JHU), Kirsten O'Hearn (JHU), Barney Pagani (UD), Melanie Palomares (JHU), Jay Reiss (UD), and Andrea Zukowski (UD). Each of these people contributed enormously to the project as they started their careers. Over the years, as people finished their Ph.D.s or postdoctoral fellowships, they moved on to independent scientific careers; all are flourishing. It is an understatement to say that we are proud to have worked with each of these people.

Also crucial to the project over the years have been the outstanding lab managers who worked tirelessly to recruit and help design materials and test our participants, coordinate the numerous studies going on at any one point in time, and provide general support for the many aspects of the project. These lab managers include Megan Chen, Gitana Chunyo, Molly Dillon, Kate Kelliher, Whitney Street, and Andrea Zukowski. Not only did they each bring special skills to the project—ranging from theoretical linguistics to graphic arts—they were unfailingly of good cheer, amazing intellect, and dedication. Special thanks go to each of these remarkable people. Andrea Zukowski was our first lab manager, brilliantly coordinating all of our studies while simultaneously working on her dissertation in linguistics and then moving on to an academic research position in linguistics. Gitana Chunyo managed the first JHU lab, setting up our eye trackers and working on syntax and semantics in WS before moving to the Czech Republic to teach. Whitney Street was able to manage the project at its most complex time while simultaneously knitting scarves, hats, and cell phone holders in her spare time before moving on to graduate school in psychology. Megan Chen then took over and held the fort, tying up loose ends and ably assisting with new studies before moving on to graduate school in public health. Molly Dillon came to the project as the book was being written, and took on the daunting task of creating the complete set of figures in the book. Her creativity, thoughtfulness, patience, and extreme graphic arts skills were evident as she worked through a year of creating, editing, coloring, texturizing, and sometimes even trashing figures for better ones, before she, too, moved on to graduate school in psychology. Kate Kelliher is in charge today, ably handling the many details required to get our book out the door.

We have been very fortunate to have great colleagues, many of whom have shared our fascination with Williams syndrome and the research that has helped us understand the syndrome and its relationship to normal development. Over the years, we naturally engaged many of them in discussion and debate about the nature of language and spatial representation, their brain and cognitive bases. They include Susan Courtney, Howard Egeth, Lisa Feigenson, Jon Flombaum, Apostolos Georgopoulos, Justin Halberda, Helene Intraub, Mike McCloskey, Julien Musolino, Brenda Rapp, Amy Shelton, and Takashi Yoshioka. Other JHU collaborators who allowed us to work with them on issues of brain structure include Andreia Faria and Susumu Mori. Several colleagues from the community of WS scientists provided key support in the early phases of the project, by helping us establish connections with WS groups, helping us to understand some of the key characteristics of the population, and/or simply giving us a "reality check" with respect to what kinds of experimental procedures might or might not work. These include Paige

Kaplan, Carolyn Mervis, and Helen Tager-Flusberg. Finally, several colleagues read portions of the manuscript; we are especially indebted to Lucy Osborne for her careful reading of Chapter 2, and Julien Musolino for his reading of Chapter 6.

We consider ourselves extremely fortunate to have received continual funding for the WS project. We are grateful to the following organizations for this support: The March of Dimes Foundation (Grants 12 FY0446, 12 FY0187, and 12 F 0194 to BL), the National Science Foundation (Grants SBR-9808585 and BCS 0117744 to BL and JEH), and the National Institutes of Health (1R55 NS37923 and NINDS RO1 050876 to BL and JEH). The Johns Hopkins University School of Medicine General Clinical Research Center provided funding for studies of brain structure and function in WS (M01-RR00052 to BL). Finally, the John Simon Guggenheim Memorial Foundation and the Krieger School of Arts and Sciences of the Johns Hopkins University provided support for Landau's sabbatical year, during which she was able to dedicate herself full time to work on this book.

We have already noted that it took a village to carry out this project. But the village goes far beyond those colleagues and collaborators whom we have already acknowledged. The most important contributors, by far, have been the participants with Williams syndrome and their families, who have always made time in their busy schedules to visit with us in our lab over the years. These visits have always been an occasion for good cheer: Our participants are unfailingly upbeat and happy to be with us, wonderfully cooperative, and generally a delight for us to host. Similarly, their families have always shown a cheerful and upbeat attitude about the visits and a deep interest in the science of what we are doing and why. Many of the WS participants and their families have become our friends; we enjoy catching up with them on family events, successes in the Special Olympics, the challenges of making sure that children with WS are provided with appropriate schooling, the stresses of raising adolescents, college courses to be planned and taken, and so on. Many of our families are involved in the Williams Syndrome Association, and we would also like to especially note this remarkable organization of families with WS. Their active pursuit and support of scientific study of people with WS has made our research possible. Over the years, the WSA has facilitated our research by connecting us with potential participant families, and by hosting our research at their biennial conference. To both the WSA organization and our participants and families, we gratefully acknowledge their hard work, their enthusiasm for our research, and their unflagging dedication to understanding as much as they possibly can about Williams syndrome. We hope that the results of our project will ultimately make a difference for these people.

Barbara Landau, Johns Hopkins University, Baltimore, MD
James E. Hoffman, University of Delaware, Newark, DE
December 2011

I

The Puzzle of Williams Syndrome

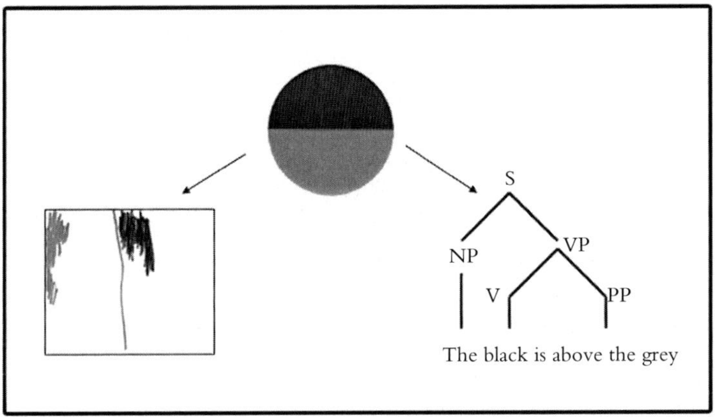

Our experience of the spatial world is seamless. We look around and see a unified layout in which objects occupy positions relative to each other and move along coherent spatial paths. We ourselves are part of this layout, and many of our everyday activities involve negotiating the space around us. These negotiations depend on our representations of space—the ways that our mind and brain encode, store and use spatial information about the world. When we get dressed in the morning we know how to find our clothes, how to insert which body parts into which openings, and how the parts of the clothing need to be fitted together by buttoning or zipping. Eating breakfast engages yet another set of skills that depends on our knowledge of space: We know how to use forks and cups to eat and drink, pushing food onto the fork and tipping the cup at the proper angle with skill. As the day moves on, we navigate the spaces of home, school, work, using well-known routes and easily taking detours if the hallway is blocked or the bridge is out.

Much of our spatial understanding likely shares its foundation with other species. But there is one additional capacity that is held by humans alone: We have language. This capacity allows us to talk about our thoughts and experiences, both spatial and nonspatial. Like our spatial knowledge, language is produced and understood in seamless fashion, allowing us to convert thoughts into sentences—formal structures of exquisite complexity. The reach of language is so broad that it can express virtually any meaning that a human being can conceive of, including, of course, meanings expressing aspects of our spatial experience.

These two systems of knowledge—space and language—arguably form two of the most important systems of human understanding. Both are systems of remarkable complexity—so complex that no machine can yet recognize objects, navigate through space, or talk and understand a simple conversation as well as a child. Both systems are broad and deep, spanning virtually every aspect of our daily lives and representing the most foundational aspects of human experience. Both systems come to us naturally—they develop early in life without formal tutoring and are used effortlessly and unconsciously.

It seems easy to imagine that these two systems have evolved under the control of the roughly 20,000 protein-coding genes in the human genome (see Clamp et al., 2007, for a recent estimate). A more surprising possibility is that the two systems might be under the control of different sets of genes—genes that target cognitive systems such that a deficit or change in one or more genes could cause a change in one system but not the other. Yet this is precisely the possibility that was presented to cognitive scientists several decades ago when they learned of the unusual case of people with Williams syndrome—a relatively rare genetic deficit in which roughly 25 genes are missing on chromosome 7, leading to a cognitive profile that includes severely impaired spatial understanding together with striking strength in language. People with Williams syndrome are verbally fluent, producing and understanding well-formed sentences that convey coherent meanings through appropriate linguistic devices provided by their native language. But, as the image at the opening of our chapter shows, a person with Williams syndrome cannot copy a simple figure better than an average 4- or 5-year-old child; he can also have difficulty tying his shoes, and is likely to be severely impaired in some navigation tasks.

Could this syndrome represent a clear and simple case of a link between genes and cognition? Could the absence of roughly 25 genes on one chromosome cause the derailment of one major system of knowledge while leaving another intact? If so, what could be the developmental mechanisms by which a genetic change could selectively affect specific cognitive systems?

This book is about the possibility that a genetic deficit can selectively affect certain systems of knowledge but not others, and how that selective developmental deficit might come about. We focus on spatial representations as a case study, and closely consider how one would dissect the human spatial representational system to determine whether and how selective damage could occur. Although language will not be the focus of our book, we will eventually need to consider what the linguistic system is like in people with Williams syndrome, since the contrast between language and spatial representation is one of the oft-cited hallmarks of this syndrome. As it will turn out, the explanation for the spatial-cognitive profile of people with WS may account not only for the severe deficit in the spatial domain, but also the observed strength in language. Moreover, we will propose that the same principles that help explain this unusual profile will be important in explaining normal development—that is, principles of normal spatial-cognitive development are required to understand unusual development.

In the remainder of this chapter, we set up a framework for examining the nature of the spatial deficit in people with Williams syndrome, and how this fits with the profile for the same capacities in normally developing children. This framework requires three steps. First, we lay out the striking hallmark characteristics of the cognitive profile in people with WS including observations on the spatial deficit and the strength in language. Next, we turn to the "puzzle" of Williams syndrome—how a genetic deficit could lead to such an unusual cognitive profile. In this section, we first explore the question of how we should think about the relationship between genes and cognition, emphasizing the importance of the cognitive end of the equation. We then flesh out the discussion by considering the cognitive domain that is the main topic of our book—the nature of human spatial representation—focusing especially on normal cognitive architecture in this domain, and the ramifications of this architecture for potential patterns of breakdown in people with WS. We also raise the crucial role of development in any attempt to understand how a genetic deficit could result in profound spatial impairment. Finally, we present our approach to thinking about how spatial-cognitive impairment could be produced by genetic change.

1.1 Hallmarks of the WS Cognitive Profile

Some of the earliest observations on people with WS suggested that this syndrome could represent a straightforward case in which the absence of roughly 25 genes causes severe deficits in the spatial system while leaving language completely untouched. Such a case would constitute a dramatic example of how a small set of genes could fairly directly be responsible for the development of a complete knowledge system. As an example, Ursula Bellugi and colleagues, who provided many of the observations picked up by the cognitive science community, noted "a marked dissociation between linguistic and spatial cognition in WMS" (1994, p. 36). This "dramatic dissociation" was illustrated by the case of an 18-year-old with an IQ of 49, who was asked to both draw and describe an elephant. The results are shown in Figure 1.1.

Contrast between visuo-spatial and language
abilities in Williams syndrome

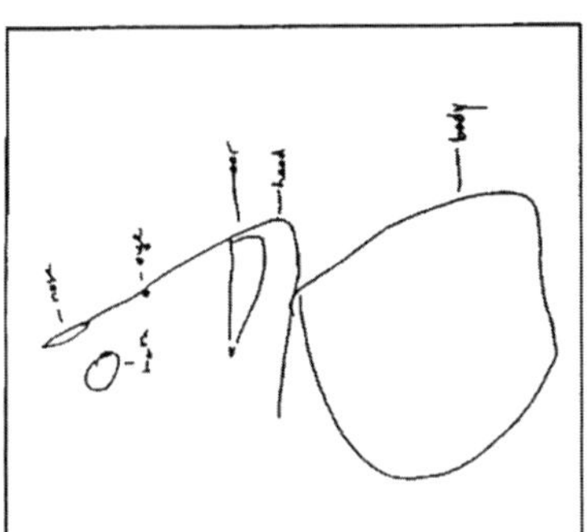

And what an elephant is, it is one of the animals. And what the elephant does, it lives in the jungle. It can also live in the zoo. And what it has, it has long gray ears, fan ears, ears that can blow in the wind. It has a long trunk that can pick up grass, or pick up hay.... if they're in a bad mood it can be terrible... if the elephant gets mad it could stomp; It could charge, like a bull can charge, they have long big tusks. They can damage a car... It could be dangerous. When they're in a pinch, when they're in a bad mood it can be terrible. You don't want an elephant as a pet. You want a cat or a dog or a bird....

Figure 1.1. Bellugi's sample comparison of drawing and language in a person with Williams syndrome, age 18, IQ of 49 (Bellugi, Wang, & Jernigan, 1994). The person was asked to draw an elephant and separately, to tell what an elephant is. Reprinted from Bellugi, Wang, and Jernigan (1994), with permission of Lawrence Erlbaum Associates.

As Bellugi et al. observed, the drawing by itself would be unrecognizable without some of the language that accompanies it, but the young man's linguistic description is quite fluent, informative, and well formed both in terms of meaning and form. Moreover, the contrast between the drawing and the linguistic description is even more marked when one factors in the person's IQ—which was 49. How could a person with this IQ produce such a deficient drawing? How could a person with an IQ of 49 produce such a complex and articulate linguistic description? And how could a deficit in the person's genome cause this unusual cognitive profile?

The central components of the Williams syndrome cognitive profile have been borne out in many studies: People with WS do, indeed, have scores on standardized IQ tests that fall in the category "mild-moderate" retardation. People with WS do, indeed, have severe deficits in certain classes of spatial tasks. They have severe problems in drawing objects from memory (as in the example shown in Figure 1.1); they also have severe problems in copying figures that are perceptually present. And people with WS are indeed verbally fluent and engage even quite complex linguistic structures when they speak and understand others.

To provide some concrete examples of the spatial impairment observed in copying tasks, consider Figure 1.2, which displays simple figures copied by two 11-year-old children with WS who visited our lab over the years. The target figures are presented at the top of the panel, and the copies are shown in the two panels below. When asked to copy these figures, these individuals were offered colored pens and shown the target figure adjacent to a blank page, on which they were to copy it. As is clear from the copies, the colors are perfectly preserved, as are many of the elements of the model figures. Just as obvious is the lack of spatial organization of the elements that make up the overall model figure.

Strikingly, several of the WS copies show a clear sensitivity to geometric elements of the model—several show a clear line separating the blue and red regions; another shows each of the colored elements of the model with their appropriate textures. But in both cases, the elements are misarranged—the blue and red halves are separated by a vertical line (not a horizontal one), and the textured/colored elements are placed in separate groupings, but the groups themselves are arranged in a close to haphazard fashion. One immediately wonders: Do these people know

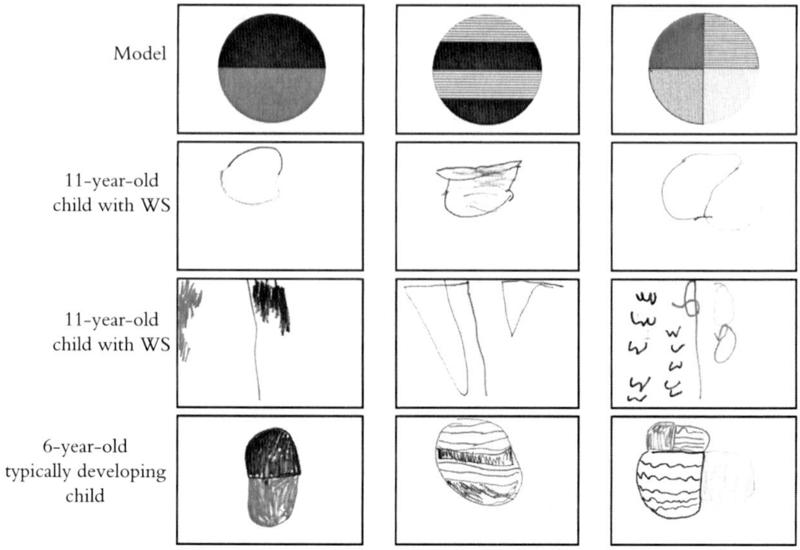

Figure 1.2. Copies of target models by two children with WS and one typically developing child who were seen in our lab. The models were visually present while the children made their copies. Reprinted from Dilks, Hoffman, and Landau (2008), with permission of John Wiley and Sons. (*See* color insert.)

that they are performing poorly on this task? Do they know that their drawings are not good representations of the model? The answer is emphatically yes: Especially for older children, adolescents, and adults, people with WS often voice concern as they carry out their copy, telling us that they know they are "not good at this kind of thing." Perhaps more striking, when we asked several children to "describe the (model) to your mother," we hear answers such as "Well, it's a circle split in half with blue on top and red on the bottom." Clearly, the linguistic description fits the model quite well, and without the evidence from copying, one wouldn't necessarily suspect that the person was incapable of copying the pattern.

Block construction tasks offer similar evidence. These tasks—widely included in standardized IQ tests including the Wechsler Adult Intelligence Scale (WAIS) and the Differential Abilities Scale (DAS; Elliott, 1990)—require people to duplicate a target pattern that is composed of multiple blocks, by using replicas of the individual blocks. Figure 1.3 shows three

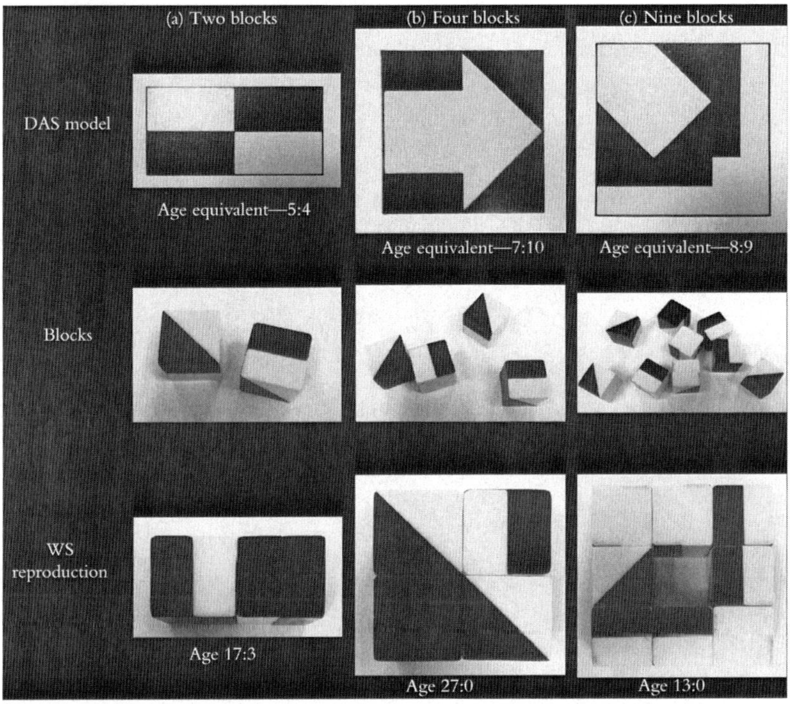

Figure 1.3. Representative model patterns from the Differential Abilities Scale (Elliott, 1990), and sample copies by people with WS tested in our lab. The top row displays the model shown to the participant. Age equivalents represent the 50th percentile for normally developing children. The middle row shows the blocks given to the person, in order to copy the model. All blocks have the same six sides, including vertical, horizontal, and diagonal splits over two colors. The bottom row shows three illustrative copies produced by people with WS, along with their chronological ages. Note that in all cases, there is severe compromise in the accuracy of the copies, even though the chronological ages for the WS participants are far higher than the age equivalent for normally developing individuals. (*See* color insert.)

versions of the task: one simple (two-block), one moderately complex (four-block), and one quite complex version (nine-block).

In the two-block version (a), the model pattern contains two blocks, each split in half by color. The person's task is to use the set of two blocks provided to copy the pattern. Each block has six sides, each with a different pattern (e.g., one side solid yellow, another vertically split by color).

To copy the pattern, the person must first turn over each block until he finds a pattern that corresponds to the pattern on one of the model blocks. Having correctly identified the two component patterns (one on each block), he must arrange them correctly (usually on a table top). This item can typically be copied correctly by children between the ages of 5 and 6 (50th percentile for this item is 5 years, 4 months in the DAS). In the four-block version (b), the model is composed of four blocks, each with a distinct pattern. Again, the participant must find sides of the four available blocks that match the components of the model. When put together, the four blocks form a design in which the borders of the most salient aspect of the pattern—here, an arrow—violate the borders of the blocks themselves. The age at which 50% of children pass this item is 7 years, 10 months. In the nine-block version (c), the same processes hold and this type of item is not accurately copied by normally developing children until they are roughly 8–9 years old. The copies by people with WS, shown in Figure 1.3, indicate that they have severe difficulties copying the models accurately, and a pressing issue is to figure out what it is that causes them such difficulty. We return to this issue in detail later in the book, but for the time being, suffice it to say that people with Williams syndrome—even adults—suffer from severe deficits in these tasks; and this means that there is a severe deficit in some important aspect or aspects of their representation of the spatial world.

The story on language provides a compelling contrast. Earliest observations showed that—at least anecdotally—people with WS exhibit surprising fluency, range of vocabulary, and control over grammar, including both syntactic and semantic structures. Additional early evidence on language production and judgment tasks suggested that lexical and grammatical abilities of adolescents with WS are remarkably strong, especially in view of the other characteristics of their cognitive profile, such as their retardation (Bellugi & Marks, 1993; Bellugi et al., 1994). For example, Bellugi and colleagues (1994) tested people with WS on comprehension of sentences such as "The horse is chased by the man" and their completion of tag questions, such as "John and Mary like apples, (don't they?)." Both of these require considerable syntactic knowledge. Bellugi's participants performed at ceiling levels, indicating that—on an absolute scale—these syntactic structures could be computed with sufficient detail to produce and understand grammatical English sentences of some complexity. Bellugi and colleagues' early observations also suggested a strong vocabulary (1994). In particular they reported that, given the standardized Peabody Picture Vocabulary Test:

> WMS subjects were often able to correctly match a word to one of four possible pictures, even with advanced items such as "abrasive" "cooperation" and "solemn." . . . [T]he WMS subjects characteristically score above their mental age, while the (Down syndrome) DNS counterparts typically score below their mental age, accentuating the differences between the two groups. . . . When asked to name as many animals as they can in a minute, WMS subjects provide significantly more responses than DNS subjects do. . . . Whereas DNS responses are typically fewer, and more often involve perseverations or category errors (e.g. "horsie, dog, ice cream"), WMS responses are nearly all within category; moreover, they are peppered with unusual items such as "weasel," "newt," "salamander," "chihuahua" "ibex" and "yak." We have found that WMS adolescents give a larger number of uncommon responses than do control children who are matched on the number of common responses. (p. 12)

The observation of strength in the vocabulary has persisted in recent studies, although strength is greater in the concrete vocabulary than in relational terms such as spatial terms (e.g., "under," "over") or other comparatives (e.g., "bigger," "longer"; see Mervis & John, 2008). The observation of "unusual" vocabulary has been widely cited (e.g., Pinker, 1994); however, later, more well-controlled studies have shown that people with WS do not tend to produce more low frequency words as once thought (see Chapter 6 for discussion). In general, the vocabulary of people with WS does not contain an especially high proportion of unusual words, though again, it is striking to hear them use words such as "ibex" or "yak" when one knows that their standardized IQ is around 60 or 70. However, a number of other studies have since shown that people with WS do control some aspects of linguistic structure that are remarkably rich and subtle. For example, Zukowski (2009) reported that adolescents with WS could produce complex sentences with relative clauses (e.g., "Max is looking at the cow that the boy is pointing to") under appropriately felicitous conditions. Musolino, Chunyo, and Landau (2010) have shown that children and adults with WS can comprehend and respond correctly to the truth value of target sentences as complex as the following, shown along with the corresponding true situations in Figure 1.4:

(a) "The cat who meows will not be given a fish or milk" (true if the cat did not get either one).

(b) "The cat who does not meow will be given a fish or milk" (true if the cat got either one or the other).

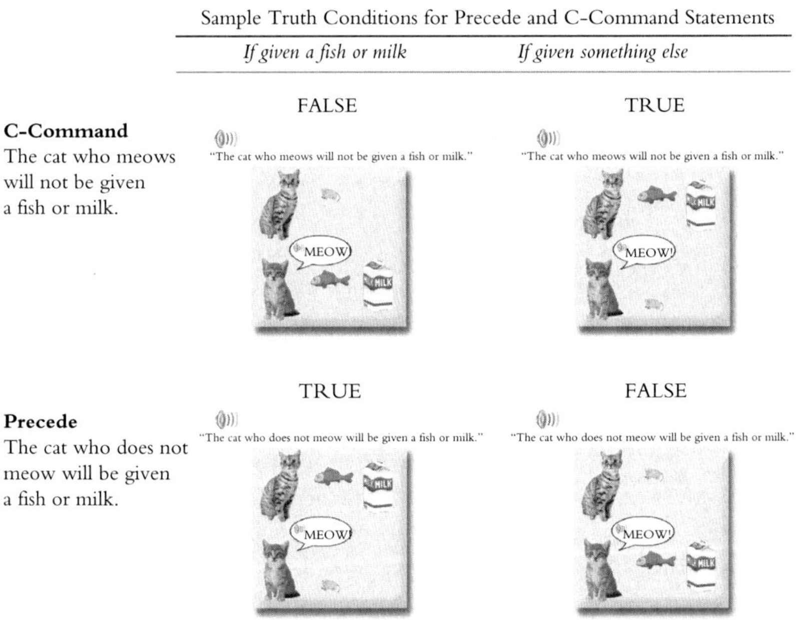

Figure 1.4. Complex sentences and their truth conditions. Adolescents with WS can comprehend the complex sentences shown at the left, and can judge them to be true or false under each condition shown. Note that even though the two sentences are superficially quite similar, the truth conditions vary depending on the hierarchical relationship between the "not" and the "or"; technically, the difference between a relationship of "C-command" versus "Precede." Processing complex sentences such as these attests to the rich grammatical knowledge in people with WS. After Musolino, Chunyo, and Landau (2010); see Chapter 6 for discussion.

Understanding the difference between the two target sentences entails understanding that the combination of negation (not) and disjunction (or) gives rise to entailments that are different, depending on where in the syntactic structure the two elements occur (see Chapter 6 for discussion). The strong performance of people with WS in tasks such as these attests to the fact that their genetic deficit does not in any serious way derail the ability to learn and use complex and rich principles of syntax and semantics that are considered by modern linguists to be foundational to human knowledge of language.

These observations on the representation of space and language form the core of the puzzle of Williams syndrome: The cognitive profile appears to be strikingly "imbalanced," with knowledge of complex linguistic structure attested along with apparent failure to represent and/or deploy what would seem to be fairly basic aspects of spatial organization for a simple copying task. This profile appears in people who do not have frank neurological damage to the brain—imaging studies show an absence of clear lesions in people with WS—but the functional consequences of their genetic deficit include striking differences in the degree to which different cognitive systems are damaged. Clearly the absence of roughly 25 genes in some sense causes this cognitive profile. How is this possible?

In order to think about this problem, we now introduce three different issues.

- First, we consider what it might mean for genes to *cause* such a cognitive profile, asking how we should think about the relationship between genes and cognition. We will argue that genes (or the absence thereof) can indeed target cognitive systems, but that the causal chain between genes and cognition is extremely complex and indirect, making it crucial for us to choose a clear level of analysis as our focus. We will argue for the importance of *cognition* in understanding the WS spatial deficit.
- Second, we focus on theoretical models of spatial-cognitive architecture, and what they can tell us about the ways in which a cognitive system such as spatial representation might be organized such that a *damaged* system could lead to severe impairments in copying

and block construction tasks. We emphasize the importance of specialization of function within the broader cognitive architecture.

- Third, we argue that development—in particular, *normal* development—will play a crucial role in understanding how a cognitive system can emerge with such a characteristic profile. We will ask how we can compare the unusual cognitive profile of people with WS to the profile of nonaffected individuals, arguing that the comparative analysis of unusual and more typical cases of development provide complementary insights into the nature of spatial-cognitive architecture and its development.

Pursuing these three issues will provide a framework—or set of principles—for examining the spatial profile of people with Williams syndrome. We will use these principles to guide our presentation in the rest of the book, as we present evidence regarding the nature of spatial representation and its development. These principles will in turn allow us to construct a theory that explains how the spatial profile could possibly emerge from the absence of a small number of genes. In the end, we will argue that the explanation for the spatial profile can also account for the empirical facts about language in people with Williams syndrome.

1.2 Three Principles for Solving the Puzzle

We will argue shortly that understanding the spatial cognitive deficit in people with WS requires embracing three tenets: that there are indirect and complex causal chains between genes and cognition; that cognitive architecture is important in any theory of spatial representation and its breakdown; and that the role of development is crucial in understanding how unusual cognitive profiles might emerge under genetic change.

1.2.1 How Can Genes Cause Cognitive Deficits? Complexity of the Chain and the Importance of Cognition

In some sense, it is trivially true that the absence of genes in people with Williams syndrome *causes* the cognitive profile, including severe spatial impairment and preserved language. It is commonplace to hear that genes are implicated in the development and manifestation of structure, mechanism, and behavior. For example, we know that the gene for *Pax6* is crucial for the development of the vertebrate eye (Mathers, Grinberg, Mahon, & Jamrich, 1997); without the gene, the structural characteristics of the eye do not develop properly. Studies of twins have shown that human fingerprint ridge count has a heritability ratio of .97 (Bouchard et al., 1990); that is, almost all of the variance between members of identical twin pairs is accounted for by their genetic similarity. Increasingly, genetic variation is being linked to behavior, from the genetics of socially "outgoing" mice (Li et al., 2009) to the possibility that the severe deficits in autism may be linked to changes across multiple genes (Glessner et al., 2009). But there is a large leap from knowing that certain genes are missing to understanding how this genetic change might *cause* a specific cognitive deficit. So how should we approach the study of spatial deficit caused by a genetic disorder?

It is useful to start with an approach suggested by John Morton (2004), in his important book *Understanding Developmental Disorders: A Causal Modeling Approach*. Morton begins by asking us to think about the nature of explanation, and, in particular, how we can spell out the links in the causal chain for cognitive deficits. As an exercise, he asks us to consider what *caused* Romeo's death. He reports that people provide a variety of answers to this question, including the following: that Romeo's death was caused by Juliet's apparent death; that it was caused by an underlying depressive state that ran in his family; that it was the feud between their families; and that it was the slow mail service between Verona and Mantua (p. 6). He then considers two plausible hypotheses. The first is this:

(a) Romeo was killed by the poison that he took.

He points out that this hypothesis is certainly a reasonable one, and that it is scientifically acceptable in that it allows us to identify the gaps in the causal chain—which poison it was, how it operated on the body, how long it took, and so forth—that could potentially be filled by scientific study. But he also suggests that this hypothesis somehow misses the mark. While it is true that Romeo was killed by the poison that he took, it is unlikely that anyone would consider this a good causal account of his death.

Another hypothesis is at the other end of the spectrum:

(b) Romeo's genes caused him to commit suicide.

Morton suggests that even if we were to assume that suicides ran in Romeo's family and that suicide was heritable, this hypothesis would be deeply unsatisfying because the gaps in the causal chain are so large that they do not really explain why Romeo died. Clearly, the act of committing suicide is not coded in the genes, and to claim that this is an explanation is to miss the point that causal chains need to be well specified to be useful. Morton points out that what we really want is an explanation that spans neither too much nor too little space in the chain of events. A satisfying causal explanation will allow us to identify and describe the mechanistic and proximal steps between cause and effect; or, if we cannot do this, then at least to identify where in the chain we are missing information, and how we could in principle discover what belongs in the gap.

The same arguments apply to thinking about how genes might cause an unusual cognitive profile such as that characterizing Williams syndrome. If we simply say "Genes cause the profile," this is deeply unsatisfying. For one thing, it is trivially true; as it is true that genes—and their heritability—are in some way partially responsible for almost every aspect of our lives, including hair and eye color, fingerprint ridge count, and religiosity (Bouchard et al., 1990). In this sense, saying that the deficit is caused by missing genes is simply uninformative. At the other end of the spectrum, saying that genes cause the WS profile is unsatisfying because the gap between cause and cognition—and its manifestation in behavior—is so large as to lack any scientific utility.

The assumption that genes "target" cognitive systems is not an easy one, and cautionary tales abound. Although FOXP2 has been described as "the grammar gene" (Gopnik, 1990, Gopnik & Crago, 1991; see Pinker, 1994), we now know that damage to this gene causes a broad range of developmental deficits in humans beyond language and is also known to be present in nonhuman species that have no language. In fact, the mechanism by which this gene may affect language may be rooted in a quite general function of the brain such as complex motor control (Fisher, 2006; Vargha-Khadem et al., 2005). Similarly, although WS is characterized by a set of missing genes, and has severe spatial cognitive deficits as its hallmark, a range of other genetic and chromosomal deficits including Fragile X syndrome, Turner syndrome, and chromosome 22q11.2 deletion or velocardiofacial syndrome (Simon, 2007) also present with spatial deficits. Thus the link between a single gene or a cluster of genes and the final cognitive outcome is unlikely to be a one-to-one relationship (see Chapter 2 for review of some individual gene functions in the WS region of deletion). Still, there must be some causal chain that leads from genes to cognition and the question is how to use that fact in our science.

Once we understand the scientific limits of the simple statement that the absence of 25 genes causes the WS cognitive profile, we need to ask how to proceed. A number of writers have pointed out that fully understanding the effects of genes on cognition will require that we coordinate efforts focusing on two different ends of the causal chain. At the genetic end, we need to understand the role of genes, exactly what they do at the molecular levels, and how these molecular events begin the causal chain leading from genetic specification—including cases of deficit—to development of brain and mind. Understanding the genetic end of the equation is not the topic of this book, and indeed, we will have virtually nothing to say about this issue, except to review the critical candidate genes for WS and the limited speculation on their links to behavior (see Chapter 2).

At the other end of the causal chain is cognition, and it is this end that will be our focus. As Ramus (2006) discusses, the causal chain between genes and cognition is anchored in both ends; but the genetic analysis of any disorder "can only be as good as the characterization of the phenotype, and cognitive phenotyping is (or should be) in the hands of cognitive scientists" (p. 249). Making good on characterizing the cognitive phenotype is also Morton's (2004) emphasis, as he points out that understanding developmental deficits such as autism and dyslexia require substantive models of cognitive architecture that can make predictions about behavior based on damage to components of the cognitive system and/or their interactions.

So how should we think about the relationship between genes and cognitive deficits? The naive statement for the cases reviewed above—that there is a "gene *for* language" or a set of genes "*for*" dyslexia—can be questioned in part because they have been shown to be false (FOXP2) and in part because the distance between cause and effect is so large as to be a gap the size of a chasm (in Morton's terms). The same holds for the idea that among the missing genes in people with Williams syndrome, there is a gene or even a few genes "*for*" space. At the same time, the profile for Williams syndrome is in many ways qualitatively different from that of other syndromes. Indeed, the early work by Bellugi and colleagues showed repeatedly that there are clear differences in cognitive performance between people with WS and people with Down syndrome. Clearly, genes are in the causal chain for cognitive deficits—they just cannot, by themselves, *explain* the deficit.

What all this means is that the gene-to-cognition causal chain is likely to be enormously complex; at present it is vastly underspecified at many points. Progress can be made by being clear about exactly what part of the causal chain is being studied—and at what level of description—and by laying out the mechanisms involved as clearly as possible. Since we intend to focus on the cognitive end of the explanatory chain, it will be crucial to understand the mature organization of the target cognitive system. This means understanding the cognitive architecture of spatial representation in adults. Without this understanding, we would be unable to interpret any patterns of deficit among people with WS. Accordingly, we now turn to current evidence on the architecture of spatial representation, and its ramifications for understanding spatial impairment in people with WS.

1.2.2 The Cognitive Architecture of Space: The Importance of Specialization of Function

The seamless way in which we perceive, act on, manipulate, and talk about space underlies the naïve intuition that the core of human spatial knowledge is governed by a single unitary system of spatial representation. Such a global, unspecialized system would be consistent with the idea that the cognitive computations involved in any kind of spatial cognition should be largely equivalent. For example, there might be a single global mechanism that computes spatial relationships—whether they are needed to support our recognition of the spatial relationships within parts of an object, the landmarks and routes across a navigational arena, or the relationship between the hand and a tool that it will reach for, grasp, and use. The idea that there is a single system called "spatial cognition" is one that is implicitly accepted when we read of "deficits in spatial cognition" that are caused by brain damage to the adult brain, or by genetic or environmental insult to the developing brain. Developmental deficits such as Turner syndrome, Fragile X syndrome, or chromosome 22q11.2 deletion have been characterized in terms of spatial deficits, and sometimes in terms of brain areas that contribute to these functions, but there is little theoretical dissection of the spatial cognitive system to help us understand what aspects of spatial representation are in fact damaged (see Simon, 2007, for discussion). The idea of a general "spatial disorder" is also consistent with a general approach to cognition that emphasizes domain-general mechanisms of learning—mechanisms that could, for instance, guide the development of object recognition, visual-manual control, or spatial language equally well.

But many decades of research on spatial representation in normal and brain-damaged humans as well as other species challenge this approach. Rather than engaging a single monolithic system of spatial representation, human spatial understanding appears to be the product of multiple systems of representation, each of which is dedicated to representing a particular cognitive function or set of functions (Kanwisher, 2010; Milner & Goodale, 1995; Ungerleider & Mishkin, 1982). This specialization—or division of labor—within the broader system of spatial representation can be established in two different and complementary ways (see Figure 1.5).

First one can consider each spatial-cognitive domain in terms of the functions it must carry out, whether it be recognizing objects, faces, or places, carrying out visual-manual actions on objects, navigating through space, or talking about our spatial experiences. These different functions (among others) are distinguished by the kinds of computations that are carried out, and there is striking evidence that these distinct functions are associated with different regions of the brain (Burgess, 2008; Kanwisher, 2010; O'Keefe & Nadel, 1978; Palmeri & Gauthier, 2004; Reddy & Kanwisher, 2006). A second way of setting the division of labor is by considering a broader cut, grouping together regions that are part of the two major streams of visual processing in the brain—the ventral and dorsal streams. The ventral stream originates in primary visual cortex, and moves anteriorly and ventrally toward the temporal areas of

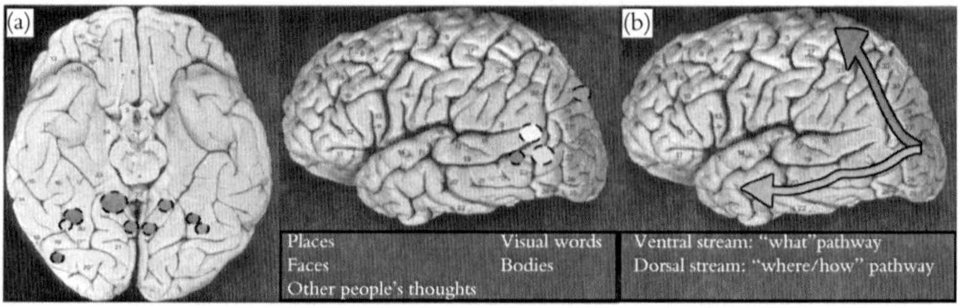

Figure 1.5. Two alternative organizations of the division of labor within spatial representations. One can consider a division of labor based on specific functional domains, such as representation of faces, places, and visual words (left and middle panel). Or one can consider a broader division of labor based on the two main pathways of the visual system (right panel), the ventral ("what") and dorsal ("where/how") pathways. Both organizations are useful in providing hypotheses about the spatial impairment in people with Williams syndrome. Figures adapted from Kanwisher (2010), with permission of PNAS. (*See* color insert.)

the brain; the dorsal stream also originates in primary visual cortex, but its path moves dorsally toward the parietal and sensorimotor areas. These two streams also have roots in even earlier parts of the visual system, with specialized cells in the retina. Both streams (and even possibly some further subdivision within the dorsal stream) have been established on the basis of anatomical and functional evidence, and provide a second way of thinking about specialization (Kravitz et al., 2011; Milner & Goodale, 1995; Ungerleider & Mishkin, 1982).

Regardless of which division of labor one considers, there are strong arguments and evidence supporting the idea that there are multiple specialized systems of spatial representation. One kind of argument is computational: The cognitive computations required to carry out different spatial "tasks"—or functions—vary considerably across the various domains. For example, object recognition appears to require computation of the object's features and/or parts and their spatial organization into an overall shape as well as its constancy over variation in viewpoint, size, lighting, and so on (see Palmeri & Gauthier, 2004, for review). These computations are sufficiently complex that machine models cannot yet accomplish object recognition as well as normal adults—for whom the process is both obligatory and is carried out extremely rapidly (Grill-Spector & Kanwisher, 2005). By contrast, the computations required to reorient oneself in a spatial layout appear to engage a geometric representation of the layout (Burgess, 2008; Cheng, 1986; Gallistel, 1990; Hermer & Spelke, 1996; O'Keefe & Nadel, 1978). The computations required to talk about space engage linguistic categories such as nouns and prepositions, and these map only loosely onto spatial categories derivable from nonlinguistic systems representing objects and layouts (Landau & Jackendoff, 1993; Talmy, 1983).

A second argument for specialization comes from empirical studies of adults who have sustained brain damage due to accident, stroke, tumor, and so on. Abundant evidence shows that damage to the normal adult brain can selectively damage different aspects of spatial representation. This functional decomposition of the broader spatial system has also been linked to the location of brain lesions. For example, adults with damage to the inferotemporal lobe can present with severe agnosia for objects, but individuals with object agnosia can have preserved ability to recognize faces (Farah, 2004; Moscovitch, Winocur, & Behrmann, 1997). Damage to the fusiform face area (FFA) area early in life can lead to developmental prosopagnosia—lifelong impairment in face perception (Farah, Rabinowitz, Quinn, & Liu, 2000); face and object perception can also be dissociated in individuals with developmental prosopagnosia (Duchaine & Nakayama, 2005). The ability to smoothly reach for and grasp common objects can be damaged independently of the ability to recognize objects, and vice versa, possibly reflecting the functional division of labor between the dorsal and ventral streams of the brain (Milner & Goodale, 1995). Topographical memory for spatial layouts is severely impaired in patients with damage to the hippocampus, although nonspatial processing is spared (Hartley, Bird, Chan, Cipolotti, Husain, Vargha-Khadem, & Burgess, 2007).

The results of such studies with adults who have sustained brain damage are consistent with recent imaging studies of the normal adult brain during tasks that tap different spatial functions. For example, distinct regions of the brain appear to be engaged when adults passively view faces, places, and bodies (Kanwisher, 2010); the first two regions are quite similar to those that have been identified through patient studies. Regions including the hippocampus, parahippocampal cortex, and entorhinal cortex areas are thought to underlie representation of environment layouts and navigation through them (Epstein & Kanwisher,

1998; Maguire et al., 2000), and these areas are engaged as people view movies that simulate their own movement through spatial layouts (Jacobs, Kahana, Ekstrom, Mollison, & Fried, 2010).

The principle of specialization also has consequences for how we think about both normal development and development under conditions of genetic deficit. The two different divisions of labor within the broader system of spatial representation again offer two broad possibilities for the case of Williams syndrome. The first is that, given selectivity in the mature mind/brain's representations of space, genetic developmental disorders such as WS might also present with patterns of impairment that cleave along the lines of normal cognitive architecture. Natural cleavage might be observed by impairment showing selectivity over domains (e.g., faces, not objects; navigation but not visual-manual action), or selectivity between streams of processing (e.g., dorsal impairment but not ventral stream impairment, or vice versa). The idea of domain selectivity is roughly consistent with the original hypothesis put forward by Bellugi et al. (1994) suggesting that spatial representations in people with WS are severely impaired but language is intact, and it is also consistent with work showing that some aspects of face processing in adults with WS are commensurate with age-matched controls (Tager-Flusberg et al., 2003), even though other spatial functions are severely impaired. The idea of selectivity along streams of processing has been suggested as an organizing principle for thinking about the normal development of spatial functions (Johnson, Mareschal, Csibra, 2008) as well as a possible explanation for the distinctive cognitive profile of people with WS (Atkinson et al., 2003; Wang, Doherty, Rourke, & Bellugi, 1995), a point we take up in more detail in Chapter 2.

But some have argued that even though the adult mind and brain have specialized spatial systems, the developing mind and brain need not. That is, the starting point for development may not embody specialization, and specificity in the mature brain may be largely a product of experience and development (Karmiloff-Smith, 1998, 2007). If this hypothesis were true, it would lead us to expect that genetic disorders in general—and WS in particular—could give rise to cognitive impairments that do not necessarily respect the lines of normal cognitive architecture. For example, spatial representations might cleave along lines that are quite different from those typically shown in a normally developing system, and spatial-cognitive performance in any particular domain might reflect different principles of organization than the normally developing child. Clearly, whether specialization is reflected in the developing system of people with WS is an empirical question, and one that we aim to address in this book. Concretely, we will ask whether the WS spatial deficit ranges quite generally over the various spatial subsystems, with a "flat" profile of equal compromise across the systems, or whether the impairment is highly selective, with "peaks and valleys" across different spatial functions. Crucially, we need to determine why any peaks and valleys exist—whether they are the product of normal or abnormal developmental processes.

Thinking about these possibilities highlights the fact that understanding unusual development will require that we also consider the role that development itself plays in producing the spatial impairment. A quite strong version of the specialization hypothesis would predict that the pattern of impairment typical of people with WS should echo the patterns that have been observed among adults who have sustained brain damage. But WS is a developmental disorder, and this requires that we understand how the spatial systems in question normally develop. As it turns out, the issue of development is itself complex, with ramifications for theories of normal spatial cognitive architecture, theories of its breakdown and impairment under genetic deficit in WS, and even for the straightforward empirical question of who should form our comparison groups. We now turn to these issues.

1.2.3 Timing Matters: The Importance of Normal Development

Williams syndrome is a genetic deficit that is identifiable at birth, through phenotypic characteristics and/or chromosomal analysis. Because the deficit is present at birth, the syndrome is, by definition, developmental in origin. The very fact that cognition unfolds over development means that any hypotheses about the nature of the spatial deficit will have to take into consideration aspects of developmental process. This point has been made eloquently by Annette Karmiloff-Smith (1998), who argues for the crucial role of *development* in our theories of cognition under genetic deficit.

There are two different views of why development matters. One is that development itself changes cognitive structure, and abnormal cases of development will inevitably engage different developmental processes, making comparison to normal development and the mature state an un-telling case of "apples and oranges." The second view is that normal development embodies change, and we cannot evaluate what we mean by developmental cognitive deficit unless we have a firm handle on what the normally developing spatial system looks like. We will discuss both views but endorse only the second.

The first view reflects a recent trend in the developmental literature that focuses strongly on the role that development plays in changing cognitive structure (Elman et al., 1996; Karmiloff-Smith, 2007). With this focus in mind, some have argued that we can never understand the nature of developmental cognitive deficits unless we examine the emerging cognitive profile (Karmiloff-Smith, 1998). For example, systems that appear modular in adults may not start out as modular, but could *become* modular over development, by continued application of the same cognitive processes to the same kinds of information. Karmiloff-Smith considers cases such as Williams syndrome, and argues that such a genetic deficit will inevitably result in a brain that has somewhat different organization from a normally developing brain. This altered brain structure will lead to altered mechanisms of learning and, ultimately, altered knowledge representations. The strong view predicts that these representations are qualitatively different from those emerging in the normally developing brain and mind. For example, on this view, the representations and processing of faces should be qualitatively different among people with WS, compared to normally developing individuals (Deruelle et al., 1999).

On this view, examining spatial impairment in Williams syndrome would be unlikely to shed much on normal spatial representations, simply because it will inevitably be the end product of abnormal developmental mechanisms, resulting in abnormal representations (Karmiloff-Smith, 1998). This view would also suggest that the mature model of spatial specialization we have described will not be a relevant target for investigation, since genetic abnormalities will inevitably alter the developmental mechanisms leading to brain and cognitive structure, resulting in qualitatively different brain structures, different mechanisms of learning, and, consequently, different cognitive end states. That is, spatial-cognitive systems produced through abnormal development should look quite different from systems produced under normal development.

The second view—which we endorse—is quite different. While we agree that studies of developmental deficits must engage discussion of development—and not prejudge representation solely by what is known from cases of adult brain damage—we also believe that there are extremely strong constraints on what a spatial representational system could look like. Indeed, we have so far argued that the normal mature systems of spatial representation are specialized, that is, they are characterized by different kinds of representations and computations required for different tasks, including object recognition, face recognition, visual-manual action, and navigation, among others. And these arguments have been based largely on evidence from the adult brain and mind. But we believe that the fact that damage to the mature brain quite often results in well-organized breakdown renders plausible the idea that the same might hold for cases of developmental impairment of genetic origin. This would be the case if spatial systems normally develop from origins that themselves embody strong constraints on their architecture—an idea embodied in the notion that there are "core" aspects of human knowledge, such as object, space, number, and social understanding, that emerge very early in development and under tight experiential constraints (Carey, 2009; Spelke, 2000). In this framework, one might predict that developmental impairments stemming from genetic deficits should—like cases of lesions to the adult brain—reflect breakdown or cleavage along the lines of a normally structured cognitive system. In the case of spatial representations, one would predict that the impairment should reflect the properties of normally structured spatial systems.

Distinguishing between these possibilities will not be easy, and much will depend on how we will determine whether the system in people with WS is similar to or different from the norm. But the two views do make different predictions. The strong view of difference would suggest that the abnormally developing system should be *qualitatively different* from the normal system. This would mean that the spatial systems should cleave along lines quite different from those in the normal system, and/or that they should exhibit patterns of performance and error types that suggest not just less efficient computations, but truly different ones. In contrast, the strong view of similarity suggests that there should be clear specialization of spatial systems, with any peaks and valleys reflecting the lines of normal architecture, including characteristic patterns of error or vulnerability.

Clearly, these are empirical questions, which we will address through detailed examination of overall performance as well as error patterns in the performance of people with WS compared to nonaffected people. We can do this in two ways. Looking *across* spatial systems, we can ask whether the peaks and valleys observed across these systems respect normal cognitive architecture—in terms of either content domains (e.g., objects, faces, navigation) or streams of processing (dorsal versus ventral stream functions). Does the impairment reflect a domain-oriented cleavage, or one that is better thought of as a stream-oriented breakdown? Looking *within* spatial systems, we can ask whether the structure of performance reflects *quantitative* or *qualitative* changes from a normal profile.

Importantly, our framework and its predictions for unusual development do *not* entail giving up the idea that development itself is important. In fact, as we now argue, examining developmental trajectories among normal individuals is a crucial part of understanding what the spatial deficit in WS is about, and by inference, how it might emerge.

Throughout our discussion, we have asked whether the spatial impairment in people with WS reflects the properties of *normal* cognitive architecture. But what we have not yet addressed is the question of how to make the appropriate comparisons. What is the correct control group? This turns out to be a crucial question in thinking about the WS spatial impairment.

Since the earliest research on cognition in people with WS, much research has been framed in terms of the complementary hypotheses of "sparing" and "deficit" across different cognitive domains. Indeed, the earliest theoretical descriptions of the WS cognitive profile embraced the possibility that this syndrome could be strong evidence for cognitive modularity, wherein one system (language) was "spared" while the other (space) was profoundly impaired (Bellugi et al., 1994). Since this time, many if not most studies of cognition in WS have been framed in terms of the possibility that parts of the cognitive system are "intact"—or not damaged—while other parts are severely damaged.

In its strongest form, a hypothesis of *sparing* or *intact* cognitive structure might predict that people with WS should perform both quantitatively and qualitatively the same as nonaffected people of the same chronological age—known as chronological age (CA) matches. The hypothesis of sparing thus appears to require that we use CA matches as our control group. But because one of the characteristics of the syndrome is mild to moderate retardation (Mervis et al., 2000), such a comparison will almost inevitably mean that the CA matches will have an overall IQ higher than the individuals with WS (though see Meyer-Lindenberg et al., 2006, for studies of WS individuals with IQs in the normal range). Thus the strategy of using a CA-matched group may be setting the bar inappropriately high. Clearly, if people with WS perform more poorly than their CA matches on one or more tasks, this could be due to mild retardation rather than to differences in the nature of the cognitive representation itself.

For this reason, researchers have often tried to control for the effects of retardation by matching WS individuals to nonaffected individuals on the basis of "mental age" (MA matches). In principle, determining who constitutes a MA match is neither simple nor straightforward, since it requires the dubious assumption that we actually understand what we mean by "mental age" (outside of the obvious psychometric meaning of score *X* at age *Y*). In practice, determining an MA match is usually done by establishing equivalent performance on a presumably independent control measure—usually a standardized IQ test. The resulting MA controls will often be chronologically younger than the WS individual with whom they are matched, and they will likely have a higher overall IQ (since this is a function of one's score relative to one's chronological age).

Although the most common approach in the scientific literature is to match using either CA and/or MA control groups, there is a serious theoretical question of whether matching of either kind will provide a telling comparison. On the one hand, matching on the basis of CA assumes that one system can be completely intact, including its core representations and computations *along with* all of the more general cognitive mechanisms that must generally be engaged in carrying out any cognitive task—working memory, attention, vigilance, and so on. This is a questionable assumption, especially since mental retardation surely reflects some general effects on mental processing. If our interest is in the structure of knowledge representations, we would want to factor out any consequences of poor working memory or general attention. On the other hand, matching on the basis of "mental age" makes little sense, given that we know precious little about what either overall IQ or mental age actually measures. Even when scientists use more refined measures to match groups—for example, an overall language measure to match if one is testing some aspect of language, a general visual-spatial measure to match if one is testing some aspect of spatial processing—this still presents us with the problem that we do not necessarily know which of an infinite number of possible language tests is the "right" one, that is, the one that best reflects language capacity. Another serious problem is that different capacities develop at different rates, so it is very difficult to infer what should be the "equivalence" score on some target variable, even if we match carefully on the control variable (see Mervis & Klein-Tasman, 2004, for an excellent discussion of these and other problems in group-matching designs.)

Our own approach is quite different, but is generally consistent with the developmental approach to cognitive impairment first discussed by Zigler (1967) in the context of mental retardation. Zigler's view assumed that mental retardation represents the lower end of the normal curve; hence cognition in a retarded individual should be similar to a normally developing individual, just "less," at any given point. Our approach is similar with respect to the nature of spatial impairment. We will *not* prejudge what the equivalence level should be—whether it should be the same as a person of the same chronological age, the same overall mental age, or even the same mental age on some particular task. Rather, we will determine cognitive equivalence by comparing performance among people with WS to the developmental curves generated by normally developing children (and sometimes, adults) on the tasks of interest. Some of these individuals will be CA matches, and some will be MA matches; and these can be useful for a first look at relative strengths and weaknesses. However, the more important comparison will be found in examining the developmental trajectory generated by individuals over a broad age range—in our case, from ages 4 through 12. Normal adults will also serve as the benchmark for mature performance. This broad developmental age range allows us to generate normal developmental curves for different aspects of spatial cognition, onto which we can map the performance of people with WS. From this, we can establish equivalents across spatial subsystems, and gain insight into the overall pattern of performance among people with WS compared to normally developing individuals.

This approach is particularly important in the case of a broad investigation into spatial representations, because different spatial subsystems might *normally* develop at different rates and, therefore, might mature at different points in developmental time. In addition, there are likely to be different developmental timetables for different capacities. For example, language develops on a fairly uniform timetable, with 4-year-olds showing the capacity to produce and understand complex structures. But 4-year-olds still have difficulty tying their shoes—a patently spatial task with a substantial action component. Although the uneven cognitive profile of people with WS demands that we understand how different cognitive systems develop relative to each other, the field offers us remarkably little insight into the *relative* developmental timetables for different spatial functions—whether they grow at the same pace or are on completely separate developmental trajectories, and whether this changes as each system becomes more mature. Although there is evidence on developmental trajectories for some aspects of brain development (Casey et al., 2005; Gogtay et al., 2004; Huttenlocher, 2002) and the development of selected aspects of spatial functioning (e.g., Newcombe & Huttenlocher, 2000), there is little evidence on the normal developmental timetables *across* a broad range of different *kinds* of spatial representations, including, for example, object representation, motion perception, action, imaginal and spatial transformations, spatial language. Recent studies of the development of ventral stream functions such as object and face processing have begun to suggest that there may be considerable developmental change *across* different spatial domains, even those thought to be housed in one visual processing stream of the brain (Golarai et al., 2007; Scherf et al., 2007). In addition, it appears that functions as basic as attention to the global versus local aspects of a pattern undergo significant development, not reaching mature levels until adolescence (Scherf et al., 2009). In contrast, other visual-spatial functions, such as perceiving illusions, appear to function at adult levels by age 3 or 4 (Palomares, Ogbonna, Landau, & Egeth, 2009), and many signatures of mature face processing are present shortly after birth (McKone et al., 2009; Turati et al., 2008). Understanding the spatial impairment in people with Williams syndrome requires that we understand a broad range of spatial representational functions, and their *normal* developmental trajectories. Without understanding the nature of normal spatial-developmental timetables, it is impossible to evaluate the nature or meaning of what appears to be a strikingly unusual cognitive profile.

Our approach, therefore, will be to compare our findings from people with WS against a trajectory of normally developing individuals. In most cases, a subset of these normal individuals will be, in fact, matched to our participants with WS on the basis of mental age; sometimes they will be equivalent on the basis of chronological age. But the crucial comparisons will be people with WS against the developmental (i.e., age-based) trajectory of *normally developing children*, who themselves exhibit quite different strengths and weaknesses across different tasks—which fall sometimes into different spatial domains and sometimes across different streams of visual processing.

We will ask, for each task, domain, and stream of processing, whether the WS pattern of performance in some task(s) mirrors that of normally developing children *at some age*. Importantly, the trajectories shown by normally developing children will inform our theories of spatial architecture, our theories of development, as well as our theories of what has gone wrong when roughly 25 genes are missing from chromosome 7, as in the case of Williams syndrome.

1.3 Summary

In our introduction to the puzzle of Williams syndrome, we have made three general points.

- First, we have argued that understanding how genes *cause* the unusual cognitive profile observed in WS involves an extremely complex causal chain, and that scientific progress can be made only by clearly defining the target level of explanation. We will be concerned with the level of *cognition* in order to understand the spatial profile.

- Second, we have argued that understanding the spatial deficit will require understanding the nature of the cognitive architecture underlying normal spatial representation in humans—and that all evidence points to specialization within spatial systems. That is, human spatial representation includes a set of spatial subsystems with qualitatively different kinds of representations and functions.
- Third, we have argued that any understanding of spatial impairment stemming from a genetic difference will have to involve a discussion of normal development. In particular, we have suggested that the right strategy is to examine the *normal* trajectory of spatial development—both quantitatively and qualitatively—focusing on the possibility that there may be different trajectories for different spatial functions.

The developmental issue is crucial because, as we have noted, many genetic conditions are developmental in nature—that is, they manifest themselves early in life, and therefore might have quite different repercussions on the end state than might be revealed by studying damage to a mature brain. Only by comparing the unusual spatial profile of people with WS to the spatial profile of normally developing children of different ages will we be able to understand the nature of the WS spatial impairment. Is there global breakdown in the system, or do the contours of impairment respect the normal boundaries of spatial-cognitive architecture? Are these boundaries best characterized by the same subsystems as have been revealed through studies of adult brain damage? Or is there a different organization of impairment than any observed in the mature brain? Are some subsystems more affected than others, or is there a "flat" profile across the systems? And how does this pattern of impairment compare to the profile that would emerge under normal development? In short, we agree that understanding the cognitive consequences of a genetic deficit such as Williams syndrome requires that we take seriously the idea of development itself. Our proposal is that the key is thinking about developmental timetables *across* different spatial functions, how these functions look in normal development, and how they might change under genetic deficit.

In the next chapter, we move toward a hypothesis about the nature of the spatial impairment in people with Williams syndrome. We first review what is known about the genetic foundation of the impairment and its effects on structure and function in the brain, using findings from recent brain imaging studies. We then turn back to the hallmark of the spatial profile, analyzing in detail the cognitive requirements of the block construction task and tying this to known cognitive and brain functions of normal adults and developing children, as well as people with WS. Using this information, we propose a hypothesis about the nature of the spatial impairment in Williams syndrome—which we then test (in succeeding chapters) against the evidence from our lab and that of others.

2

Background on the Problem

Genes, Brains, and the Hallmark Spatial Profile

In this chapter, we examine in detail the hallmark spatial profile of people with WS in the context of what is currently known about their genetic profile and associated structural and functional characteristics of the brain. As we argued in Chapter 1, it is a long causal chain from genes to brains to cognition, but because Williams syndrome is a genetic deficit, a complete account will inevitably consider which genes are missing, and therefore might be candidates implicated in the cognitive profile. As we will see, our understanding of the link between the deleted genes and the cognitive profile is at present only suggestive, with one area of particular promise—the link between genes and spatial navigation. Our understanding of the brains of people with WS is growing rapidly and we now know that there are some definite abnormalities in both structure and function of the brain among adults with WS. The nature of the documented abnormalities fits well with more general findings on brain and cognitive function in humans, suggesting possible loci in the brain for the spatial disorder.

Crucial to the picture, of course, is a thorough understanding of how the spatial-cognitive systems work, and how key aspects of spatial representation might be abnormal in people with WS. The current limits in our understanding of the causal chain across gene, brain, and cognition reinforce our belief that understanding the nature of the spatial-cognitive profile in people with Williams syndrome is a crucial piece of the larger puzzle—the piece that we contribute in this book. Therefore, after a brief review of what is known about the genetic and brain profile of people with WS, we will set out to examine in detail the hallmark spatial profile, focusing on an in-depth analysis of visuospatial construction tasks that are most often offered as a key diagnostic of the WS spatial profile. These tasks include drawing and copying, and—most often cited—block construction tasks.

In the block construction task, people are asked to copy a target pattern by assembling individual blocks so that they duplicate an overall pattern they see (see Figure 2.1, for example). The pattern construction task of the Differential Abilities Scale (Elliott, 1990) has been the most widely used block construction task in studies of people with WS. Performance on this task has been used as the benchmark for diagnosing the spatial component of the classic WS profile, which includes severe impairment in this task and significantly worse performance on it than on a verbal task from the same battery (Mervis, Robinson, Bertrand, Morris, Klein-Tasman, & Armstrong, 2000).

Although the block construction task (and its relatives in other standardized test batteries) is generally used as a shorthand measure of spatial ability, careful scrutiny of the task reveals that it is extremely complex, drawing on many capacities that are likely to engage quite basic but distinct functions of the human spatial representational systems. Indeed, in our early studies, we came to realize that the task is so successful as a proxy for overall spatial ability exactly because it does draw on many basic spatial functions. As we will see, the analysis of the components of the block construction task dovetails in an interesting way with what is known about brain abnormalities in people with WS, suggesting a first hypothesis about the nature of their spatial impairment.

We now turn to a brief review of the current evidence on the genetic profile of people with WS, followed by what is known about

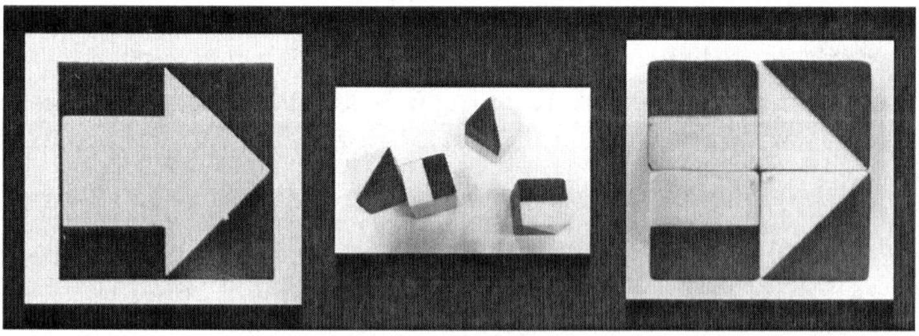

Figure 2.1. Sample model from the Differential Abilities Scales, Pattern Construction subtest (Elliott, 1990). The left panel shows the model pattern as shown to participants. The middle panel shows the four blocks they are given, which they must use to copy the model. The right panel shows a model that has been accurately assembled using the four available blocks. (*See* color insert.)

brain structure and function, and finally—but most crucially—the detailed nature of the hallmark visual-spatial construction task which points to some possible components of the a marked spatial disorder observed in WS.

2.1 Genes and the WS Profile

Williams-Beuren syndrome was first brought to the attention of the medical community in the 1960s by two physicians who reported a constellation of features associated with the heart condition supravalvular aortic stenosis (SVAS; Beuren, Apitz, & Harmjanz, 1962; Williams, Barratt-Boyes, & Lowe, 1961). Yet it was not until the late 1980s that the attention of cognitive scientists was drawn to the syndrome for its unusual and striking cognitive profile (Bellugi, Sabo, & Vaid, 1988). At that point, the syndrome was known to be a multisystem disorder, with phenotypic characteristics including SVAS (occurring in roughly 75% of WS patients; Osborne & Mervis, 2007), hoarse voice, stellate irises, various disorders of connective tissue, and a characteristic facial profile including full cheeks, small chin, and short upturned nose, as well as the unusual cognitive profile (see Morris, 2006a, 2006b, for review). Further progress was made when the syndrome was shown to result from a microdeletion on chromosome 7q11.23 (Ewart et al., 1993; see Figure 2.2 for illustration). The incidence of WS is currently estimated to be 1 in 7,500 (Stromme et al., 2002), making it a relatively rare disorder, but the estimates have changed (toward increasing incidence) as diagnostic methods have improved. WS is usually diagnosed by a combination of phenotypic characteristics plus fluorescent in situ hybridization (FISH) tests, which allow a probe of the deleted region of chromosome 7.

More than 95% of people who are clinically diagnosed with WS show a deletion in the so-called Williams-Beuren syndrome (WBS) region, typically spanning approximately 1.5 Mb of deleted genetic material, encompassing about 26 missing genes (Scherer & Osborne, 2007). The size of the deletion is not directly related to the phenotype, though the lower limit for appearance of the WS phenotype appears to be 10–12 missing genes (Scherer & Osborne, 2007). Longer than

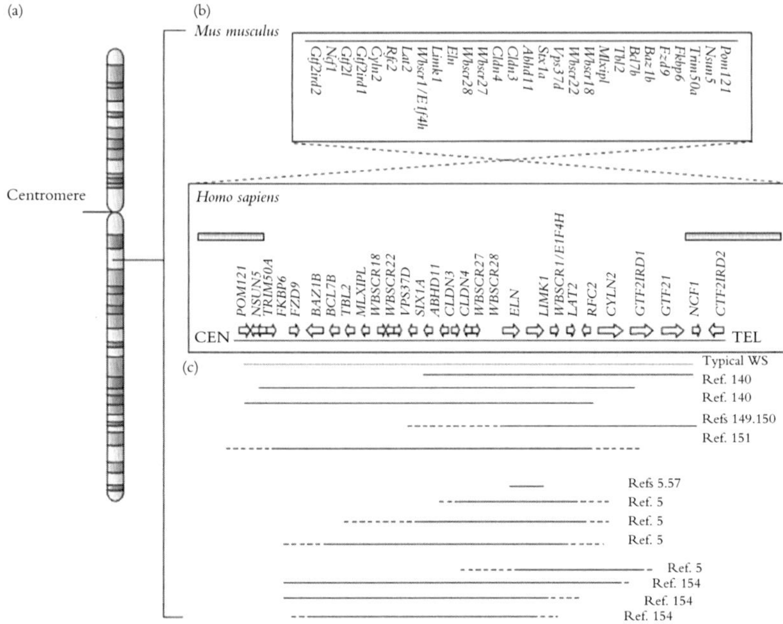

Figure 2.2. (a) Chromosomal location of the hemideleted region. (b) Map of the region in humans (center) and the homologous region in mice (top). Location of low copy repeat regions marked by bars. (c) Extent of typical Williams syndrome deletion and examples of small (atypical) deletions. Dashed lines indicate uncertain extent of the deletion in that portion. Reprinted from Meyer-Lindenberg et al. (2006), with permission of Nature Publishing Group and adapted from American Academy for the Advancement of Science (2005).

typical deletions predispose people to considerably lower cognitive functioning (Morris, 2006b); shorter than typical deletions are rare, but are important because they can be used to test hypotheses about the role of individual genes. For example, people with SVAS typically have point mutations in elastin, but do not have the cognitive profile for WS, thus ruling out a direct role for elastin in the cognitive profile (Frangiskakis et al., 1996; see Morris, 2006b, for review). Interestingly, the region of deletion in WS is generally predisposed to a number of different rearrangements, including both deletions (as in WS) and duplications, the latter of which leads to a pattern of severe language disorder—quite unlike the pattern for people with WS, who show strength in language (Osborne & Mervis, 2007).

Since the discovery of the microdeletion, genetic studies of WS have pursued two questions that are relevant to understanding the cognitive profile: Which genes are deleted in people with WS? And what is the relationship between these genes and the cognitive profile, especially the impairment in visual-spatial cognition? Methods to probe the latter question have included studying mouse models of the deletion (made possible by the fact that a region on mouse chromosome 5 contains the same string of genes as the WS critical region; see Figure 2.2), and studies of people with deletions smaller than the 1.5 Mb span characteristic of the "classic" WS deletion. These smaller deletions afford scientists the opportunity to isolate cases in which only one or several genes are deleted, thereby determining their role in producing different aspects of the WS phenotype, including the cognitive outcome.

By now, most of the roughly 26 genes in the typical deletion region have been identified (Scherer & Osborne, 2007; Osborne, 2006). Of these genes, about 15 are considered to be unlikely candidates for any aspect of the WS phenotype (at least given current understanding). Several others are known to be critical to the WS diagnosis but are unlikely candidates for playing a causal role in the cognitive profile. The clearest such case is ELN—the gene for elastin—which is the only gene conclusively linked to a particular aspect of the WS phenotype (Osborne, 2006). Elastin deletions are known to be related to various connective tissue abnormalities, and to cause the heart condition SVAS; indeed, people with autosomal dominant SVAS have point mutations in elastin, but do not have any other characteristics of WS (Morris, 2006b). Thus the elastin deletion is not sufficient for WS. Nor is it necessary, as only about 96% of people who are phenotypically diagnosed with WS have a deletion of the elastin gene (Lowery, Morris, Ewart, Brothman, Zhu, Leonard, Carey, Keating, & Brothman, 1995). Most important for our purposes, elastin is an unlikely candidate for playing a role in the cognitive profile, because it is not expressed in the brain (Frangiskakis et al., 1996).

In contrast, two commonly deleted genes have been suspected to play a causal role in some aspect of the WS cognitive profile. But even here, the story is complex and indirect and, at present, quite incomplete. The gene GTF2I, which is expressed in the brain, has been linked to mental retardation, which is a common (though not inevitable) symptom associated with WS. The link is, however, independent of other primary characteristics of the WS cognitive profile (Morris, 2006b). This was shown by Morris et al. (2003), who studied five families with small deletions in the WS critical region, none including a deletion of GTF2I. The patients had SVAS and some had the WS cognitive profile of relative strength in verbal measures and relative weakness in visual-spatial construction, but none were mentally retarded. Thus the WS cognitive profile can exist without retardation, a fact that has led some researchers to study this select group of people (see Section 2.2 on brain structure and function).

The other gene that is a candidate for linking to the WS cognitive profile is LIMK1—a gene that is expressed in the mouse developing nervous system and adult brain, and is involved in cell morphogenesis and growth of neuronal axons (Osborne, 2006). Importantly, LIMK1 is the only single gene that has been linked to the visual-spatial deficit in people with WS. Even this link, however, is tenuous and points to the importance of understanding the complexity of the causal chain, as well as the complexity of the spatial-cognitive profile itself. The details of studies attempting to link LIMK1 to the visual-spatial deficit are worth describing.

2.1.1 LIMK1 and the Spatial Deficit

The first paper suggesting a link between LIMK1 and the visual-spatial deficit link was a report on the cognitive profile of two families with a partial WS phenotype (Frangiskakis et al., 1996), including heart disease common to people with WS and the WS cognitive profile—defined as weakness in visual-spatial construction (as measured by the block construction task), and relative strength in a verbal measure. The family members typically had smaller deletions than the classic deletion (of roughly 1.5 Mb), which afforded investigators the opportunity to see whether quite small deletions—of just a few genes—still result in spatial impairment. Results showed a common impairment even in individuals who had extremely small deletions (83.6 kb); these deletions encompassed the sites for ELN and LIMK1. Because elastin is known to be responsible for connective tissue abnormalities (including SVAS) but is not expressed in the brain, the investigators proposed LIMK1 as a clear candidate implicated in the WS spatial-cognitive profile.

This exciting proposal has been followed up with rather more sobering empirical results. In one study, mice were bred to be homozygous knockouts for LIMK1; that is, this gene was deleted in both copies of mouse chromosome 5, which contains a region with the same genes as the deletion site in human chromosome 7 (Meng et al., 2002; see Figure 2.2 for mouse chromosome 5 region).[1] Brains of the mice showed abnormalities of spine morphology in both hippocampal and cortical neurons, as well as abnormal syntactic transmission in hippocampus. Behaviorally, the mice also showed differences from control mice in the Morris water maze, a classic task used to study animals' ability to learn places (see Knierim & Hamilton, 2011, for review). In this task (most often used with rats), the animal is trained in a circular pool to find a platform that is submerged below the water (see Figure 2.3). Once it learns to reliably find the platform, it is removed, and the animal is tested in "probe trials" on its ability to swim to the location where the platform was. Swimming to the location of the platform shows that the animal has built up a representation of the location of the platform, and conditions are varied in order to discover what kinds of cues the animal had used to define the platform's location. For example, the pool may be rotated within the larger environment (i.e., room), and one can ask whether the animal defined the location in terms of local cues such as parts of the pool's edge, or more distal cues such as landmarks present in the larger room. (Both appear to be important, as we review in Chapter 5.)

In Meng et al.'s (2002) study, mice were trained to find the submerged platform in the pool; over 5 days of training, the lengths of their paths to the platform declined, consistent with the idea that they were learning the location of the platform. On this measure, knockout mice and control mice did not differ. Nor did they differ in probe trials following the acquisition phase. Both groups of mice initially swam to the location where the platform had been. The main difference occurred during a third phase—reversal learning—which tested the animal's

[1] People with WS have deletions on only one copy of chromosome 7. Knockout mice have deletions on both copies of chromosome 5.

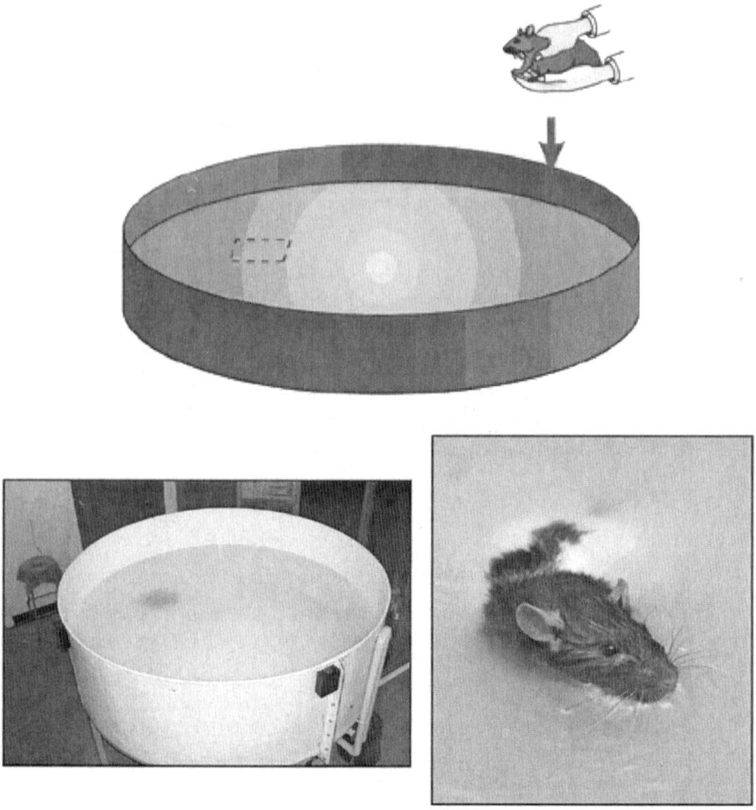

Figure 2.3. Setup for the Morris water maze task. In the task, the animal is trained to swim to a submerged platform in a pool. After this is learned, the platform is removed, and animals are tested on their ability to swim to the location where the platform had been. Meng et al. (2002) found that LIMK1 knockout mice could learn the first location for the platform, but then showed difficulty in reversal learning, where they had to learn a new location for the platform. Top panel adapted from Eichenbaum (2000), with permission from Nature Publishing Group.

ability to find the platform when it had been placed in a new location. This phase took place 48 hours after the initial learning phase. Here, the knockout mice showed longer paths than controls as they acquired the new position of the platform; in addition, the controls showed steady improvement over 4 days of testing, but the knockouts showed improvement only for the first two days, after which their performance simply leveled off.

Although this experiment reveals some deficits in the spatial behavior of the knockout mice, there are several possible explanations for the results. For example, as the authors note, it is possible that the reversal learning difference was due to the knockout mice having learned the initial platform location better than the controls; it is also possible that the deficits in new learning were not specific to spatial behavior, or that the observed deficits were due to perseveration, which could be generally increased in the knockout mice, without being specific to spatial tasks. Such problems of interpretation can be resolved with additional experimentation, and experiments on spatial behavior in such genetically altered mice will be an important part of the effort to understand the spatial profile in people with Williams syndrome. The initial findings are especially intriguing insofar as we observe abnormalities in some aspects of navigation among people with WS, possibly linked to abnormalities in the hippocampus and parietal areas (see Section 2.2 and Chapter 5). At the same time, we must be cautious in our inferences from the mouse knockout studies, since it is clearly difficult to directly translate the mouse's deficit in place learning to the complex spatial profile observed in people with WS.

An additional approach to evaluating the possible role of LIMK1 in the WS cognitive profile is used in studies of individuals with very small genetic deletions in the classic site, that is, deletions restricted to just one or several genes (rather than the 25 or so genes associated with the class WS deletion region). As with the original Frangiskakis et al. (1996) study, one can use the case of such small deletions to determine whether a single gene is either necessary or sufficient for a particular aspect of the profile.

Using this approach, Gray, Karmiloff-Smith, Funnell, and Tassabehji (2006) studied two adults with deletions of only LIMK1 and ELN, and compared these individuals to two adults who had a clear diagnosis of WS based on a more typical (larger) deletion. Gray et al. administered 16 perceptual and visual-spatial tasks, including construction tasks, and found that the adults with the classic WS deletion were clearly impaired on the spatial tasks as a whole, but that the two individuals with deletions of only LIMK1 and ELN were not. The two people with the classic WS genetic profile had problems in almost every spatial task that was administered, including the construction tasks, a task requiring that they match the orientation of a card to its slot, and a task requiring that they simply reach and grasp a visible object (see Chapter 4 for performance of groups of WS individuals on similar tasks). These findings reinforce the conclusion that LIMK1 is not sufficient for the profile of spatial impairment observed in people with WS, consistent with reports of other patients with quite small deletions in this region, who do not show the WS cognitive profile (Tassabehji et al., 1999).

The failure to find obvious links between LIMK1 and the visual-spatial cognitive profile of people with WS can be disappointing only if one assumes a simple link between individual genes and complex spatial behavior. This, of course, is exactly the kind of assumption that we have argued against. At present, we have little understanding of how individual genes work to produce complex behavior. This is not to say that there will never be an answer to how genes modulate behavior. Evidence to date, however, suggests that this story will be complex, involving multiple genes interacting with one another.

Moreover, what becomes very clear from considering these attempts to connect a specific gene with a spatial profile is that the correct characterization of the spatial profile in question is itself a significant part of the problem in establishing a causal chain. We need to understand the cognitive endophenotype—the overall cognitive profile, including the range of basic spatial functions that are compromised in people with WS, and how they interact to produce the striking impairment in visuospatial construction tasks. If—as we suspect—the deficit in block construction and copying tasks is itself complex and naturally decomposes into multiple components, it may be fruitless to start by trying to link individual genes with performance in such a complex task. Put quite coarsely, there is not likely to be a single gene for visual-spatial construction abilities as a whole, since such tasks are likely the result of "cobbling together" many more fundamental spatial capacities. On the other hand, the exciting prospect of linking genes and cognition would be improved if we were able to identify the basic cognitive components that, together, result in complex behavior. In a nutshell, to make progress, we will need to better understand the natural component structure of human spatial representation. As we argued in Chapter 1, this is likely to reflect separate specialized systems that could themselves be differentially affected by genetic conditions.

2.2 Brain Structure and Function

Genetic deficits involving genes that are expressed in the brain are likely to have widespread ramifications for brain development. A crucial part of the puzzle, therefore, is to determine whether and how the brains of people with Williams syndrome differ from the normally developed and normally developing brain. Although the WS brain does not show any frank lesions (as would be the case for adult cases of brain damage due to stroke, e.g.), there is growing evidence that there are many abnormalities in brain structure and function among people with WS. In addition, for some of these abnormalities, there is suggestive evidence for possible links to the WS cognitive profile. As we review below, the profile of brain structure and function in WS is uneven, with some reports of normal function and other reports of clear abnormalities. Within the broad arena of spatial functions carried out by the brain, there is suggestive evidence for a profile that may echo the profile observed in spatial behavior.

2.2.1 Brain Structure

Numerous studies have shown that there are many unusual characteristics of the brains of people with WS in comparison with normal, unaffected people who are matched on the basis of age, and, in some cases, IQ. A list of the abnormalities is long: The brains of people with WS are typically smaller than normal, with reduced volume of gray matter (Galaburda & Bellugi, 2000; Kippenhan et al., 2005), and abnormalities in the morphology of gyri and sulci—the ridges and grooves of the cortex (Gaser et al., 2006; Jackowski & Schultz, 2005; Kippenhan et al., 2005; Van Essen et al., 2006). There are also abnormalities in the structures and mechanisms underlying connectivity, including reduction in the size and shape of the corpus callosum (Schmitt et al., 2001; Tomaiuolo et al., 2002), and unusual paths exhibited by other major white matter tracts (Faria et al., 2012; Hoeft et al., 2007; Marenco et al., 2007). The combination of abnormalities in both gray and white matter suggest that early development of the brain in WS may be substantially different from typically developing brains; some have conjectured that very early mechanisms of neuronal migration may lead to later abnormalities (Marenco et al.,

2007). As there are little data at present on the brains of very young children with WS (for an exception, see Jones et al., 2002), we do not yet know whether these brain abnormalities are present from birth or evolve as a consequence of complex cascading events related to abnormalities in early experience.

Most significant for understanding the hallmark spatial deficit is the increasingly clear picture of abnormalities in several specific regions of the brain, in particular, the parietal lobe and the hippocampus, both known to be systematically engaged in a variety of spatial functions in both humans and other species (Burgess et al., 1999). Figure 2.4 shows the major lobes of the brain and the hippocampus, located deep within the medial temporal lobe.

The parietal lobe is of interest because it is thought to be heavily involved in our ability to compute spatial relationships among objects, in order to carry out actions such as reaching and grasping and directed visual search (see, e.g., Milner & Goodale, 2008). Within the parietal lobe, the area of the intraparietal sulcus (IPS) has drawn special interest, both for its multiple functions in spatial behavior in animals and the existence of proposed homologs in humans (Grefkes & Fink, 2005). The parietal areas also have extensive connections to the hippocampus and surrounding areas; this set of regions is known to be involved in spatial navigation (Aguirre & d'Esposito, 1999; Burgess et al., 1999; Epstein & Kanwisher,

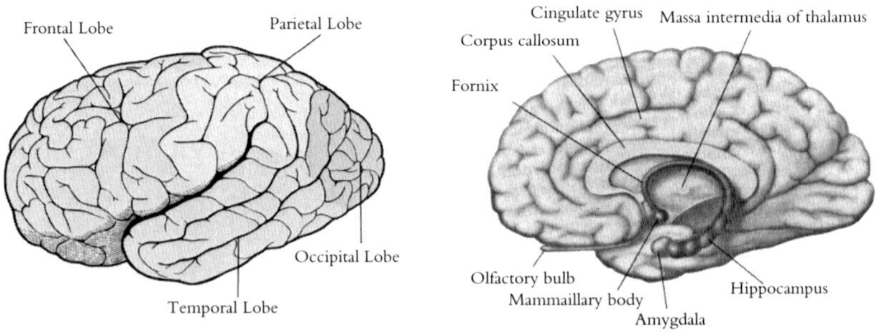

Figure 2.4. Major lobes of the brain (left panel) and hippocampus (right panel), which is buried within the medial temporal lobe. Right panel reprinted from Gazzaniga et al. (2008), with permission from W. W. Norton & Company. (*See* color insert.)

1998). Both the parietal and hippocampal areas are likely to be engaged in a wide range of spatial behaviors.

The parietal areas, and especially the IPS, have been reported to show structural abnormalities in people with WS. Several investigators have reported that people with WS show reduced volume of the right and left superior parietal areas, even after controlling for the overall reduced gray matter typical in this population (Eckert et al., 2005; Meyer-Lindenberg et al., 2004; Reiss et al., 2004). Reduction in gray matter in the parietal-occipital region has also been found in children with WS (*M* age = 11), compared to age-matched controls, suggesting that this abnormality may be present relatively early in development (Boddaert et al., 2006), although studies of much younger children would be needed to confirm this. Reported abnormalities in the IPS include reductions in sulcal depth (Kippenhan et al., 2005) and qualitatively abnormal white matter tracts connecting to the IPS (Marenco et al., 2007). Studies of nonhuman primates suggest that the IPS bears much of the responsibility for computing information about the locations of objects, the positions of body parts, eye movements, and properties of objects that are particularly relevant for actions such as reaching and grasping, in both animals and humans (Grefkes & Fink, 2005). The IPS also appears to be engaged in number processing, suggesting a link between space and number (Hubbard, Piazza, Pinel, & Dehaene, 2005), and raising the possibility that weakness in number knowledge among people with WS (Ansari, Donlan, & Karmiloff-Smith, 2007; O'Hearn & Landau, 2007) might be related to abnormalities in this part of the brain.

In addition to these abnormalities, unusual morphology of the hippocampus has been documented. Although the size of the hippocampus is not different from normal individuals matched for age, gender, and IQ, there are subtle differences in shape (Meyer-Lindenberg et al., 2005; see Figure 2.5). Moreover, Marenco et al. (2007) found clear abnormalities in the white matter tracts connecting to the hippocampal complex through the ventral cingulate (see Figure 2.5).

These structural abnormalities of the WS brain are suggestive, but more important are the functional studies that can help us understand what aspects of cognitive functioning might be linked to these abnormalities. We turn to these next.

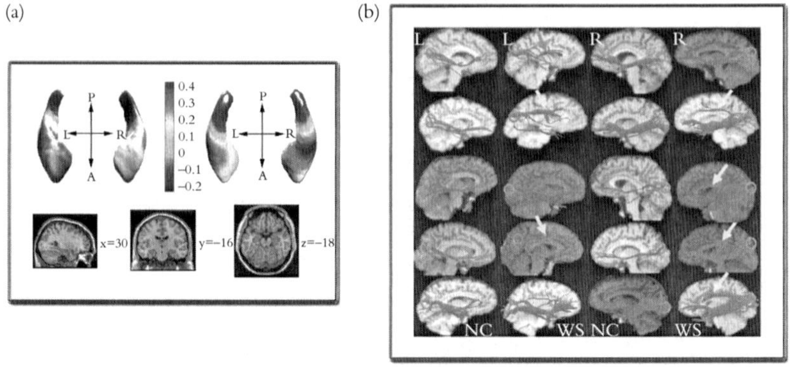

Figure 2.5. (a) Differences in the shape of the HF in WS and normal controls. Shape change is rendered on an average age (between groups) template of the HF. Top left: anterior view; top right: posterior view. Color scale correlates to the degree of deformation. Units are arbitrary. Negative values reflect local volume reduction in WS patients relative to controls. Positive values reflect local volume expansion in WS patients relative to controls. Double arrow marked A-P shows anterior-posterior direction. Double arrow marked L-R shows left-right direction. Significant findings ($P < 0.05$, corrected at the voxel level using small volume correction for the hippocampus ROI) were positive and greater than 0.3 and located in the mid/anterior section of the HF. Bottom: Same template shown superimposed on a representative single-subject MRI for orientation purposes. Coordinates x, y, and z are given in mm distance from the anterior commissure. (b) Differences between controls and WS in tracks connecting to the IPS (intraparietal sulcus) and VCING (ventral cingulate). Fiber tracking was performed with DTI studio seeding tracts from all voxels in the brain and then displaying only fibers that traversed the IPS ROI (illustrated as a blue circle) and a coronal plane at the center of the thalamus. The yellow arrows indicate the fiber tracts coursing rostrally to the corpus callosum, which were never present in controls (normal control, NC, first and third columns) but present in four of the five individuals with WS (second and fourth columns), especially in the right hemisphere (Mann-Whitney U = 2.5 $P < 0.05$). The blue arrow indicates fibers connecting the IPS to the thalamus, observed in the left hemisphere of one individual with WS. Reprinted from Meyer-Lindenberg et al. (2005), with permission of the American Society of Clinical Investigation (this is for Fig 2.5a). Reprinted from Marenco et al., copyright © 2007 National Academy of Sciences, U.S.A. (this is for Fig 2.5b). (*See* color insert.)

2.2.2 Brain Function

Several recent studies involving functional brain imaging (fMRI) have begun to paint a picture of spatial functioning that suggests a profile of peaks and valleys including normal structure and function in primary visual cortex (V1) and in several functions beyond V1 along the brain's ventral stream, but definite functional abnormalities in the parietal regions (including the IPS) as well as the hippocampus and its surrounding regions.

A first question is whether early visual processing—in primary visual cortex (V1)—is abnormal, possibly promoting abnormalities further upstream in the visual system. The primary visual cortex is the area of the brain that first processes incoming information from the retina and lateral geniculate nucleus (LGN); visual processes carried out in this area include grouping of elements, a mechanism that is crucial to perceiving objects (see Chapter 3). Notably, one of the earliest hypotheses about the spatial deficit in people with WS focused on their difficulty in one of the hallmark tasks—copying figures that contain both local and global elements (for example, a large M made up of small Hs). Bihrle et al. (1989) proposed that people with WS had a "global processing deficit," resulting in failure to group local elements into a coherent spatial whole and possibly accounting for their difficulty in reproducing spatially organized copies. Although the hypothesis itself has not proven to be true (see Chapter 3), it would be possible for subtle abnormalities of early visual processing to contribute to the copying deficit.

However, the results of a recent study suggest that these early visual areas are functionally and structurally normal. Olsen et al. (2009) carried out a functional imaging study of the early visual areas of adults with WS in comparison to age- and IQ-matched controls. Olsen et al. took the unusual approach of testing an exceptional group of adults with WS who had measured IQs within the normal range, thus both eliminating possible confounds due to mental retardation, and allowing comparisons to normal unaffected adults who were matched on the basis of both age and IQ (see also Meyer-Lindenberg et al., 2004, 2005; Sarpal et al., 2008). The people they studied had also participated in other brain imaging studies, and were known to show abnormal processing in the IPS during tasks related to the hallmark block construction task (Meyer-Lindenberg et al., 2004).

Olsen et al. used a standard method for retinotopic mapping of V1: People passively viewed rotating hemicircles and expanding rings, displays known to activate the primary visual cortex in normal individuals. When people with WS viewed these stimuli, their primary visual cortex was also activated, and Olsen et al. measured the size and location of the activated region as well as its center of gravity. Although the area itself was smaller in absolute size (consistent with smaller overall brain volume, also reported), the ratio of V1 to hemispheric volume was no different from that of the normal controls. In addition, the centers of gravity for V1 were quite similar between people with WS and controls. The only difference Olsen et al. found was that the borders of V1 were somewhat more variable for the WS group compared to the normal controls.

Another study has examined activation patterns in people with WS for selective areas of the brain that lie beyond V1 and compose the ventral stream, in particular, those that are typically activated when people view faces (fusiform face area, FFA) and houses (parahippocampal gyrus, parahippocampal place area, PPA), as established by Kanwisher and others (see Kanwisher, 2010, for review). Sarpal et al. (2008) had people with WS (who had IQs in the normal range) passively view faces and houses. Controls were normal age- and IQ-matched individuals. Sarpal et al. looked for characteristic activation patterns in the task, as well as connectivity with other regions. They reported that both groups showed similar overall activation of the target regions (FFA and PPA), and that each participant with WS showed activation in these regions. There were no differences across groups (WS versus normal controls) in activation when people viewed faces, compared to when they viewed scrambled images. Other recent results have shown that the FFA region in adults with WS is roughly twice as large as that of normal individuals of about the same age (Golarai et al., 2010); it is unclear why these results are different from those of Sarpal et al.

Sarpal et al. also found that when people viewed houses compared to scrambled images, people with WS showed lower activation than controls in more dorsal regions of the brain. Sarpal et al. also found some abnormalities in the links between the FFA and PPA and other brain areas, specifically, the link between the FFA and the amygdala (which is related to emotion processing) and the link between the PPA and parietal areas—which are strongly implicated in a variety of spatial computations.

Similar findings emerged from another study examining functional activity in the ventral stream of people with WS. O'Hearn et al. (2010) found that adolescents and adults with WS showed activation levels to faces in the FFA (compared to other objects) that were no different from chronological age matches. For houses, O'Hearn et al. also found that the people with WS also showed low activation in the PPA when they viewed houses (relative to other objects), and, indeed, that their activation level was lower than that of children who were mental age matches. O'Hearn et al. also found that the WS group showed reduced activation to houses in the parietal areas, consistent with the findings of Sarpal et al.

The general picture that emerges from these studies is one of normal activation in the WS brain for regions involved in face processing, lower but normally localized activation for regions involved in house (place) processing, and impaired or different connectivity between these areas and other regions of the brain. These results suggest strikingly different profiles for the functional brain activity involved in faces versus places in people with WS, with normal patterns of activation in response to faces, but functional impairment in the representations of places—a point to which we return when we discuss navigation (see Chapter 5).

Compared to the findings of normal activations shown in V1 and the ventral stream for faces (and from Sarpal, houses), the picture is quite different for areas that lie in the dorsal stream, in particular the IPS. In the first functional imaging study that tested people with WS, Meyer-Lindenberg and colleagues (2004) examined brain activation as people carried out visual-spatial construction tasks. As noted earlier, these people had normal IQs, and were compared to age- and IQ-matched controls. People underwent brain scanning while they carried out two different tasks. In one, they were shown two complex shapes and asked whether they matched or not (match task); because these stimuli were distinguished by relative orientation of parts, the authors anticipated dorsal as well as ventral stream activation. In the second task, people were shown the same shapes, but were asked whether they could be assembled to form a square (construction task). This task was expected to primarily activate the dorsal stream.

No group differences were found in activation levels for the ventral stream in either task. However, there were clear differences in dorsal stream activation, especially for the construction task. For the match task, comparing activation to baseline (simple motor press), Meyer-Lindenberg et al. found greater activation of the dorsal stream among normal individuals than people with WS. For the construction task, comparing activation for the square completion question relative to the match task, normal individuals showed significant activation in the dorsal stream, but individuals with WS showed no significant activation. Both of these findings show hypoactivation of dorsal stream areas among people with WS, suggesting a primary deficit linked to these regions.

In a second experiment, Meyer-Lindenberg et al. showed people images of faces or houses, and asked them to attend either to the identity of these items or to their location on the screen. When asked to attend to identity, people with WS showed activation in ventral stream areas that was no different from controls; in addition, faces activated classical areas known to be engaged in normal children and adults (FFA for faces, BA18 and 19d for houses; see Golarai et al., 2007, for developmental evidence on ventral stream). However, when asked to attend to location, significant differences across groups were found, with the WS group showing reduced activation in the dorsal stream compared to controls. The locus of this hypoactivation was similar to that observed in the construction and match tasks. Structural imaging of the WS participants showed reductions of gray matter in the area of the dorsal occipital-parietal and intraparietal sulci, consistent with the functional abnormalities observed.

Meyer-Lindenberg et al. hypothesized that, given the hierarchical structure of the visual system, the anatomical changes in the IPS might impair the processing of information further along in the dorsal stream (see Figure 2.6). To test this idea, they used the data from the face/house task and applied a path analysis to model the flow of information from early visual areas to the most highly activated regions of the ventral stream, the region of the IPS that they had found to be anatomically changed, and a further region of the dorsal stream that had been the site of the most pronounced differences in activation between people with WS and controls. They found only one difference: Normal controls showed a reliable path from the occipital-parietal sulcus to later dorsal

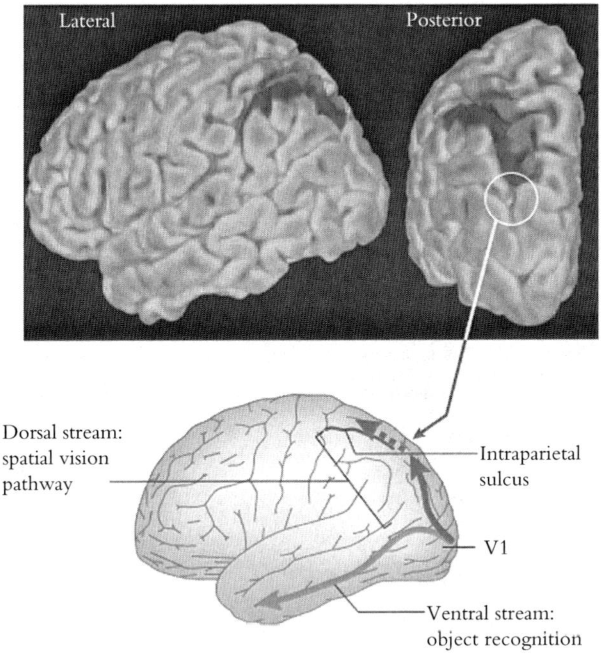

Figure 2.6. Meyer-Lindenberg et al.'s findings from brain imaging and path analysis suggest that the WS brain has structural abnormalities in the area of the intraparietal sulcus, with reduced functional processing in areas further upstream. Reprinted from Meyer-Lindenberg et al. (2006), with permission of Nature Publishing Group. (*See* color insert.)

stream areas, whereas people with WS did not. This is consistent with Meyer-Lindenberg's idea that the spatial deficit in people with WS can be traced to weakness in a functional pathway between the region of structural abnormality in the area of the occipital-parietal sulcus/intraparietal sulcus, and later processing in the dorsal stream. Overall, there appears to be a general weakness in the dorsal stream functioning, coupled with relative strength in the ventral stream.

In addition to functional abnormalities in the dorsal stream, there is evidence that the hippocampal formation (HF) shows impaired functioning (Meyer-Lindenberg, Mervis, Sarpal, et al., 2005). Although structural imaging showed no difference in volume between people with WS and normal controls, functional imaging indicated clear abnormalities that likely contribute to the overall profile of spatial disorder. Compared to normal adults matched for age and IQ, Meyer-Lindenberg et al. found that people with WS showed reductions in resting blood flow (measured by PET imaging) and evidence of reduced synaptic activity, measured by magnetic resonance spectroscopy (MRS). Moreover, they found that when normal adults viewed houses or faces, they showed activation in the hippocampal formation, with increased activation for faces compared to houses in the anterior portion of the HF. By comparison, people with WS showed no activation for either type of stimulus. This lack of functional activation along with depressed levels of energy in the hippocampus at resting state suggested to Meyer-Lindenberg and colleagues a primary dysfunction of the hippocampus in people with WS, perhaps due to functional impairment in neurons in this region. The parietal structures—also known to show abnormal functioning in people with WS—are known to have extensive connections to the hippocampal formation via the parahippocampal cortices (Aguirre, Zarahn, D'Esposito, 1998; Burgess et al., 1999; Epstein et al. 1999; Suzuki & Amaral, 1994). Poor functioning in the parietal areas and the hippocampal formation among people with WS would lead to compromise in a wide range of spatial tasks.

The profile of normal functioning in early visual areas and certain areas in the ventral stream, in combination with abnormalities in both parietal areas and hippocampal formation, may be linked to the profile of peaks and valleys of the spatial profile. In order to determine whether this is true, we need to consider the range of spatial functions that might pose problems for people with WS, as well as those that should not be problematic. Although patterns of brain activation in tasks such as mock block construction and passive viewing are an important start, we believe that a deeper understanding of the spatial deficit must start with a cognitive level explanation of the spatial profile. Can we think about the cognitive components of spatial tasks in a way that can shed light on the nature of the peaks and valleys in the WS profile?

In order to do this, we now take a step back, and begin to analyze the problem by considering in detail the requirements of the spatial task used most often to document the severe spatial deficit in people with WS—the block construction task.

2.3 Understanding the Block Construction Task and Why It Might Be So Difficult

The WS spatial profile has been most often characterized as a deficit in visuospatial construction tasks, including copying of figures (using a writing instrument) and block construction tasks (using a set of squares or cubes to reproduce a target design). In our lab, we have carried out both kinds of tasks, using the Beery Test of Visuo-Motor Integration (VMI; Beery & Buktenica, 1967; see Georgopoulos et al., 2004), and the Pattern Construction subtest of the Differential Abilities Scale (DAS; Elliott, 1990). Results from the VMI show the hallmark deficit among people with WS; two examples of VMI figures and their copies by 10 children with WS are shown in Figure 2.7. These children were on average 10 years old (*M* age = 119.9 months, *SE* = 8.8 months), and clearly reproduced the local elements of figures, but often failed to preserve the spatial relationships among elements, as was first noted by Bihrle et al. (1989).

Results from the pattern construction task also show severe deficits. In the DAS version of this task (which we use in our lab), participants are shown a two-dimensional pattern that they must replicate using a set of wooden blocks each having a different solid color or a vertically, horizontally, or diagonally split two-colored pattern. Depending on the complexity of the puzzle, it may require assembly using two, four, six, or nine blocks. The correct number of blocks is given to the participant, and he or she must assemble the blocks to recreate the target pattern. Figure 2.8 shows three sample puzzles and reproductions by people with WS.

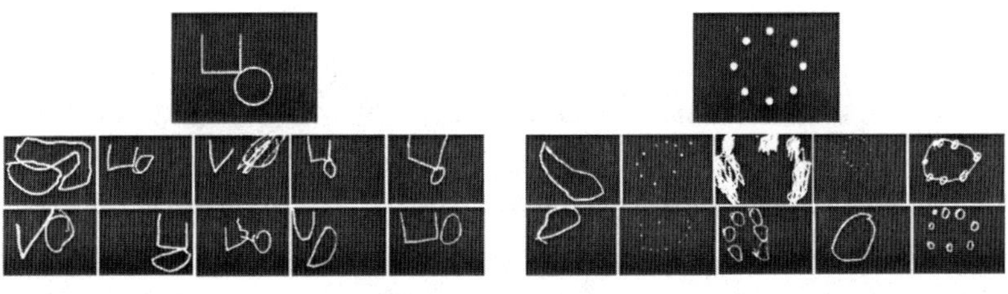

Figure 2.7. Copies of two model figures from the VMI (Beery & Buktenica, 1967) by 10 children with WS (*M* age = 10), who were tested in our lab. Models are shown above their respective copies (see Georgopoulos et al., 2004, for data and discussion). Adapted from Georgopoulos et al. (2004) with permission from Springer.

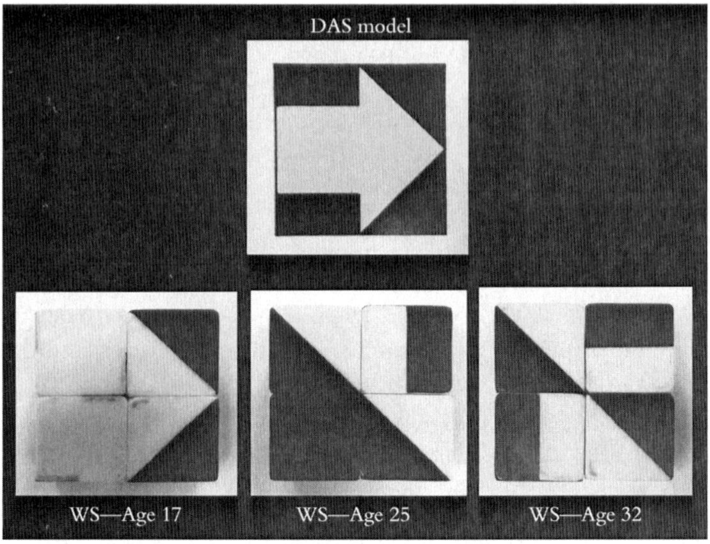

Figure 2.8. Sample model from the pattern construction task (DAS; Elliot, 1990) and sample copies by three participants in our studies. (*See* color insert.)

Consistent with these sample reproductions, extensive evidence from several labs shows that people with WS have severe difficulties in constructing accurate copies, with age equivalents on the task often around 4 or 5 years, and below the 3rd percentile for their age, comparable with other reports in the literature (Bellugi, Sabo, et al., 1998; Mervis et al., 2000; see Hoffman, Landau, & Pagani, 2003). Clearly, block construction poses a serious challenge to people with WS.

Why is copying so difficult for people with WS? An early hypothesis proposed that people with Williams syndrome suffered from a deficit in "global processing" (Bellugi et al., 1994; Bihrle et al., 1989). However, this hypothesis has not proven to be true. A number of studies have shown that visual grouping processes—which allow observers to perceive global configurations that are integrated from local units—operate quite well in people with WS, sometimes at levels remarkably like unaffected adults (see Chapter 3 for discussion). For example, Pani et al. (1999) showed that adults with WS can use global cues for "grouping" to facilitate search for letters, and they do so at levels similar to normal adults. Palomares et al. (2009) found that people with WS can detect the presence and location of a "line" that is assembled from local orientation elements at levels similar to normal adults. And Farran et al. (2003) found that people with WS can *match* configurations on the basis of both local elements and global configurations, even though they have great difficulty *copying* the global configuration (see Chapter 3).

Perhaps more important, the hypothesis of global processing deficit fails to account for the WS spatial deficit because it does not take into account the remarkable complexity of visual-spatial construction tasks. Perceptual processing of local and/or global elements is surely a component of these tasks, but it is just as surely not a complete characterization of the component processes required by these tasks. To illustrate, we now consider in detail the cognitive requirements of the block construction task.

2.3.1 The Cognitive Requirements of the Block Construction Task

To explore why the block task is so difficult for people with Williams syndrome, we created a computerized version of the task, and examined performance on this task in detail (Hoffman, Landau, & Pagani, 2003). To illustrate, Figure 2.8 shows a model pattern that we adapted from the Pattern Construction subtest of the DAS (Elliott, 1990). Based on DAS norms, this pattern is solved by 50% of typically developing children at the age of 7 years, 10 months; but it proves to be quite difficult even for older children and adolescents with WS. In our lab, the average age at which this problem was solved was 19 years, 5 months (out of 67 test sessions); the youngest person with WS who solved it was 10 years, 5 months, and some individuals as old as 42 did not solve it. The complete set of puzzles used in the Hoffman et al. study is shown in Figure 2.9; these included what we called "simple" and "complex" puzzles. The simple puzzles used block faces that were solid-colored only, resulting in emergent boundaries in the puzzle that fit individual blocks. Complex puzzles primarily used block faces that were nonsolid (i.e., with internal structure), resulting in emergent boundaries in the puzzle that violated the boundaries of individual blocks. Figure 2.9 also shows two version of each puzzle that were used: The *standard format* presented models with blocks immediately adjacent to each other, while the *segmented format* presented the models with blocks slightly separated from each other.

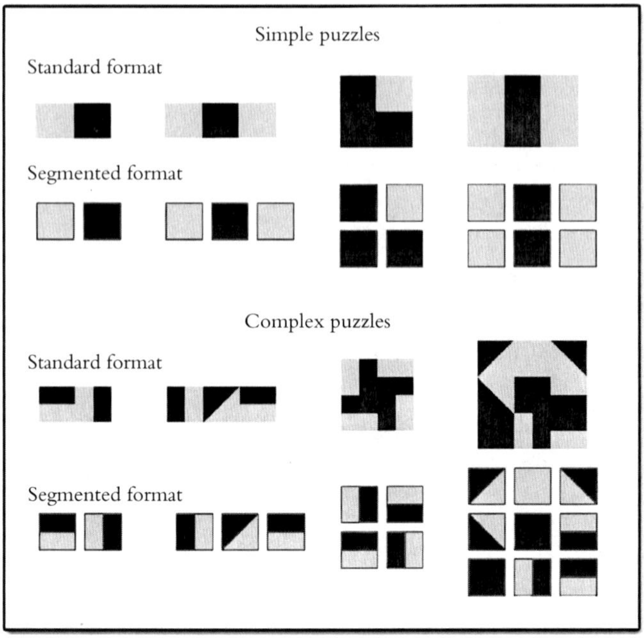

Figure 2.9. Simple and complex puzzles used in study by Hoffman et al. (2003). Simple puzzles required using block faces that were solid colors. Complex puzzles required using block faces that were not solid, in other words, with internal structure of vertical, horizontal, or diagonal splits by color. In simple puzzles, the borders of each block are consistent with the emergent patterns; in complex puzzles, however, the borders of each block may span more than one component of the emergent pattern of the puzzle. Hoffman et al. presented these puzzles in two formats: The standard format was the same as is used in the pattern construction task (DAS; Elliot, 1990). The segmented format displayed models with the individual component blocks slighted separated from each other. We predicted that this format would enhance performance by people with WS, and it did. Adapted from Hoffman et al. (2003), with permission from Elsevier; see text for discussion. (*See* color insert.)

In our study, we tested eight children with WS (*M* age = 9;5, range = 7–13;11) and eight normally developing children matched for mental age (*M* age = 5;3, range = 5;1–6;4), giving them eight puzzles as shown in Figure 2.9. The entire problem space was shown on a standard-sized computer screen, and the participants used the computer mouse to move blocks around the screen. As shown in Figure 2.10, the target model appeared in the upper left of the panel, the "copy area" appeared on the upper right, and the parts blocks were shown in the lower half of the display. By using a mouse to move individual blocks from the "parts area" into the copy area, people could construct a copy of the model pattern. In addition, with this method, people could easily move blocks in and out of the copy space, correcting themselves if they wished, as they solved the problem.

Although the task mimics many of the features of the standard block assembly task (e.g., from the DAS), there are clearly some differences: The blocks are two-dimensional showing only one exposed face, and the computer screen shows a well-defined "copy" space into which the blocks must be placed. By contrast, in the pattern construction task of the DAS, observers must use a set of six-sided blocks that they must pick up, examine, and rotate to select the correct side; in addition, the copy area is simply a uniform table top with no explicit "copy" grid. We simplified the process of moving and positioning blocks; they could not be rotated in place, and when a block was released in the target section of the copy area, it "snapped" into place in the nearest block location.

Despite the differences between the standardized pattern assembly task and our computerized version, performance on our task was strongly correlated with people's performance on the DAS pattern assembly task ($r = .70$). Simple puzzles were solved quite often; individual blocks were correctly placed in the copy space at least 89% of the time by children with WS; normally developing children matched for mental age (around age 5) dropped blocks correctly at least 96% of the time. Complex puzzles were much more difficult. Children with WS still solved the two-block puzzles at very high rates (greater than around 85% of trials), and normal 5-year-olds performed slightly better (greater than around 90%). However, once the children reached the four- and nine-block problems, performance by children with WS dropped precipitously, with only about 50% correct solutions for four-block puzzles and 10% for nine-block puzzles. Normal 5-year-olds constructed correct solutions about 90% of the time for four-block puzzles and about 50% of the time for nine-block puzzles. The range of performance, and especially the comparison between simple and complex puzzles,

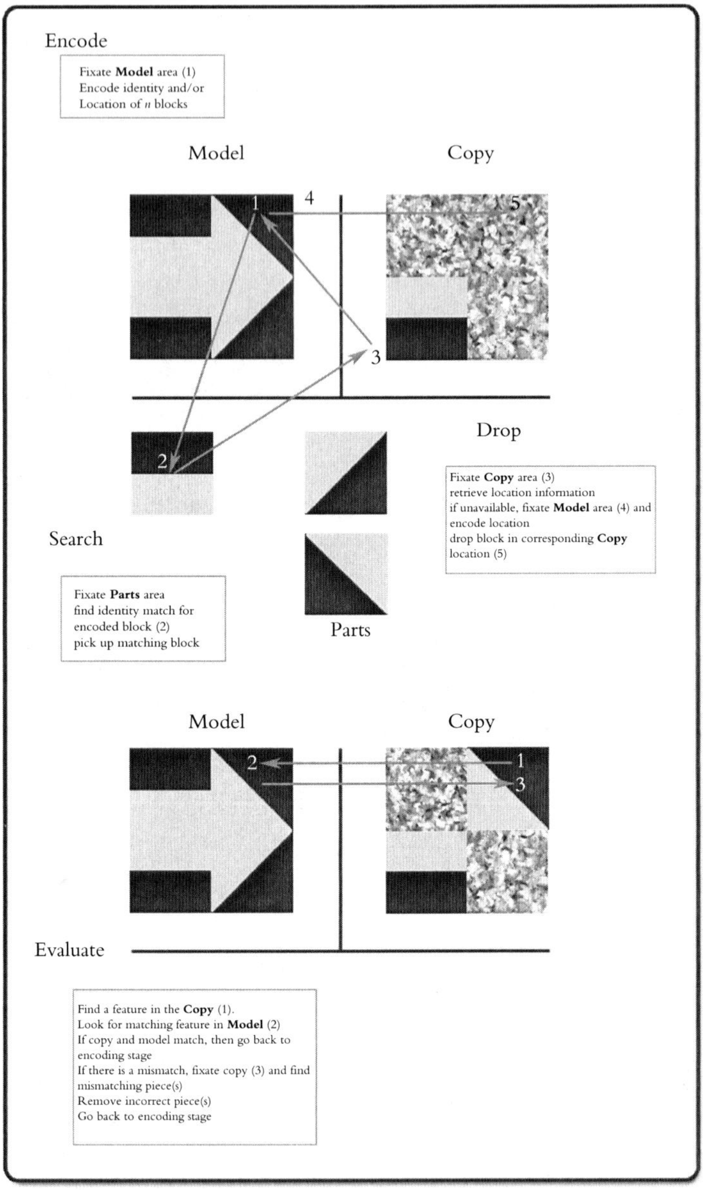
Encode
Fixate Model area (1)
Encode identity and/or
Location of n blocks
Model
Copy
1
4
5
3
2
Drop
Fixate Copy area (3)
retrieve location information
if unavailable, fixate Model area (4) and
encode location
drop block in corresponding Copy
location (5)
Search
Fixate Parts area
find identity match for
encoded block (2)
pick up matching block
Parts
Model
Copy
2
1
3
Evaluate
Find a feature in the Copy (1).
Look for matching feature in Model (2)
If copy and model match, then go back to
encoding stage
If there is a mismatch, fixate copy (3) and find
mismatching piece(s)
Remove incorrect piece(s)
Go back to encoding stage

◀ Figure 2.10. A computational analysis of the block construction task, adapted from Hoffman et al. (2003). Upper panel: The observer encodes the identity of a candidate block in the model, by fixating the model area (1). This step requires *segmenting* the model into candidate blocks, which are not obvious in the model. The observer then moves his gaze to the parts area (2) to find a *match* for the encoded block. This step requires representing the internal structure of the candidate block and successfully selecting it among the alternatives. The observer then moves his gaze to the copy area (3) in order to place the block. If necessary, he moves his gaze back to the model (4) to pick up information about the block's location in the puzzle. He then *places* the block into the copy area (5)—in this case, in the wrong location. Lower panel: The observer *evaluates* his copy by fixating the block he placed (1), then looking for the matching block in the model (2). If the copy and model match, then he can go back to the encoding stage (1, upper panel). If he detects a mismatch, then he can remove the incorrect block and start over again. See text for discussion of segmenting the model, choosing parts, and placing the blocks in the correct location. See text for discussion of problems among people with Williams syndrome in segmenting, matching, and placing blocks. Adapted from Hoffman et al. (2003) with permission from Elsevier. (*See* color insert.)

afforded us the opportunity to closely examine the difficulties children had in carrying out our version of the task.

2.3.2 Components of the Block Task

Based on people's performance on our task and related ones (to be reviewed below), we argued that the block construction task requires several steps, each of which engages a different set of cognitive processes. Our analysis built on a proposal by Ballard, Hayhoe, Pook, and Rao (1997) that was designed to account for normal adults' performance, when they solve block construction tasks that are quite similar to the one we used with our WS group. Based on computational considerations for how one *could* solve the block task, Ballard et al. suggested that the task can be broken down into several subgoals. In addition, they introduced the important idea that the sequence in which these subgoals are satisfied can be visualized by examining the sequence of eye fixations that observers make on different locations in the problem space. Most surprisingly, they proposed that normal adults do not typically solve the block construction task in one large step, in other words, by looking at the model, selecting all the candidate blocks, and then accurately assembling them into an entire design. Rather, adults tend to solve the puzzles in piecemeal fashion, "one block at a time."

An illustration of the component processes is shown in Figure 2.10. The observer first encodes a block. To do this, he looks at the model, selecting a particular portion of the puzzle he will begin with, fixating a particular part of the puzzle, and segmenting to "create" a block-sized chunk. The observer then creates a representation of the block's "identity"—that is, the spatial arrangement of the two colors on the block. According to Ballard et al.'s analysis, this fixation also establishes a mental "pointer" to the block in the puzzle; this pointer carries no specific information about the block's identity or location in the puzzle, but merely serves as an index that will allow the observer to go back to the same block later on, in order to access information about its location in the model. The observer then searches for the matching block; he moves his or her gaze to the parts area, and selects the matching block. In order to retrieve the location of the block, he then returns his gaze to the pointer he set on the model block. He copies by dropping the block into the corresponding location in the copy area. After setting several blocks, the observer can evaluate his copy using additional fixations between the model and copy. Copies can be modified if the observer detects a mismatch.

Following this general framework, we proposed that errors in the block construction domain could arise from two distinct kinds of cognitive processes: People might be impaired in their *spatial representations*, including representing and remembering the spatial identity and location of the block they are working on, or they might be impaired in the *executive processes* that guide solution strategies. These strategies might include deciding on how many blocks to place after each fixation on the model, how often to check whether the emerging copy matches the model, and so on. For example, unlike normal adults, people with WS may simply look once at the model, and then try to assemble the entire puzzle without referring back to the model at all. This might be a faulty strategy that leads to errors if the number of blocks being stored after each fixation exceeded the limits of working memory. As we will see, our analysis and follow-up experiments show that the severe deficit shown by people with WS can be largely attributable to failures in several *spatial* components of the task, culminating in a cascade of deficits that results in severe breakdown of the ability to accurately copy the entire pattern. We now review the task in terms of its spatial requirements.

1. *Mental segmentation of the model into component parts—in this case, individual blocks.* A first step is for the observer to mentally analyze the target model into candidate blocks: Which chunks in the model are represented by which individual blocks? Although this might be relatively simple in cases such as a pattern composed of four solid blocks assembled in a row, many of the target models in the DAS have an emergent design that is not coincident with the block-sized pieces that will ultimately form the pattern. For example, Figure 2.8 shows a model that—on first glance—looks like a yellow arrow on a black background. But the set of candidate blocks nowhere contains a yellow arrow; in fact, the blocks are limited to solid yellow or black, or yellow/black splits along a vertical, horizontal, or diagonal axis of the block. In order to even determine which blocks to select (or in the case of real blocks, which sides of each block to use), a person must use some voluntary selective attention processes to visually segment the model into the relevant block-sized pieces.

Segmentation itself proves to be difficult for people with WS, as well as normally developing children. This is shown by the fact that pre-segmenting the puzzles for WS participants significantly improves their performance (Hoffman et al., 2003; Key, Pani, & Mervis, 1998). In our study, we presented the models either in their original form (e.g., as shown in Figure 2.8), or with the model segmented into its candidate block components, presenting each block slightly separated from every other, but in the same spatial arrangement (Figure 2.9). We found that the children with WS showed an advantage of about 20% correct placement of individual blocks when they were solving four-block segmented puzzles compared to nonsegmented ones. Normally developing children matched for mental age also showed a significant reduction in errors of about 15% on the four-block segmented puzzles; they also showed a substantial improvement on the much more difficult nine-block puzzles when the puzzles were segmented, compared to nonsegmented. WS children did not show any advantage for the segmented nine-block puzzles, which suggests that added complexity (i.e., moving from a four- to nine-block puzzle) at some point outweighs any possible advantage of having a pre-segmented puzzle.

2. *"Marking" individual blocks in the model, for return visits.* Ballard et al. (1997) argue that when normal adults carry out a block copy task, they move through cycles in which they first fixate the model, selecting a block for focus, and picking up information about its identity (e.g., color); they then move to select a block; and then return their gaze to the model, picking up information about the block's location in the puzzle. People use this information to drop the block into the copy area, followed by a return fixation on the model to check that the drop is correct. Ballard et al. argue that this process of breaking down the task in this way is advantageous, as it reduces the memory load that would be required to carry information about one or more block's identity and location.

Using this logic, we tracked children's fixations as they carried out the computer version of the block assembly puzzle. We first looked to see whether children were fixating the model before they dropped each block; Ballard et al. had found that in about 90% of these "drop cycles," normal adults did show at least one fixation on the model. The remaining drop cycles were assumed to be cases where the identity and location of the block being dropped had actually been encoded on the previous trial (therefore waiving the requirement to glance back at the model).

When we examined the percent of drop cycles containing at least one fixation on the model, we found that for "simple" puzzles (those using only solid colored blocks), there were no differences between the children with WS compared to either mental age matched children (around 5 years of age) or even normal adults. However, fixations for the "complex" puzzles showed a distinctly different pattern. While children with WS and normally developing 5-year-olds showed roughly the same number of fixations on the model (and even the same as normal adults), the fixations of children with WS varied considerably as a function of the size of the puzzle. For puzzles with two or three blocks, all three groups of participants fixated the model on between 60% to 70% of the drop cycles. But for the four- or nine-block puzzles, normally developing children and normal adults increased their fixations on the model, while the children with WS showed a large decline. The fact that fixations on models containing two or three blocks looked quite similar across groups suggests that the children with WS may be able to set up to three "markers" as they move through assembling the puzzle.

We asked whether the lower levels of fixation by children with WS were the cause of their impaired performance for the four-block, and especially the nine-block puzzles (which were solved with only 10% accuracy). For example, if the children were failing to adequately fixate the model in the nine-block puzzles, they might not have had the information needed for accurate copying. Alternatively, it could be that failure to fixate the model could be driven by the fact that the children are somehow aware that they have severe difficulty in these complex puzzles, and hence just do not even attempt to gather much information. The latter turned out to be the case: Even when we examined only trials where a block was placed after the child fixated the model, the children with WS performed more poorly in placing blocks correctly than the normally developing 5-year-old children.

We asked whether the poorer performance of WS children (relative to normal 5-year-olds) could be explained by their failure to check their block placement as they constructed their copies. One way of finding out is to look at whether participants checked their completed copy against the model, in other words whether they fixated the model after dropping the final block. Looking at the complex puzzles only, we found that the children with WS, the normally developing controls, and the normal adults checked their completed puzzles 61%, 60%, and 64% of the time, respectively. This suggests that the children with WS were checking their final product about as often as even normal adults.

Next we looked at checks on the model that occurred while people were carrying out their solution. Both normal adults and children increased their checks on the model for nine-block puzzles, relative to four-block puzzles. Children with WS showed a slight decline of these intermediate checks when they were doing the most difficult puzzles—surprisingly, since they also perform more poorly and might be expected to be more vigilant. However, we also found that the children with WS—like normal children—initiated corrections (i.e., removing a block from the copy area and replacing it with another) when they had, in fact, placed a block incorrectly. This suggests that both children with WS and normal children were equally able to assess whether they had placed a block correctly or not—again, by checking the model—and that they knew how to initiate a repair once that happened.

Remarkably, the children with WS were about as poor, relative to normally developing 5-year-olds, in fixing an erroneously placed block as they were in first placing a block. In other words, when children detected an error, and removed a block, they then began the process all over again, sometimes making the same kinds of mistakes on the repair as they had on their initial placement. Figure 2.11 shows a sequence of shots from one such erroneous sequence: The WS child who carried out this sequence first placed the two blocks in the wrong positions, then removed both, and effectively recreated the erroneous positions. We observed this kind of cycle on numerous occasions with WS children. The upshot of this cycle is that the children perpetuated errors to

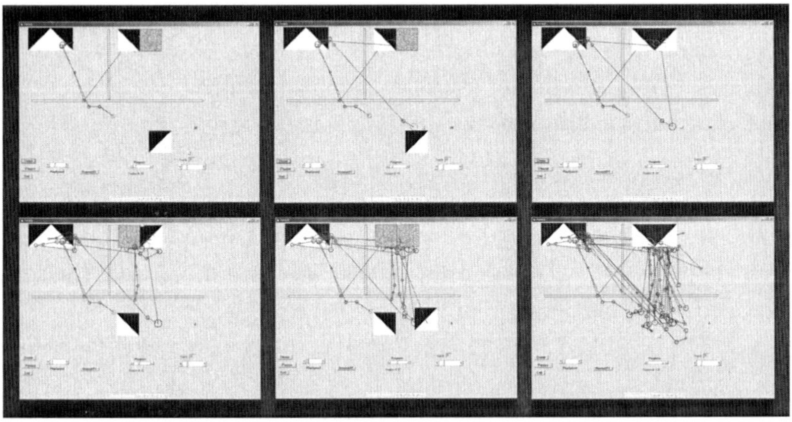

Figure 2.11. Sample screen shots showing a WS child's sequence of fixations for a two-block puzzle. This sequence (top row, left to right, then bottom row) shows that the child was fixating the relevant regions as he/she progressed through the puzzle, even checking on the final product (e.g., top row, right), then removing blocks to redo the puzzle (bottom row, left and middle). Despite this, the child continues to place the two blocks in the incorrect positions. Circles represent fixations; lines indicate trajectory of saccades between fixations.

a larger degree than normally developing 5-year-olds—simply because they could not correctly select and position a block in the first place.

Overall, the evidence from eye fixations suggests several things. First, the children with WS as well as normal children and adults do seem to carry out the block construction task cyclically, using the model as a place to "return" and check on what they have done. This fits well with Ballard et al.'s idea that this task is done in somewhat piecemeal fashion, off-loading some complexity from memory by working one block at a time, and checking and repairing along the way. What is especially striking about the pattern for children with WS is that much of their eye-fixation patterns look quite similar to that of normal 5-year-olds, and in some cases, even normal adults. What is different, of course, is their final performance for complex puzzles, especially for larger puzzles. The error detection and repair cycles suggest that what is amiss is not the *executive processes* that tell a person that they should check, nor that they have made an error, nor that they should initiate a repair—but rather, the mechanisms by which they can select the correct block from the options and correctly represent its location in the copy area. These key mechanisms rely on accurate spatial representations, which we turn to next.

3. *Individual blocks must be accurately selected from the available set.* Suppose the overall model is correctly segmented. In our task, the observer must now move his or her gaze to the area displaying individual blocks, and select the correct one. This step requires that he accurately represent the individual block that he or she will be seeking, and hold it in working memory while scanning the set of block choices for selection. In the version of the block task shown in Figure 2.8, accurately choosing the block entails representing the geometry of each target block (whether it is split vertically, horizontally, or diagonally) and the relative locations of the two colors in the halves of the block (in the figure, yellow and black).

The process of representing and retaining these block properties is also a problem for people with WS. As a follow-up to our main block construction study, we carried out a matching task that was similar to the full construction task, except that people were required only to select a block that matched one that was specifically marked with a clear dot in the design (see Figure 2.12a). We found that the children with WS performed reliably more poorly than the normally developing children matched for mental age. Moreover, the errors of both groups tended to preserve geometric structure (i.e., vertical, horizontal, or diagonal split), but err on the location of each color, systematically resulting in errors of reflection. For example, if the marked block was vertically split with black on the left and yellow on the right, children would most often err by choosing a vertically split block whose colors were reversed. Although both groups of children showed the same qualitative pattern, performance overall was much poorer among the children with WS, indicating that they experience significant problems in representing and holding in working memory the combination of color and location (though not overall geometry) within a single block. This difficulty suggests that part of the problem experienced by people with WS is in correctly representing and remembering (even if only for a few seconds) the correct block. We take this up further in Chapter 3.

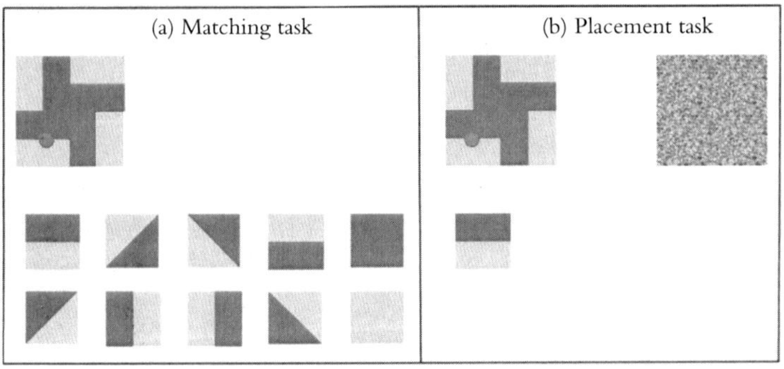

Figure 2.12. (a) Matching task. Children were shown a model with a pink dot located in the center of one of the blocks, and were asked to find the block that was exactly the same in the block bin below. (b) Placement task. Children were shown a model with a pink dot located in the center of one of the blocks, and were told that the block below was the same one. They were asked to place it in the copy area in exactly the same place as the one in the model. The matching and the placement tasks are components of the full block construction task. Children with WS performed more poorly than normally developing mental-age-matched children (on average 5 years old). See text for discussion. (*See* color insert.)

4. *Individual blocks must be placed in the correct locations in the copy space.* Suppose now that the observer has selected the correct block from the parts area. He or she must now place that block into the copy space in a location that is the *same* as in the model. The meaning of "same location" can vary, and is determined in part by the reference system that is used to define the object's location. In our task (or any similar block copy task), placing the block in the *same location* in the copy as in the model means coding it in terms of an object-centered reference system, centered on the model For example, in Figure 2.10, the block being fixated is in the upper right part of the model, and the same location (upper right of the copy area) must be used for placing the block in the copy. Note that, given this setup for the task, using other reference frames will not result in an accurate copy. For example, a person cannot use his own body's frame of reference to accurately place the block in the copy space: Assuming that the model is slightly to the person's left and the copy to his right, any location defined with respect to one's own body, head, or eye will result in erroneous placement of the block. A person cannot use a frame of reference centered on the screen itself either, for similar reasons—the block's location in the model and its location in the copy will be in different locations relative to the screen. The only frame of reference that will work is the object-based system, and this system defined with respect to the model must be converted into a parallel object-based system centered on the outline of the copy in the copy space. Thus making an accurate copy requires representing the location of each block accurately in terms of an object-centered frame of reference and suppressing any tendency to encode and use a representation centered on one's body, the screen, the room, or any of many other possibilities.

In Chapter 4, we return to this problem in more detail. For now, we note that children with WS have difficulty with this step as well. We carried out a placement task similar to the full construction task, except that children were shown the entire puzzle with one block marked, and a replica of the target block was positioned below the model. Children were asked to move this replica block into the correct location in the copy space (see Figure 2.12b). Again, children with WS performed more poorly than normally developing children who were matched in mental age, and their errors were often placements in another column (but not in another row). For example, a block that was located to the left of the model's midline might now be placed to the right of the copy's midline.

2.3.3 Summary of the Cognitive Components of the Block Construction Task and Reflections on Possible Brain Correlates

The foregoing sections highlight that the block construction task engages at least four crucial spatial-cognitive mechanisms. First, selective attention must be used to segment the design into block-sized chunks. Second, individual blocks or regions in the model must be "marked" so that a person can return to the target block to check whether a correct block has been selected, and whether it has been placed in the proper region in the copy area. Third, a person must be able to accurately represent the spatial identity of the individual blocks—their geometric structure, and the relative locations of colors within this structure. This representation must be held in working memory at least over the time of one or more fixations, as the person searches the candidate blocks and selects one. Fourth, the observer must be able to accurately represent the spatial location of the blocks in the model space (in an object-based reference system) and must be capable of mapping this representation onto the copy space (another object-based reference system), while ignoring other reference systems such as the body or screen-based ones.

This analysis of the block construction task is consistent with the analysis proposed by Ballard et al. (1997) and suggests that the mechanisms that allow children with WS or normally developing children to carry out the task are similar to those employed by normal adults. What is striking, of course, is that somehow the deployment of these mechanisms results in extremely poor copies by children with WS—poorer even than normally developing children who are on average about 5 or 6 years old and are matched for mental age. Our analysis of the task and the results we have reported already suggest that children with WS suffer impairments in each of the components we have described. The next several chapters will explore in detail these impairments.

The analysis also raises questions about whether and how the WS impairment in the block construction task relates to what is known about spatial functions in the brain. Are there any ties between the cognitive components of the block construction task and their realization in the brain—ties that might suggest a more general hypothesis about the WS spatial impairment?

In fact, there is striking evidence from studies of construction abilities in monkeys that provide us with a hint about the locus of damage in the brain that could be correlated with failures in the block construction task. Studies by Chafee and colleagues (2005) suggest that specific areas of the parietal cortex are responsible for the monkey's ability to represent locations of "missing elements" while they are carrying out tasks that are closely related to traditional block construction tasks. In essence Chafee et al. trained monkeys to replicate a model pattern by selecting and placing a block into a second "copy" design to create an exact replica of the model. Chafee et al. examined the patterns of brain activation that occur as the monkey carries out these tasks, and found that areas of the parietal cortex—especially the intraparietal sulcus—are activated during the construction task.

This is consistent with the idea that a homologous area of the human brain, the parietal lobe, including the IPS, might be involved in the spatial construction deficit of people with Williams syndrome, consistent with the findings of Meyer-Lindenberg et al. (2004). These areas are known to also be important in regulating visual attention in both monkeys and humans (Colby & Goldberg, 1999), and they are engaged during visual-manual action in both monkeys (Chafee et al., 2005) and humans (Milner & Goodale, 1995, 2008). Recalling our earlier discussion, we proposed that several processes were crucially involved in the block construction task. Attentional processes are important in segmenting the overall design of the puzzle into block-sized chunks. Representing the objects (blocks) correctly is crucial to selecting the correct target block(s). Representing the object-based location of an individual block (and ignoring its egocentric or screen-based location) is crucial in placing the block into its correct space in the copy area. Clearly, carrying out the action of placing the block is also an important ingredient in copying the puzzle. As we will see in the next two chapters, many of these component processes are impaired in people with Williams syndrome, providing strong convergence with the monkey work and suggesting definite involvement of the parietal areas of the brain in the WS spatial deficit.

2.4 Toward a Hypothesis: Weakness in the Dorsal Stream/Parietal Lobe Functions, Strength in Ventral Stream Functions?

The studies we have reviewed point to a hypothesis about the hallmark deficit in Williams syndrome: Spatial functions supported by the parietal cortex may be damaged. If so, this would predict that a range of spatial-cognitive functions that normally engage these areas might be impaired in people with Williams syndrome. We also reviewed evidence for some possible functional damage to the hippocampal formation. The extensive connections between the parietal and hippocampal areas might converge in predicting a host of impairments linked to these sites of damage. The studies we have reviewed also point to a complementary possibility—that spatial functions carried by the ventral stream might be strong, even spared.

The hypothesis that WS can be characterized as a deficit in dorsal stream functions and relative strength in ventral stream functions has been suggested by others (Atkinson et al., 2003; Wang et al., 1995), and the evidence we reviewed earlier (Section 2.2) is certainly consistent with it. But several key questions must be answered before concluding that the deficit is best characterized in this way.

A first question concerns the degree to which there are severe impairments across a wide range of spatial-cognitive functions that engage the dorsal stream only, as would be predicted by the dorsal stream deficit view. The block construction task has provided first and foremost clear evidence of severe spatial impairment in people with WS. And our analysis of this task certainly suggests that it is composed of several different kinds of spatial processes, pointing to the possibility that there is quite a broad deficit in spatial-cognitive functions. But our cognitive systems carry out many different spatial functions, and some of them do not appear to engage the parietal areas or the dorsal stream, at least not as their primary site. For example, our remarkable ability to perceive biological motion depends on the spatial integration of a set of moving dots to create the percept of a moving animate being. This ability is highly spatial and computationally complex, and appears to involve some areas, such as the superior temporal sulcus, that are normally considered part of the ventral stream. As another example, our ability to recognize objects surely depends in some sense on the spatial representation of individual component parts and their arrangement. Yet the perception of objects is known to depend on areas of the ventral stream, particularly the inferotemporal cortex.

Do people with WS suffer from severe impairment in only those spatial capacities that engage the dorsal stream, or is there more widespread impairment? Is there variation within each of the streams, perhaps reflecting the strength of selective specialized domains (e.g., faces)? How can we best characterize the range of strengths and/or impairments that we see?

Studies of spatial-cognitive functions carried by each stream have generally proceeded independently of each other in the literature. Consequently, we have limited understanding of whether the overall set of spatial functions pattern similarly or are quite distinct. This is true whether we adopt the hypothesis of dorsal stream deficit or the hypothesis of deficit and strength that reflects more specialized domains. Moreover, as we have argued in Chapter 1, it is hard to evaluate whether a particular spatial function is "poor" or "strong" without considering the lens of normal development.

This brings us to a final point. Our understanding of the spatial deficit in people with WS can be examined only through a systematic study of a range of spatial functions that span each of the two streams, that tap different domains, and that vary the cognitive requirements of the task. Moreover, determining whether there is truly a deficit in the dorsal stream and strength in the ventral stream will require comparing the profiles in people with WS with those of normally developing individuals. As we will see, the normal developmental profiles vary considerably across a broad range of spatial functions—some visual-spatial functions appear to reach adult levels quite early in development, while others take many years to reach maturity. Understanding the profile of an unusual population requires the backdrop of normal development. The picture that emerges when one does this kind of comparison can be quite surprising and illuminating.

We now turn to Chapters 3 and 4, in which we lay out a wide range of experimental findings examining first the representation of objects (usually assumed to engage the ventral stream), and then the representation of places (often engaging dorsal stream functions). These two chapters will set the stage for Chapter 5, which examines a quite different spatial function—navigation. In the final empirical chapter (Chapter 6), we will return to a crucial question for the WS cognitive profile: How do the facts about language in people with WS fit into what we know about space?

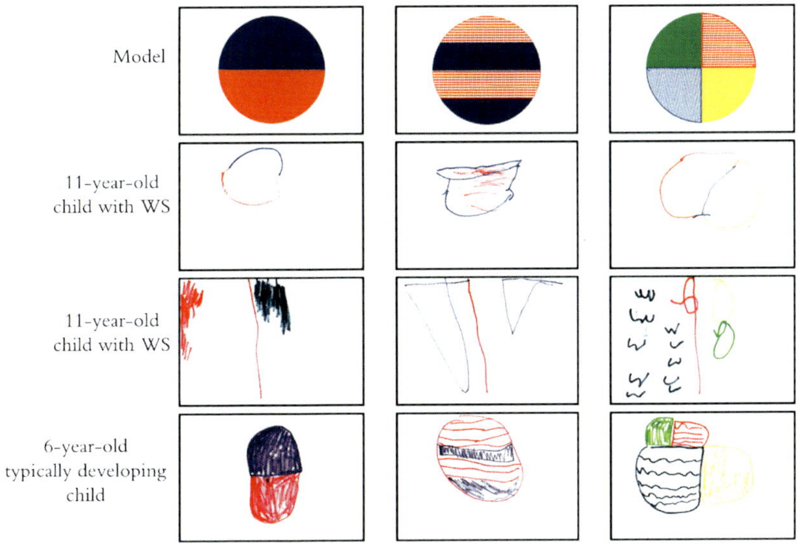

Figure 1.2. Copies of target models by two children with WS and one typically developing child who were seen in our lab. The models were visually present while the children made their copies. Reprinted from Dilks, Hoffman, and Landau (2008), with permission of John Wiley and Sons.

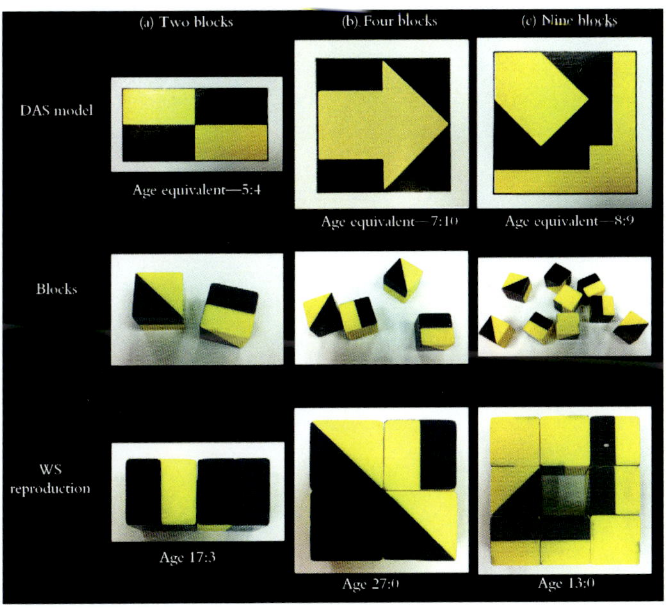

Figure 1.3. Representative model patterns from the Differential Abilities Scale (Elliott, 1990), and sample copies by people with WS tested in our lab. The top row displays the model shown to the participant. Age equivalents represent the 50th percentile for normally developing children. The middle row shows the blocks given to the person, in order to copy the model. All blocks have the same six sides, including vertical, horizontal, and diagonal splits over two colors. The bottom row shows three illustrative copies produced by people with WS, along with their chronological ages. Note that in all cases, there is severe compromise in the accuracy of the copies, even though the chronological ages for the WS participants are far higher than the age equivalent for normally developing individuals.

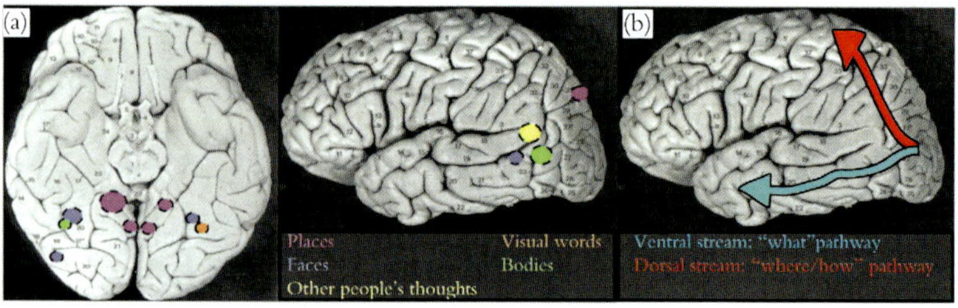

Figure 1.5. Two alternative organizations of the division of labor within spatial representations. One can consider a division of labor based on specific functional domains, such as representation of faces, places, and visual words (left and middle panel). Or one can consider a broader division of labor based on the two main pathways of the visual system (right panel), the ventral ("what") and dorsal ("where/how") pathways. Both organizations are useful in providing hypotheses about the spatial impairment in people with Williams syndrome. Figures adapted from Kanwisher (2010), with permission of PNAS.

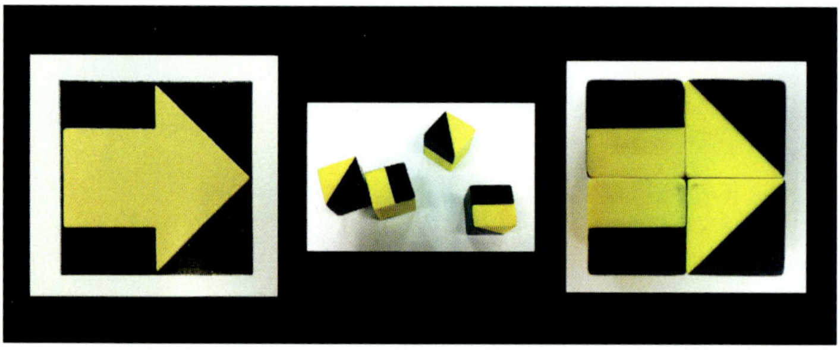

Figure 2.1. Sample model from the Differential Abilities Scales, Pattern Construction subtest (Elliott, 1990). The left panel shows the model pattern as shown to participants. The middle panel shows the four blocks they are given, which they must use to copy the model. The right panel shows a model that has been accurately assembled using the four available blocks.

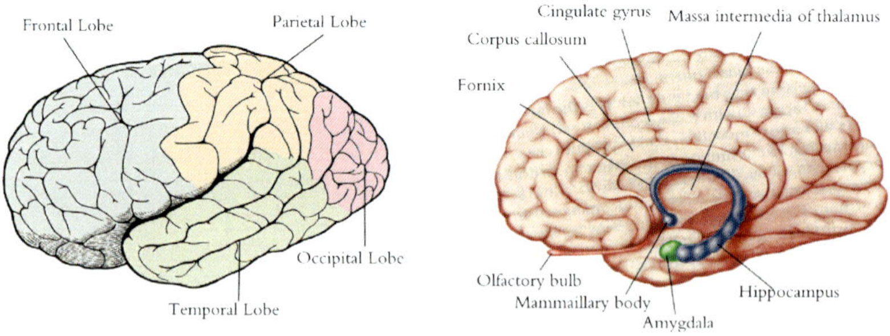

Figure 2.4. Major lobes of the brain (left panel) and hippocampus (right panel), which is buried within the medial temporal lobe. Right panel reprinted from Gazzaniga et al. (2008), with permission from W. W. Norton & Company.

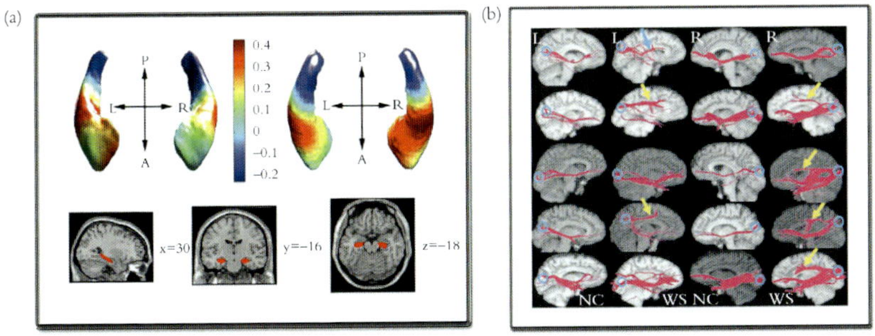

Figure 2.5. (a) Differences in the shape of the HF in WS and normal controls. Shape change is rendered on an average age (between groups) template of the HF. Top left: anterior view; top right: posterior view. Color scale correlates to the degree of deformation. Units are arbitrary. Negative values reflect local volume reduction in WS patients relative to controls. Positive values reflect local volume expansion in WS patients relative to controls. Double arrow marked A-P shows anterior-posterior direction. Double arrow marked L-R shows left-right direction. Significant findings ($P < 0.05$, corrected at the voxel level using small volume correction for the hippocampus ROI) were positive and greater than 0.3 and located in the mid/anterior section of the HF. Bottom: Same template shown superimposed on a representative single-subject MRI for orientation purposes. Coordinates x, y, and z are given in mm distance from the anterior commissure. (b) Differences between controls and WS in tracks connecting to the IPS (intraparietal sulcus) and VCING (ventral cingulate). Fiber tracking was performed with DTI studio seeding tracts from all voxels in the brain and then displaying only fibers that traversed the IPS ROI (illustrated as a blue circle) and a coronal plane at the center of the thalamus. The yellow arrows indicate the fiber tracts coursing rostrally to the corpus callosum, which were never present in controls (normal control, NC, first and third columns) but present in four of the five individuals with WS (second and fourth columns), especially in the right hemisphere (Mann-Whitney $U = 2.5$ $P < 0.05$). The blue arrow indicates fibers connecting the IPS to the thalamus, observed in the left hemisphere of one individual with WS. Reprinted from Meyer-Lindenberg et al. (2005), with permission of the American Society of Clinical Investigation (this is for Fig 2.5a). Reprinted from Marenco et al., copyright © 2007 National Academy of Sciences, U.S.A. (this is for Fig 2.5b).

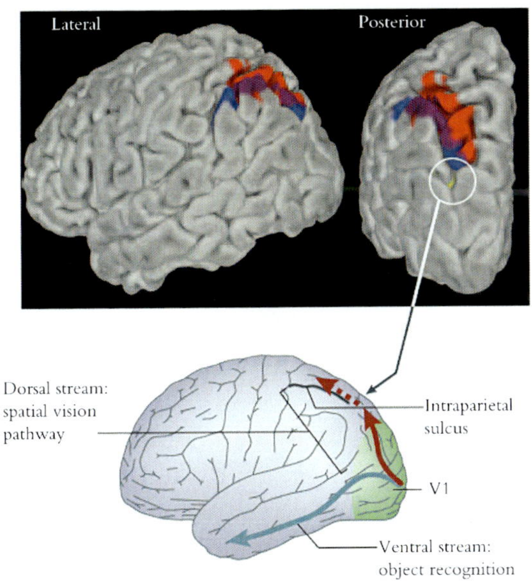

Figure 2.6. Meyer-Lindenberg et al.'s findings from brain imaging and path analysis suggest that the WS brain has structural abnormalities in the area of the intraparietal sulcus, with reduced functional processing in areas further upstream. Reprinted from Meyer-Lindenberg et al. (2006), with permission of Nature Publishing Group.

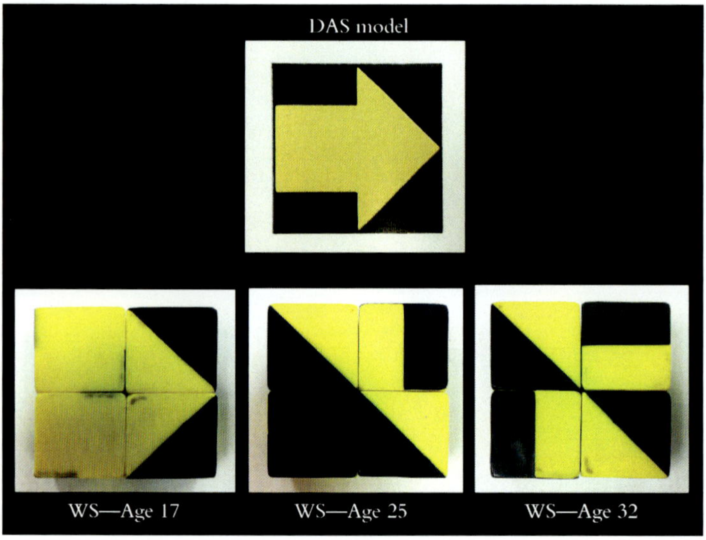

Figure 2.8. Sample model from the pattern construction task (DAS; Elliot, 1990) and sample copies by three participants in our studies.

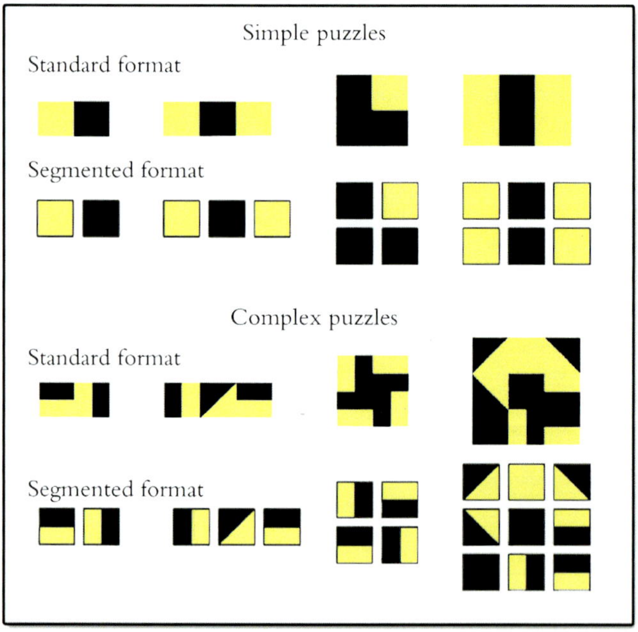

Figure 2.9. Simple and complex puzzles used in study by Hoffman et al. (2003). Simple puzzles required using block faces that were solid colors. Complex puzzles required using block faces that were not solid, in other words, with internal structure of vertical, horizontal, or diagonal splits by color. In simple puzzles, the borders of each block are consistent with the emergent patterns; in complex puzzles, however, the borders of each block may span more than one component of the emergent pattern of the puzzle. Hoffman et al. presented these puzzles in two formats: The standard format was the same as is used in the pattern construction task (DAS; Elliot, 1990). The segmented format displayed models with the individual component blocks slighted separated from each other. We predicted that this format would enhance performance by people with WS, and it did. Adapted from Hoffman et al. (2003), with permission from Elsevier; see text for discussion.

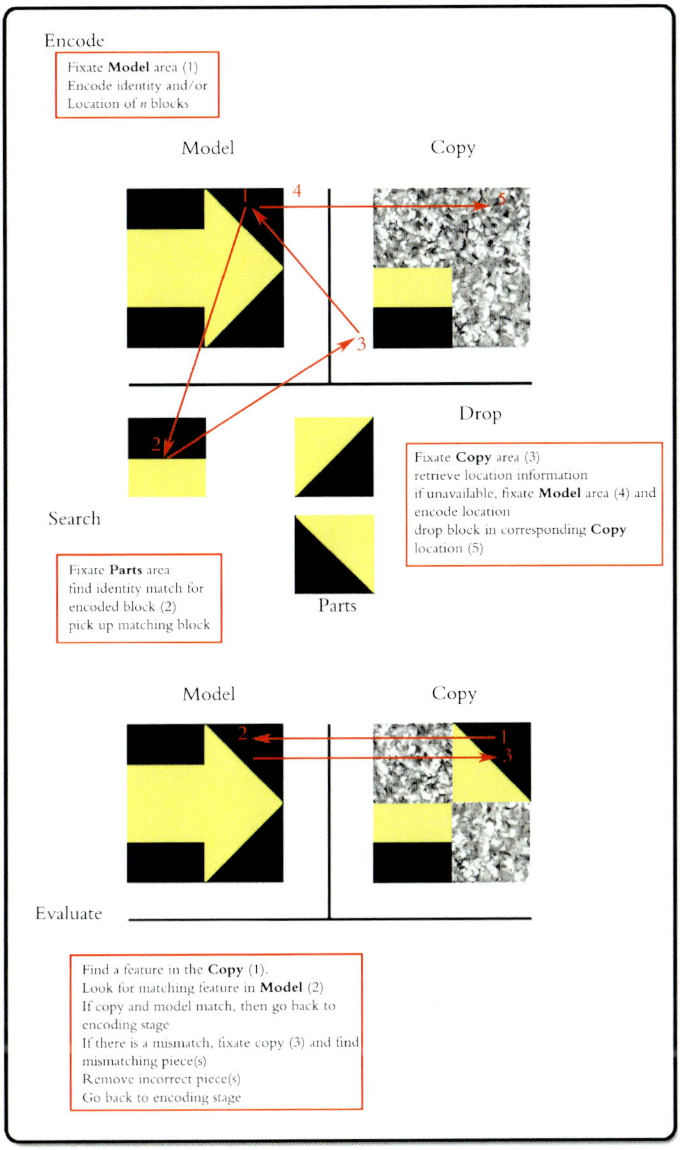

Figure 2.10. A computational analysis of the block construction task, adapted from Hoffman et al. (2003). Upper panel: The observer encodes the identity of a candidate block in the model, by fixating the model area (1). This step requires *segmenting* the model into candidate blocks, which are not obvious in the model. The observer then moves his gaze to the parts area (2) to find a *match* for the encoded block. This step requires representing the internal structure of the candidate block and successfully selecting it among the alternatives. The observer then moves his gaze to the copy area (3) in order to place the block. If necessary, he moves his gaze back to the model (4) to pick up information about the block's location in the puzzle. He then *places* the block into the copy area (5)—in this case, in the wrong location. Lower panel: The observer *evaluates* his copy by fixating the block he placed (1), then looking for the matching block in the model (2). If the copy and model match, then he can go back to the encoding stage (1, upper panel). If he detects a mismatch, then he can remove the incorrect block and start over again. See text for discussion of segmenting the model, choosing parts, and placing the blocks in the correct location. See text for discussion of problems among people with Williams syndrome in segmenting, matching, and placing blocks. Adapted from Hoffman et al. (2003) with permission from Elsevier.

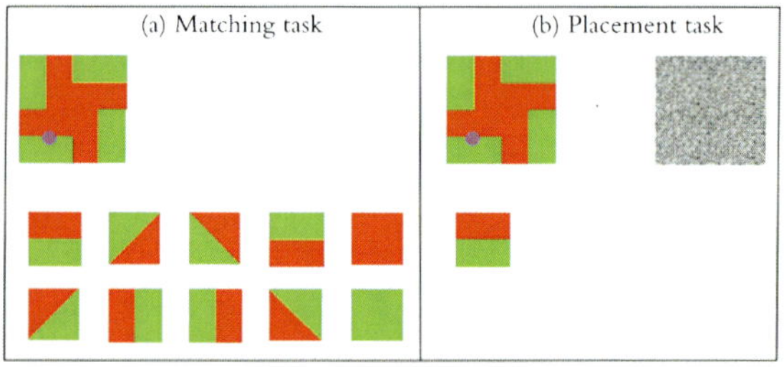

Figure 2.12. (a) Matching task. Children were shown a model with a pink dot located in the center of one of the blocks, and were asked to find the block that was exactly the same in the block bin below. (b) Placement task. Children were shown a model with a pink dot located in the center of one of the blocks, and were told that the block below was the same one. They were asked to place it in the copy area in exactly the same place as the one in the model. The matching and the placement tasks are components of the full block construction task. Children with WS performed more poorly than normally developing mental-age-matched children (on average 5 years old). See text for discussion.

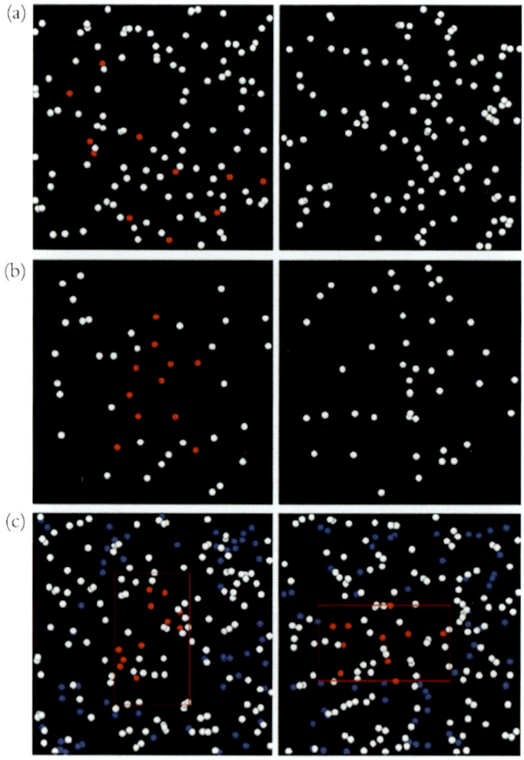

Figure 3.9. Scale illustrations of (a) motion coherence, (b) biological motion, and (c) form-from-motion displays. For illustration purposes, signal elements are indicated in red, while noise elements are colored white. The form-from-motion stimuli also included signal background elements that moved in the opposite direction of the motion of the target rectangle; these are indicated in blue. During the actual experiments, all elements (signal, noise, signal-background) appeared as white lights on a black background and no rectangles appeared in the form-from-motion displays. The participants' task was to find the panel that had dots moving together "like a school of fish" (motion coherence), to find the panel that shows a person walking "nice and upright" (biological motion), and to find the panel that has the vertical rectangle ("the tall up-and-down rectangle that looks like a door"). See text for discussion of task and results.

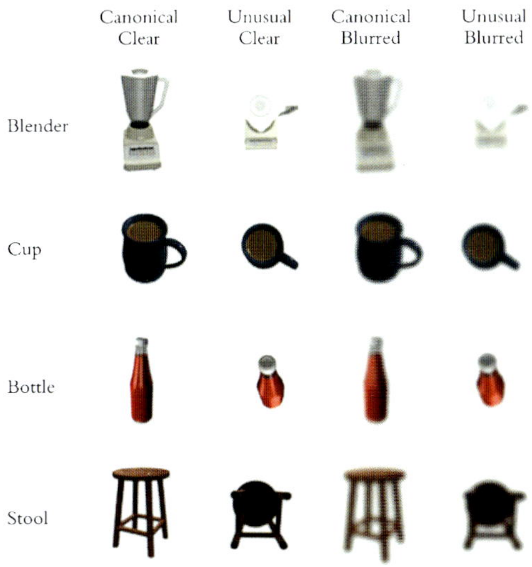

Figure 3.11. Four examples of full-color objects presented under different viewing conditions. Objects were presented from two different viewpoints (canonical and unusual), and in either clear or blurred format. Adapted from Landau et al. (2006), with permission from Elsevier.

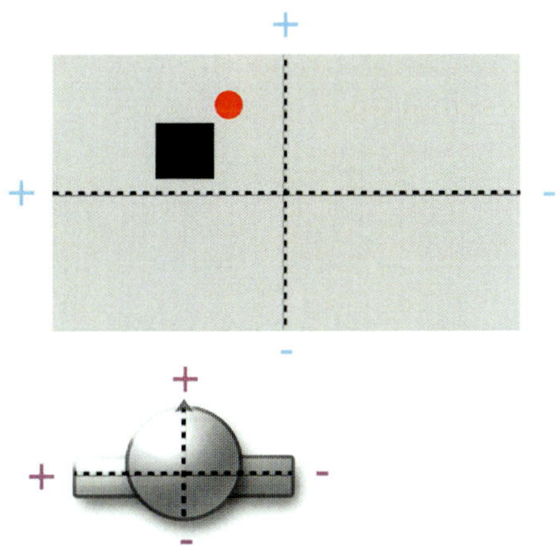

Figure 4.4. Imagine that the black square is on a gray sheet of paper positioned in front of the observer. The location of the square on the rectangular page can be defined relative to the observer's body axes, the axes of the page, or both. The dotted lines represent the axes of these two different reference systems, and the + and – represent the directions within each axis of each reference system. As one can see, the square is located *in front of* the observer, but *on the left side* of the page. These locations are defined within different reference systems—one centered on the observer, the other centered on the page itself.

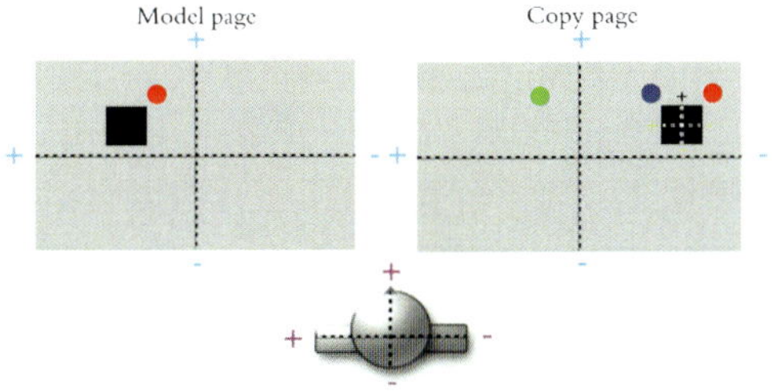

Figure 4.5. The observer can represent the location of the red dot in the model panel (left) in terms of various frames of reference. The red dot in the copy page (right) represents the "same" location using the center of the square as the origin of the reference system. The green dot represents the "same" location using the center of the page itself as the origin. The blue dot represents the "same" location using the center of the square as the origin of the reference system, but misrepresenting the direction along the horizontal axis, thereby copying the location "above and to the *left*" of the square rather than "above and to the *right*." The latter kind of error is attested in our studies of people with WS and young normally developing children.

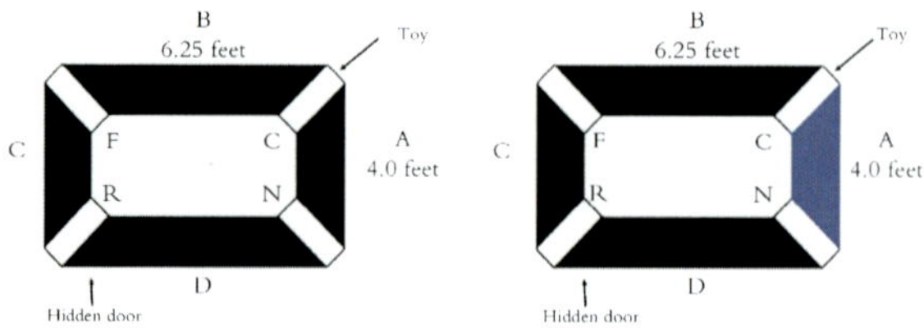

Figure 5.7. Illustration of the testing environment for reorientation experiments. A, B, C, and D denote each of the four walls. In the black wall condition (left panel), all walls were black. In the blue wall condition (right panel), wall A was blue. C, R, N, and F illustrate the four corners in which the toy was hidden (with hiding location counterbalanced across participants): C is the correct corner (i.e., corner where the toy was hidden); R, the rotationally equivalent corner (i.e., the corner that is rotationally equivalent to the correct corner); N, the near corner (i.e., the corner that is closest to the correct corner); and F, the far corner (i.e., the nonrotationally equivalent corner that is farthest from the correct corner). Adapted from Lakusta et al. (2010).

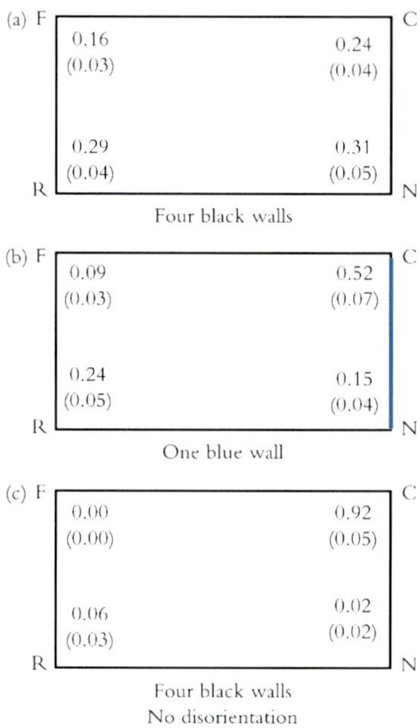

Figure 5.8. Average proportion of search (and SEs) at each corner (correct, rotationally equivalent, near, and far) for the WS participants in Experiment 1 (a, four black walls; b, one blue wall) and Experiment 2 (c, four black walls, no disorientation). Adapted from Lakusta et al. (2010).

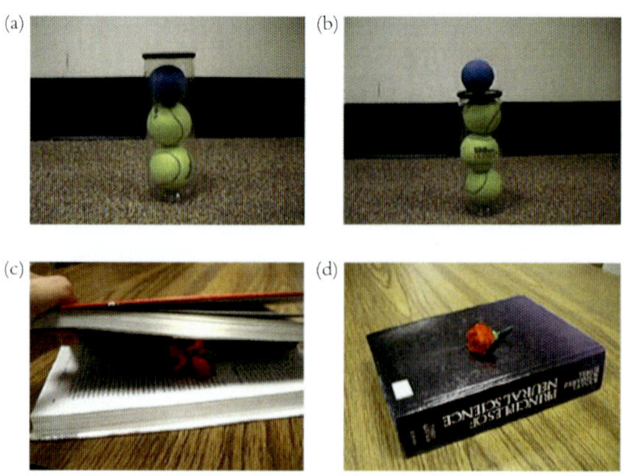

Figure 6.10. Sample of spatial semantic stimuli. Upper panel: (a) Blue ball *in* container, (b) blue ball *on* container. Lower panel: (c) Flower *in* book, (d) flower *on* book. People were given an image and were asked to complete a sentence using a spatial term. For example, they might be shown picture (a) and prompted to complete the sentence "The blue ball is ______ the container." Adapted from Munnich and Landau (2010), with permission from Taylor & Francis.

3

Objects

It might seem odd to ask about the role of object recognition in the spatial profile of people with Williams syndrome. After all, their hallmark deficit is reflected in visuospatial construction tasks such as block construction or copying figures. Still, any complete understanding of the spatial profile will necessarily entail understanding how people with WS represent objects. This is because, on all accounts, recognizing objects is at least partly a spatial affair: Formal theories of objects emphasize their shape, represented by their parts and the spatial relationships among them (Marr & Nishihara, 1978), and shape plays a crucial role in the representation of objects for children as well as adults (Kourtzi & Kanwisher, 2001; Landau, Smith, & Jones, 1998). If the WS spatial deficit is a very general one, we might expect severe deficits in at least some aspects of object representation.

Indeed, as we saw in the last chapter, people with WS show significant deficits when they are asked to merely pick out a match for one of the target blocks in the block construction task. Although these blocks are, on an intuitive level, perhaps less "object-like" than, say cups or cars, the deficit shown by WS people in that matching task raises the possibility that other aspects of their object representation are also impaired. Finally, examining object representation is required in order to test the candidate hypothesis suggested at the end of our last chapter, specifically, that WS is primarily a dorsal stream deficit. If true, then we should see relative strength among people with WS in spatial functions carried by the ventral stream—with object recognition being one of the clearest cases.

In this chapter, we will primarily deal with object recognition and the more general question of whether spatial functions in the ventral pathway show severe impairment in people with Williams syndrome. We focus on object recognition as this is crucial to making decisions about an object's category, as well as carrying out actions that are appropriate for a particular object. Cups (but not strainers) need to be recognized as things that can hold liquid; toothbrushes need to be acted upon so that one end is grasped and the other end inserted in the mouth. These two aspects of object perception—recognition and action—engage two different pathways in the visual system, with the ventral pathway playing a critical role in object recognition, and the dorsal pathway playing a large role in actions performed on objects. Object recognition is the topic for this chapter; we consider action on objects in Chapter 4.

In the following sections, we first lay out several levels of organization that are crucial for understanding object representations. We then describe research on the capacities of people with WS that fit within each of these levels, with an emphasis on the ability to group elements into single wholes (a function of "middle-level vision") and object recognition (a function of "high-level vision"). For each set of capacities, we will ask two questions. First, do people with WS show evidence that their visual systems compute the relevant spatial function? And second, how does the WS profile for each type of function fare with respect to that of normally developing children at various ages? We conclude our chapter by considering another major function carried out by the ventral stream: face recognition. This case has been hotly debated in the WS literature, and we summarize findings therein as a complement to our report on object recognition.

3.1 Object Recognition and Levels of Processing in the Visual System

Any description of our conscious visual experience would undoubtedly highlight the presence of objects, their locations, and their spatial relationships to other objects. Each object can be seen as having various features such as a particular color, size, or distance, but these are generally seen as *attributes* of the object. Apparently, objects provide a convenient way to chunk and organize the large amount of information contained in visual scenes. Nonetheless, defining what constitutes an object and discerning how the visual system represents it is anything but trivial. As David Marr (1982) pointed out, the concept of an object is a frustratingly pliable one. Is a man who is riding a horse perceived as one or two objects? One answer is that "it depends." It depends on the goals of the perceiver, which might favor the perception of a single complex object at one moment or separate conjoined objects at another. Another answer is that our percepts are driven by an abstract concept of object, which provides constraints on what we will consider "an object" (Spelke, 1990). In this chapter, we take a neutral stance on this issue of how we determine what an object is. Instead, we will assume the ability to represent objects per se, and emphasize the visual-spatial representation of objects—parts and their internal spatial structure—and the degree to which people with WS can represent that structure.

According to Marr (1982), the computations involved in visual object representation occur at several levels: early, middle, and high. At each of these levels, different questions can be posed about the object representation system in people with WS. As it turns out, we have little empirical evidence on early vision in WS—the level at which elementary features of the visual image (such as edges) are detected. We have more evidence on the level of middle vision, where "grouping" of features into objects occurs, allowing objects to be separated from their background. We also have considerable evidence on the high level of vision, where objects themselves are recognized. We proceed with a brief review of the function of each level, followed by our empirical results on object recognition in WS.

3.1.1 Levels of Visual Analysis for Objects

The level of *early vision* (resulting in what Marr, 1982, called the "primal sketch") is concerned with discovering edges in the visual input. Edges correspond to regions of the image that contain rapid changes in the color and/or intensity of light. Edges are important because they often correspond to the boundary between adjacent surfaces. In addition, the luminance and color differences that exist at edges are used to "fill in" the interior regions of bounded surfaces (Grossberg et al., 2007). The neural basis of edge detection was studied by Hubel and Wiesel (1962), who found cells in the monkey brain that responded selectively to edges of a particular orientation and size. However, these kinds of edge detectors by themselves cannot be sufficient for object recognition, as can be readily appreciated by inspecting Figure 3.1. This figure shows a Henry

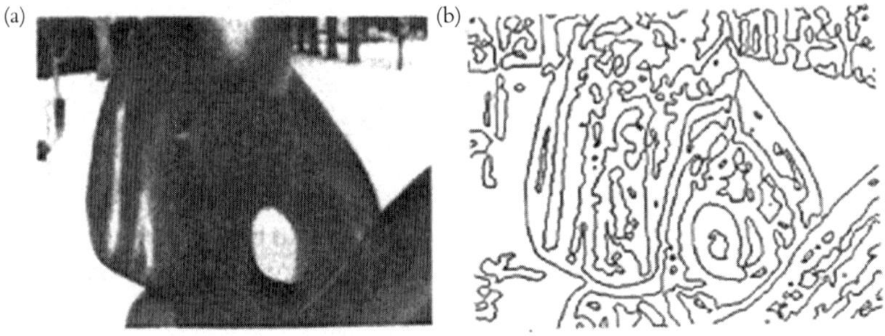

Figure 3.1. The original object (a) and the corresponding edges discovered by a computer-based edge finding algorithm (Marr, 1982). Our retinal image also contains a plethora of edges which, as in the image, do not always correspond to the object's boundaries. This makes it clear that edge detection must be supplemented by other processes, such as grouping mechanisms (see Frisby & Stone, 2010, for discussion). Reprinted from Marr (1982), with permission of W. H. Freeman & Worth.

Moore sculpture and a corresponding set of edges produced by a computer program that was designed to extract the sculpture's edges. The computer program shows that analyzing edges alone is not the only step in representing the object's shape or its part structure, because the local edges do not always correspond to the boundaries of the object. Many of the edges are simply "accidental" changes in intensity that correspond to shadows, changes in surface orientation, and irrelevant "noise." For the purpose of recognizing the object, our visual system needs to somehow ignore the irrelevant edges and combine the relevant ones into contours corresponding to the boundaries of objects. The cells in V1 that detect these edges are not up to this task as each one can only "see" a restricted part of the image. What is needed is a way to look at larger portions of the image to discover which edges should be combined. This "grouping" function is carried out by *middle vision*.

The function of *middle vision* is essentially to combine—or "group"—features into objects and separate them from the background. The well-known "Gestalt laws of organization" (Figure 3.2) represent an early attempt to provide a systematic description of the rules by which individual features can be grouped to represent objects. For example, "grouping by proximity" reflects the idea that texture

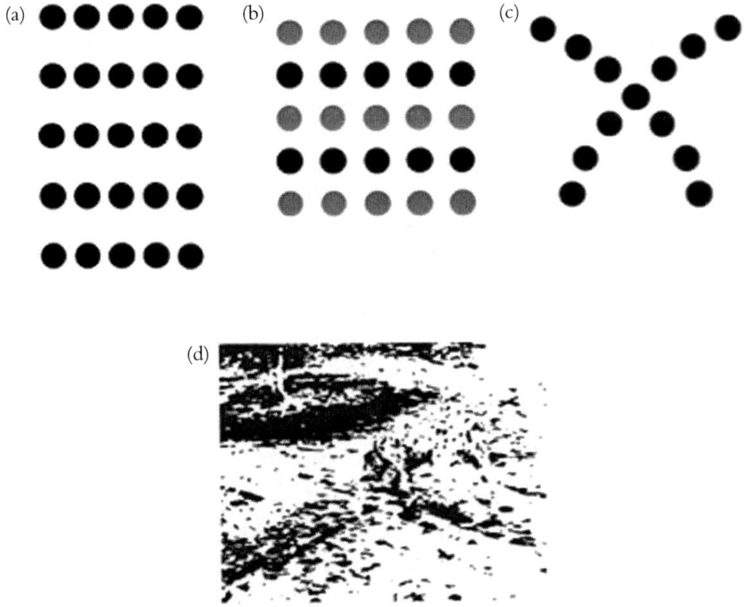

Figure 3.2. Examples of Gestalt grouping principles. (a) Grouping by proximity yields a percept of rows based on spacing. (b) Grouping by proximity also yields a percept of rows, this time based on tone. (c) Good continuation favors a percept of two crossing lines rather than two V-shaped figures. (d) The percept of a Dalmatian depends on the application of grouping principles. Dalmatian photo by R. C. James, in Gregory (1973, p. 14). Image reprinted courtesy of R. C. James.

elements that are close together probably belong to the same object. We see the array in Figure 3.2a as rows of dots rather than columns of dots, even though both percepts are equally rational. The same is true in Figure 3.2b, where similarity is based on tone; here, we seem to carry out "grouping by similarity," based on the heuristic that features belonging to the same object will generally have similar shapes, colors, and so on. In Figure 3.2c our percept is of two crossing lines, rather than two separate V's. Here, we use the principle of "good continuation," which holds that if there are multiple candidates for the continuation of a line segment, the visual system should choose the one that involves the smallest change in orientation.

These "laws" should be looked at as heuristics that will often lead to a correct bundling of features into appropriate objects but are not guaranteed to do so, particularly in cluttered environments that are typical of "real-world" scenes. The Gestalt laws reflect the operation of a very sophisticated neural network that is generally quite accurate in creating object representations; however, the nature of the brain algorithms that are responsible for this feat are still poorly understood.[1] Still, the need to group individual elements from early levels of visual processing into higher levels of organization—such as simple forms—is thought to be a critical ingredient in the representation of objects, and therefore suggests a clear question: Do people with WS show grouping processes that respect the same kinds of principles shown by people without WS, and if so, at what level of functioning? We will address this question in Section 3.2.2.

The final stage of visual processing is *high-level vision*. This system is responsible for finding a match between the bundled set of features constructed by mid-level visual processes and long-term memory (LTM) representations of familiar objects. This is a difficult task because one's current view of an object is likely to differ from previous views that have been stored in LTM on previous occasions of viewing, in terms of retinal image size, lighting, orientation, and arrangement of parts for objects whose parts are flexible. The ability of biological visual systems to recognize objects from novel views has been termed *viewpoint invariance* (Marr, 1982), and it forms the principal criterion for judging the adequacy of object recognition models.

There have been two main approaches to modeling this problem. One approach is based on *structural descriptions* of objects. That is, objects are represented in terms of a set of parts along with a list of the spatial relationships between parts. Marr and Nishihara (1978) proposed one such model that used generalized cones—volumes of different shapes—as the primitives or parts together with their spatial relationships; they further proposed that these relationships were specified in an object-based coordinate system. For example, a person could be modeled as a set of cones

[1] This is particularly the case when features from several different dimensions, such as color, shape, and motion, have to be combined. This is the so-called *binding problem*, whose solution requires the integration of information from the various cortical areas that are specialized for representing these different features. If all feature combinations were explicitly represented in terms of dedicated "conjunction detectors," the number of cells required to represent all possible combinations of basic visual features would exceed the total number of cells in the brain.

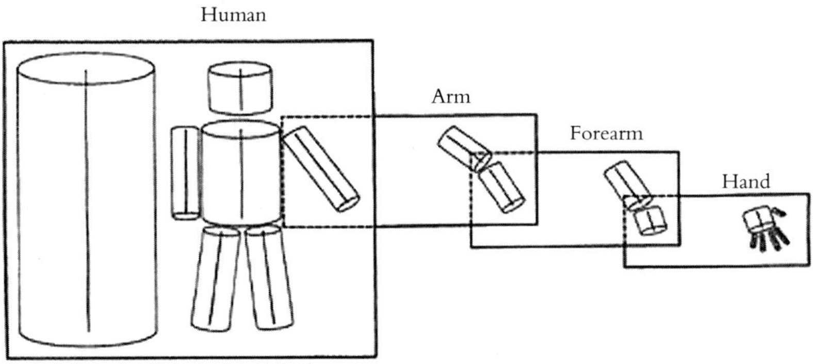

Figure 3.3. Generalized cone model of a human. The body is represented as a set of parts, each of which is subject to hierarchical decomposition. Models increase in detail from left to right. Reprinted from Marr (1982), with permission of W. H. Freeman & Worth.

representing the torso, legs, arms, and so on (see Figure 3.3). The position of each part is specified relative to the long axis of the body. In this way, objects can be recognized at novel orientations because the model is not specified in terms of the observer's viewpoint; as long as the correct parts and principal axis of the object can be recovered, the correct spatial relationships among those parts can be computed leading to successful object recognition.[2] The object-centered models have the virtue of representing objects in a highly abstract form using a small number

[2] Biederman (1987) later built on this theory in his recognition-by-components model (RBC). He extended the library of parts for building internal models of objects to 36 geons (geometrical ions) that could be assembled to represent the many thousands of objects we recognize, in the same way that a small set of phonemes can be used to recognize an unlimited number of spoken words. Importantly, geons were defined by features such as parallel lines or particular kinds of line junctions such as "arrows" that would be available in the retinal image regardless of the viewing angle of the object. Biederman proposed that the spatial arrangement of parts was specified by *qualitative relations* such as above versus below rather than metric relationships specifying fine positional detail. This allowed the model to tolerate some variations in the locations of parts. Similar to Marr and Nishihara's theory, the locations of parts were specified in an object-centered coordinate system. For example, in a representation of a person, the location of the arms would be specified with respect to the body. This approach provides for viewpoint invariance as the *object-centered locations* of an object's parts will not depend on the observer's viewpoint.

of parts, thus achieving considerable economy in storage. In addition, the claim that objects are decomposed into parts seems like a sensible approach that could capture the hierarchical nature of visual information where parts at one level of analysis are objects at another. This type of theory would predict that any viewpoint of an object should be as easy for the visual system to recognize as any other, since the representation is viewpoint-independent.

According to a second approach, the *multiple view models* (Tarr & Pinker, 1989), people store previous views of an object in memory; recognition is achieved when the person's current view of the object either matches one of the stored views or can be adjusted to provide a match with the nearest view. This model predicts some advantage to seeing an object from a viewpoint that has previously been experienced, and some penalty to seeing an object from a new viewpoint. Results of experiments are consistent with these predictions, as people's recognition time is fastest when they see an object in a viewpoint that matches a previously seen viewpoint of an object (Tarr & Pinker, 1989). These findings suggest that the human object recognition system does not always display viewpoint invariance, and, rather, is highly sensitive to the particular viewpoint of an object being processed.[3]

These two approaches make quite different predictions about our ability to recognize objects under familiar versus novel viewpoints. Clearly, recognition of objects from both of these kinds of viewpoints is a desideratum of an adequate theory of human object recognition, and therefore suggests a clear question about the object recognition system in people with WS: Do they recognize objects under novel as well as familiar viewpoints, and if so, is there a difference in their level of performance

---

[3] Critics of this approach point out that such models appear to require massive storage space that might exceed the capability of the human brain. Given the large information content of visual images and the need to store multiple views of every object that we encounter, this is a valid concern. On the other hand, a recent study (Brady et al., 2008) found that observers who viewed pictures of 2,500 objects presented over the course of 5.5 hours were able to distinguish between different poses of the previously viewed objects with 87% accuracy. This shows that the human brain has a surprisingly large capacity for remembering detailed information about the appearance of complex objects.

for the two cases? We address this question, and other related ones, in Section 3.3.

3.2 Object Recognition in People with Williams Syndrome

The severe visuospatial constructive deficit shown by people with Williams syndrome might be due to deficits in visual processing at any of the three visual processing levels we have outlined. As we noted, there is limited evidence on visual processing at the early level, but more on the middle and high levels. We discuss evidence at each level below.

3.2.1 Early Vision

The relevant evidence comes from two sources: anatomical and functional imaging studies of the relevant brain regions in people with WS; and ophthalmologic profiles of people with WS, for example, acuity and depth perception.

Evidence on characteristics of the WS brain responsible for early vision is currently mixed. On the one hand, postmortem examination of WS brains has shown overall reductions in brain volume as well as abnormal cell structure in occipital areas that are known to play a role in visuospatial processing. For example, Galaburda, Holinger, Bellugi, and Sherman (2002) reported that cells in area 17 (the earliest cortical stage in processing information arriving from the retina) were smaller and more densely packed compared to brains of age-matched controls. A later study by Reiss et al. (2004) used high-resolution magnetic resonance imaging to measure the sizes of different brain areas of adults with WS and age- and gender-matched controls. They reported that the thalamus and occipital lobe gray matter volumes were reduced in people with WS. The investigators speculated that these abnormalities observed in early visual areas might be causally related to the visual-spatial behavioral deficits observed in this population.

However, more recent studies of anatomical structure and function in early visual areas of people with WS have failed to find evidence of abnormal structure or function. As we reported in Chapter 2, Olsen et al. (2009) used structural and functional MRI (fMRI) to map area V1 in adults with WS, and found no difference in size or location of V1 compared to age- and gender-matched controls. This study used a standard method for retinotopic mapping of V1, and the findings strongly suggest normal activation patterns for basic stimulus types.

However, evidence from ophthalmologic profiles attests to a high incidence of binocular disorders, reduced acuity, and refractive errors in children with WS (Atkinson et al., 2003, 1997), suggesting that there may be abnormalities in the functioning of some early mechanisms in the visual system. Notably, though, the severity of these deficits within the WS sample did not correlate with their performance on tasks such as block construction. That is, many children showing severe deficits on block construction tasks did not have accompanying sensory deficits, suggesting that the hallmark spatial profile (construction task deficits) probably reflects deficits in higher level visual processing.

3.2.1.1 A Comment About Orientation Sensitivity

One might think that early vision could be tested by examining sensitivity to simple elements such as oriented lines that we know engage specific types of cells in V1. However, the tasks that have been used to test WS orientation perception are typically complex, and may obscure basic competencies such as orientation sensitivity. For example, several early studies suggested that children with WS showed severe deficits in judging the orientation of simple lines. Wang et al. (1995) found that people with WS were unable to pass even the initial training for the Benton judgment of line orientation test (JLO) test, which merely requires a pass on two of five "easy" orientation problems. However, as Figure 3.4 shows, the Benton test uses a somewhat complex procedure in which each of a pair of lines of different orientation have to be matched to lines with the same orientation embedded in a set of 11 differently oriented lines. Failure on this task could reflect deficits in orientation perception, but it could also stem from an inability to attend to individual lines in the choice set—which reflects deficits at higher levels of processing in the visual system.

Indeed, neuroimaging data show that the Benton JLO test activates the parietal and occipital regions, as well as more frontal areas (dorsolateral prefrontal structures), suggesting that the task engages some

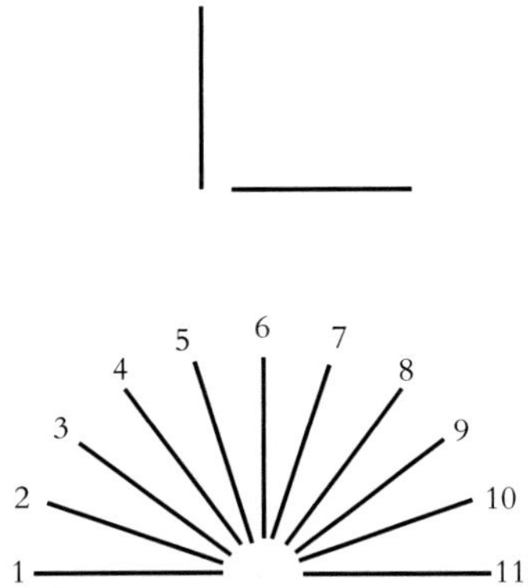

Figure 3.4. In the standard Benton test of line orientation, the observer is presented with two test lines of different orientation (top). The task is to pick out the matching orientations from a choice set of 11 lines (bottom). The correct answer in this case is lines 6 and 11. Adapted from Bellugi, Lichtenberger, Mills, Galaburda, & Korenberg (1999), with permission from Elsevier.

"executive" (i.e., planning) functions (Kesler et al., 2004). Kesler et al. also found that an easier version consisting of 5 lines instead of 11 failed to activate the prefrontal area. This raises the possibility that at least part of the difficulty that WS people have with the standard form of the JLO test might be related to deficits in executive function, rather than only or mostly reflecting a deficit at the earliest levels of the visual system.

Several sets of findings are consistent with this idea. Farran (2006) simplified the Benton test by using a smaller number of response alternatives and found that judgment of line orientation for adults with WS was now comparable to a group of mental-age-matched controls (*M* age = 5;8 years). Using another approach, Palomares, Landau, and Egeth (2009) derived thresholds for orientation matching of Gabor patches among people with WS compared to normally developing children age 3–9 years (see Figure 3.5). Performance of the WS group (average age = 18;7) was no different from normally developing 3- to 4-year old children for either oblique (45 degree) or non-oblique (0, 90 degree) orientations. Looking at Figure 3.5b, one can see that the thresholds for normally developing children decline between 3 and 9, and do not reach adult levels until even later. The performance of the WS individuals, with an average age of 18;7 and a minimum age of 11;10, does not appear to move beyond that of normally developing 3- to 4-year-olds.[4]

[4] Qualitatively, we also found that the WS observers and the 3- to 4-year-olds produced an equivalent number of mirror image errors, which were more frequent than in the older groups of typically developing children.

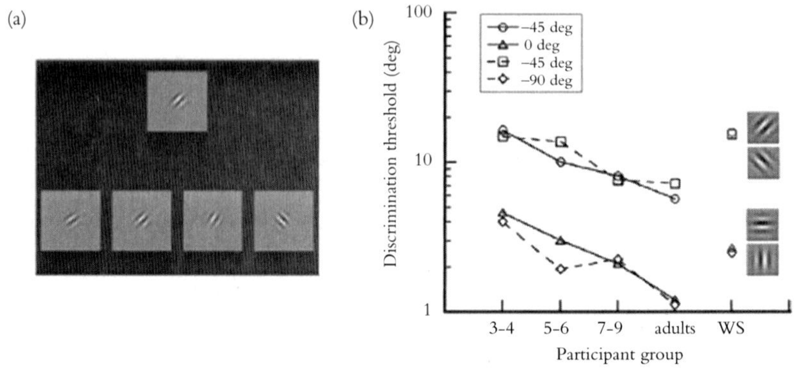

Figure 3.5. (a) A test grating and four choice gratings using by Palomares et al. (2009) to test orientation perception in people with WS and normally developing children between the ages of 3 and 9 years. People are shown the target (top) and four choices (bottom), and are asked to select the choice that matches the target. Varying the set of gratings allows one to establish individual's threshold for discrimination. (b) Mean thresholds across different target orientations for normally developing children between 3 and 9, normal adults, and people with WS. Thresholds for people with WS were no different from normal 3- to 4-year-olds for either oblique (45 degree) or non-oblique (0, 90 degree) orientations. Reprinted from Palomares et al. (2009), with permission of Elsevier.

Although these data do not directly inform us about the organization of early visual processing, they do suggest that there are deficits in the visual processing of orientation at some level. The pattern shown by Palomares et al. points to the possibility that some aspects of the visual system in people with WS may be developmentally arrested at the level of a 4-year-old normally developing child. This is a pattern we will encounter again.

3.2.1.2 Summary of Evidence on Early Visual Processing

Evidence for severe deficits at the level of early vision among people with WS is mixed. Some studies of brain organization in V1 indicate normal structure and function, while others point to abnormalities in cell packing density and overall volume. Behavioral measures show that there are some deficits in binocular disparity and acuity among people with WS. Measures of sensitivity to orientation show that people with

WS have thresholds that are no different from normally developing children who are on average 4 years of age. In normally developing children, these thresholds decrease (i.e., improve) over time between ages 3 and 9, and do not reach adult levels until later than that, suggesting that people with WS show developmental arrest in this function. The evidence on orientation sensitivity does not directly tell us about the early vision system in people with WS, because the tasks that are used are likely to involve higher levels of organization, represented by the parietal areas. But they do indicate a pattern of developmental arrest in a relatively basic visual function.

3.2.2 Middle-Level Vision

An important function of mid-level visual processes is "grouping"—the integration of information coming from earlier levels in the visual system. Deficits at this stage would be expected to result in perceptions that were fragmented, consisting of simple features that were not bundled into higher-level structures. In a sense, this sounds like the deficits associated with WS. According to the "configural deficit hypothesis" proposed by Bellugi and colleagues (2001), people with WS correctly perceive parts of objects but do not correctly combine them. This description is consistent with Bellugi et al.'s reports that during block construction, people with WS generally chose the correct parts but arranged them incorrectly. In addition, when asked to draw figures in which small letters are arranged to portray a single large letter, they correctly drew the small letters but failed to correctly represent the large letter (Bihrle et al., 1989).

A configural deficit could potentially arise from problems in mid-level visual mechanisms that are responsible for visual grouping. If this were the case, poor performance in the block construction task would actually represent a failure to correctly perceive the global structure of the model pattern. An alternative version of this hypothesis is that people with WS correctly group the local features, but they have a strong bias for accessing and attending to information at the local level.

Neither of these hypotheses turns out to be true, however. Rather, perceptual grouping appears to be present in people with WS, and performance in grouping tasks is often no different from normal adults. We will begin by reviewing studies that have examined perceptual grouping in people with WS, asking whether their grouping processes operate normally. We also ask about the normal developmental trajectory for these grouping processes. We then offer additional evidence attesting to the idea that deficits in grouping among people with WS do not underlie their deficits in block construction or copying tasks. Finally, we review evidence on a special kind of grouping process—grouping from motion.

3.2.2.1 Visual Grouping

In the earliest study of grouping by people with WS, Pani et al. (1999) asked adults with WS (*M* age = 30;9) and normal age-matched adults to search a visual display for the presence of a target letter—"T" or "F"—embedded in hybrid distractor characters (see Figure 3.6). Previous studies had shown that normal adults find the target very quickly when it is displayed spatially separated from a "group" of similar elements (Banks & Prinzmetal, 1976). Using "grouping by good form," Pani et al. varied whether the distractors formed a separate group from the target, which should reduce the time to find and identify the target. They found that both adults with WS and normal adults benefited from grouping, and, if anything, the results suggested that people with WS have some trouble switching from the global to local levels of processing. In other words, on this task, adults with WS do not appear to be "local processors."

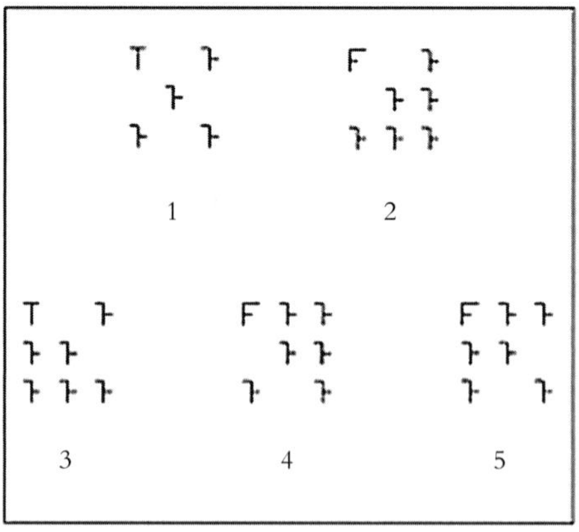

Figure 3.6. The five types of visual search display used by Pani et al. (1999). The participant's task is to indicate whether there is a T or an F in each display. "Grouping by good form" predicts that search time should be faster for Display 2 compared to Displays 1 and 5. Reprinted from Pani et al. (1999), with permission of Sage Publications.

Grouping processes may develop among normal children quite early. If so, then only comparing the WS adult performance to that of normal adults—striking as the comparison is—would not give us a complete picture. Indeed, in several studies, we have found that grouping is accomplished quite early among normally developing children, and that for these aspects of grouping, people with WS perform approximately like 4- or 5-year-old children.

In one study, we examined grouping processes by asking whether people with WS are susceptible to four common visual illusions (Palomares, Ogbonna, Landau, & Egeth, 2009; see Figure 3.7). These illusions are powerful demonstrations that the visual system in adults obligatorily integrates individual elements, causing us to incorrectly perceive the size of an object because of its surrounding context. People with WS (ages 10–41 years) along with groups of normally developing 3-, 5-, and 9-year-old children were tested on their judgments of size in illusion

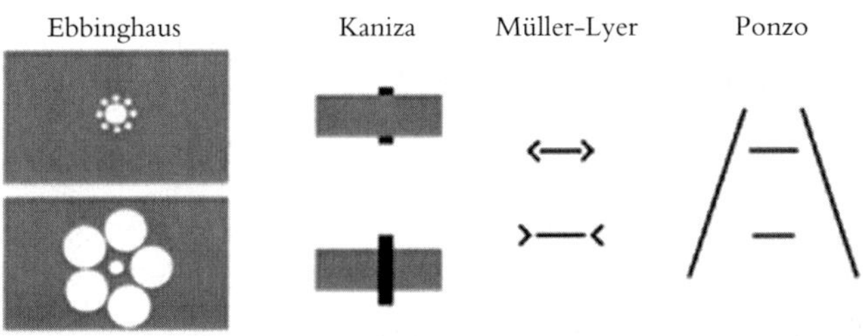

Figure 3.7. Visual illusions used by Palomares, Ogbonna, Landau, and Egeth (2009). Normal adults usually judge the sizes of the central disks (Ebbinghaus) and the lengths of the two lines (all other illusions) as different, even though they are physically the same. These illusions are due to surrounding context; when the surrounding elements are removed, people judge the two elements' sizes/lengths accurately. We found that normally developing children from the age of 3–4 years generally perceived these illusions to the same degree as normal adults. People with WS also perceived the illusions to the same degree as these groups, indicating normal grouping processes underlying these illusions. Moreover, the findings show that this type of visual integration normally develops to mature levels by age 3–4, and that people with WS attain this level. Reprinted from Palomares, Ogbonna, et al. (2009), with permission of Pion, Limited, London.

figures versus control figures—ones that appeared without a surrounding context. If people with WS have abnormal grouping mechanisms, then they should be less susceptible to the contextual influences on which these illusions depend. Instead, illusion magnitude in people with WS was found to be comparable to that of normal adults. Crucially, the magnitude of the illusion was at the adult level in normal children from age 3 onward as well, showing that this aspect of grouping emerges very early in normal development.

In a second study, we examined implicit grouping by continuation (Palomares, Landau, & Egeth, 2008). We presented observers with displays containing a square matrix of Gabor patches that varied in orientation (see Figure 3.8, upper panel). A series of adjacent Gabors that have similar orientations can be perceived as a contour embedded in the randomly oriented background items. In Figure 3.8a, one can see such a horizontal contour (a "line") near the bottom of the array formed by a series of Gabors that are aligned and have the same orientation; in Figures 3.8b and c, the contour is no longer apparent, because the aligned elements have different orientations. In this task, sensitivity can be measured as the difference in orientation that still allows the observer to detect the horizontal line.

We tested people with WS (*M* age = 18;4) and normally developing groups of children ages 3, 5, and 9. People with WS were comparable to normal adults on this task and better than normally developing 3- to 4-year-olds (Figure 3.8, lower panel). Normally developing children reached adult level by about age 5. Thus contour integration, like the perception of illusions, emerges early in normal development. There appears to be little development in the perception of illusions, and modest development between ages 3 and 5, in contour integration; at age 5, this function appears to be adult-like. People with WS are no different from adults in either magnitude of illusion or in contour integration, by these tasks, suggesting again that functions that normally emerge early are also acquired by people with WS, and reach adult levels (though at a much later age, presumably, than in a normally developing individual).

Notice that contour integration in this task depends on representing orientation and therefore we can ask how these results compare with the results on orientation perception in WS that we reported earlier. The two tasks—contour integration and orientation matching—both rely on sensitivity to orientation. However, the two tasks seem to show

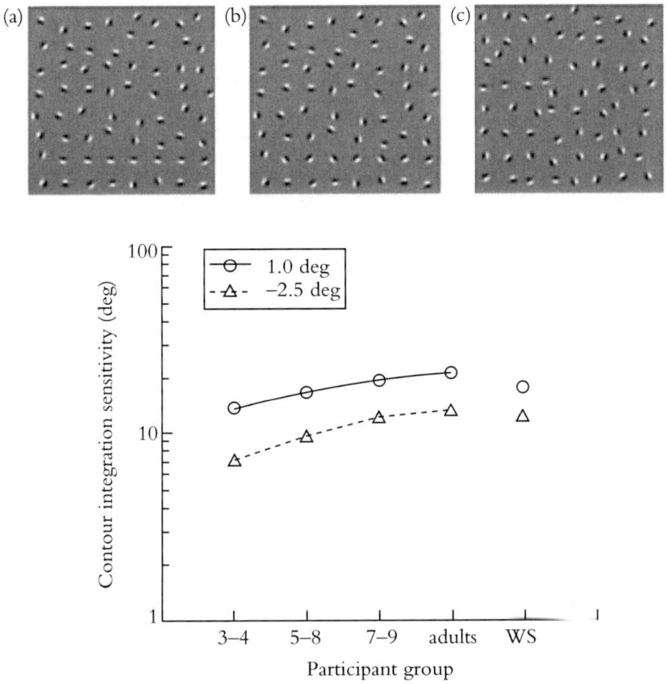

Figure 3.8. Task used in Palomares, Landau, and Egeth (2008). Upper panel: (a) Near the bottom, one can see a horizontal line made up of collinear Gabor gratings that have been the same orientation (0 deg.). Our perception of a horizontal line depends on our ability to integrate these elements. The same elements are present in (b) except that here, the collinear gratings do not have the same orientations. Part (c) shows a noise grating that does not contain a linear feature. Neither (b) nor (c) gives us a clear perception of a horizontal line. Lower panel: Thresholds for the perception of a horizontal line by normally developing children and adults, and people with WS. People with WS showed the same thresholds as 5–6-year-olds, who were no different from normal adults. Thus this type of visual integration develops to a mature level by around the age of 5–6, and people with WS attain this level. Reprinted from Palomares, Landau, and Egeth (2008), with permission of Elsevier.

somewhat different developmental profiles: Contour integration is at maturity (i.e., adult-like) by age 5, whereas orientation matching is not at full maturity even at age 9. The WS profile is remarkably consistent across the two tasks—they are adult-like in contour integration, a function that appears to mature early, with adult-like performance among normal children by age 5. And they are like normally developing 4-year-olds, and slightly worse than 5- to 6-year-olds, in orientation matching, a function that normally undergoes lengthy development, not becoming mature until age 9 or later. This comparison makes clear that what is most similar about the performance of WS people in these very different orientation tasks is their rough "normal" age equivalence, which in both cases is around age 4 or 5. The fact that the two functions undergo quite different developmental trajectories suggests an "uneven" profile in WS, but one that is most closely approximated by a normal child of around age 4 or 5.

To summarize the evidence on grouping, people with WS achieve levels of grouping that are similar to those in normal adults. However, it is important to note that these grouping functions are normally acquired quite early in development—between the ages of 3 and 5, depending on the particular measure used and the function being tested. The results suggest that middle-level functions that emerge early in development are also fully developed in adolescents and adults with WS. Our results are consistent with the original findings of Pani et al. (1999) as well as a separate study by Farran (2005), who found that adults with WS showed the same thresholds for grouping by alignment, luminance, and closure as normally developing 5-year-olds. Farran also found that the WS group performed more poorly than normal 5-year-olds for grouping by proximity, shape, and orientation; but she did not test younger children, so we do not know whether the WS performance would be consistent with normal development of 3- or 4-year-olds.

Based on the results we have reported, the original explanation of the WS spatial deficit—impairment in grouping mechanisms—seems unlikely. Grouping mechanisms seem to be intact. Further, there is now good evidence that the problem in drawing and block construction tasks is not due to a failure to correctly *perceive* the model. In several experiments, people have been presented with Navon letters (small letters arranged to compose a larger letter at the global level; Navon, 1977) and required to either construct the figure or name the local and global shapes (Farran, Jarrold, & Gathercole, 2003; Rondan, Santos, Mancini, Livet, & Deruelle, 2008). The results showed that all observers, including people with WS, performed well when asked to *name* the shapes but that the WS group had selective deficits in *arranging* the local shapes to match the global letter. If perceptual grouping were an issue, then it seems likely that one would see errors in identifying the global form.

3.2.2.2 Grouping From Motion

Although we have so far considered only mechanisms that achieve grouping through static properties of arrays, we would be remiss if we did not review the evidence on grouping mechanisms that rely on motion. One reason is that, as we have discussed, grouping mechanisms have been targeted as a possible contributor to the WS spatial deficit. Another reason is that grouping-by-motion processes are highly specialized in the human brain, raising the possibility of selective deficits among people with WS.[5] In particular, some types of grouping from motion (motion coherence) are carried out in the dorsal stream (Newsome & Pare, 1988), whereas others (biological motion) appear to engage more ventral areas as well (with the superior temporal sulcus STS one key site; Allison et al., 2000; Vaina et al., 2001).[6] On the hypothesis of general dorsal stream impairment, one might expect that motion coherence would be impaired but biological motion perception relatively spared in people with WS. As we will see, the story is not so simple, but nonetheless is quite informative.

The first set of studies on motion perception in people with WS was carried out by Atkinson et al. (1997), who examined *motion coherence*—the ability to extract a percept of motion direction over a group of moving elements. Their goal was to use the motion coherence paradigm to study the integrity of the dorsal stream. This idea was based on studies by Newsome, Britten, and Movshon (1989), who used motion coherence to learn about the motion integration properties of area MT

[5] Although motion processes start with cells in area V1 that respond selectively to motion in different directions, they are only the first stage in a motion analysis system that extends into areas MT and MTS in the dorsal stream. Cells in V1 monitor small regions of space and suffer from the "aperture problem" (Nakayama & Silverman, 1988) in which the direction of motion of extended objects seen through an aperture is often ambiguous. This ambiguity can be resolved by integrating the information from several cells in V1, and this appears to occur in dorsal area MT.

[6] This area also appears to be activated by a variety of "social stimuli," including direction of eye gaze and recognition of familiar voices (Zilbovicius, Meresse, Chabane, Brunelle, Samson, & Boddaert, 2006).

in monkeys (area V5 in humans). They showed monkeys a swarm of randomly positioned dots that moved in random directions. Embedded within this noise field was a smaller set of dots moving coherently in a single direction. They found that monkeys (and people) could detect the direction of motion when as few as 1–2 % of the total dots moved in a coherent direction. Newsome and Pare (1988) further showed that area MT was involved in this process as monkeys with damage to this area required much larger coherence values for accurate detection of motion direction.

Atkinson et al. (1997) reported that children with WS (*M* age = 9.7) were similar to normally developing children (*M* age = 8.1) on a test of global *form* perception (from motion information) but were impaired in perceiving *motion coherence*. They also reported that their WS group was more error prone in the "posting task," which requires visually guided action. These two findings are consistent with the claim that the impaired performance in visuospatial tasks in people with WS may be associated with anomalies in various dorsal stream areas, including V5 and the parietal lobe.

Atkinson et al.'s reported deficits in motion coherence would, indeed, be consistent with the hypothesis of a general dorsal stream deficit in people with WS. Nevertheless, this raises several questions. First, is the putative deficit similar for other types of motion processing such as biological motion, which is thought to involve more ventral stream processes? Second, is WS performance on the motion processing tasks in any way similar to that of younger normally developing children?

To explore these possibilities, we examined the performance of children and adults with WS on three different types of motion processing: motion coherence, biological motion, and two-dimensional form-from-motion (FfM; Reiss, Hoffman, & Landau, 2005; see also Jordan, Reiss, Hoffman, & Landau, 2002). Figure 3.9 shows stimuli for the three types of motion. Stimuli for *motion coherence* were patterned after studies such as Newsome and Pare (1988), examining how much movement information was required to perceive a single overall direction of dots. Stimuli for *form-from-motion* were designed to examine how much movement information was required for a person to extract a geometrical form from the background flow of dots. Stimuli for *biological motion* were constructed to examine their ability to extract the specific form of a human undergoing an action (walking). Johansson (1973) originally constructed biological motion stimuli by attaching lights to the major joints of human actors and filming them while they performed various actions, such as running and jumping, on a dark stage. In normal observers, these "point-light-walkers" (PLWs) evoke an immediate recognition of the portrayed action; they can even be used to discriminate gender and the affective state of the walker (Dittrich, Troscianko, Lea, & Morgan, 1996; Mather & Murdoch, 1994). This is surprising given the apparent minimalist nature of the displays and the fact that static views of the lights are not generally perceived as portraying a three-dimensional object. For each task, we used an adaptive staircase method to establish individual subject thresholds for the amount of noise required to produce a level of 71% accuracy. We tested WS children (*M* age = 14;3) and adults (*M* age = 25;3), as well as normally developing children (*M* age = 6;1) who had the same mental age as the WS children, and a group of college students (*M* age = 20;5). These groups were used to make inferences about the differences between observers with WS and normally developing groups as well as to provide information about developmental trajectories for the different motion tasks.

In the motion coherence task, observers had to detect a small number of dots moving in the same direction against a background of randomly moving dots (see Figure 3.9a). Specifically, they were asked to select which of two panels contained signal elements that moved together "like a school of fish." In the 2D form-from-motion (FfM) task, observers once again had to discriminate coherently moving dots from randomly moving noise but here there were two regions containing coherent motion (Figure 3.9c). A central rectangular area contained dots moving in one direction while the background contained coherent motion in the opposite direction. Observers had to find the panel in which the central rectangular region was oriented vertically (or horizontally). In some ways, this task is similar to the motion coherence task except that observers need to first detect motion coherence and then integrate the coherently moving dots into a surface, allowing them to determine the orientation of that surface (vertical versus horizontal). Note that this task is similar to the one used by Atkinson et al. (1997), which they simply referred to as "motion coherence." Like our 2D form-from-motion task, Atkinson et al.'s task required observers to use

(a)
(b)
(c)
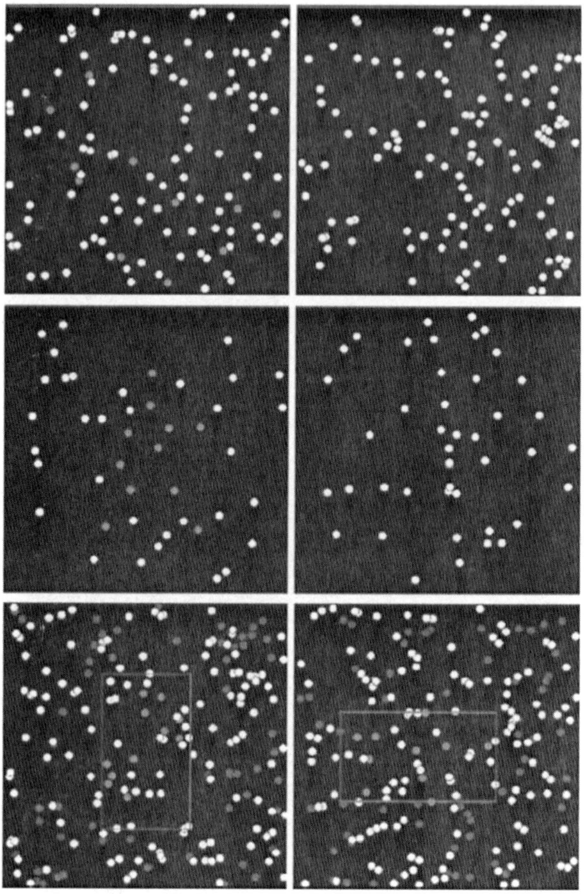

Figure 3.9. Scale illustrations of (a) motion coherence, (b) biological motion, and (c) form-from-motion displays. For illustration purposes, signal elements are indicated in red, while noise elements are colored white. The form-from-motion stimuli also included signal background elements that moved in the opposite direction of the motion of the target rectangle; these are indicated in blue. During the actual experiments, all elements (signal, noise, signal-background) appeared as white lights on a black background and no rectangles appeared in the form-from-motion displays. The participants' task was to find the panel that had dots moving together "like a school of fish" (motion coherence), to find the panel that shows a person walking "nice and upright" (biological motion), and to find the panel that has the vertical rectangle ("the tall up-and-down rectangle that looks like a door"). See text for discussion of task and results. (*See* color insert.)

motion coherence to define an embedded shape.[7] Finally, in the biological motion task (Figure 3.9b), observers had to determine which of two panels showed a person "walking nice and upright." One of the panels had a 13-point figure "walking" while embedded in noise; the other had the same display except that the 13 points of the "walker" moved out of phase relative to each other, thereby not producing a coherent walking motion. In both cases, the target 13 points remained in the center of the display (see also Jordan et al., 2002).

The results are shown in Figure 3.10. First, consider the motion coherence task. This revealed no significant differences among any of the four groups. The comparable performance for college students and normally developing 6-year-old children suggests that the neural circuits responsible for performance on this task are mature by the age of 6 (see also Freire, Lewis, Maurer, & Blake, 2006). Indeed, other research shows that adult-like performance is reached by the age of 4 (Parrish et al., 2005). This system has also reached comparable development in both of the two WS groups. This shows that at least some aspects of dorsal stream functioning are normal in people with WS by the time they reach age 14 (the mean age of our WS child group).

In contrast, the biological motion task revealed a sizeable advantage for college students over our normally developing 6-year-old controls. There was no difference between WS children and WS adults, with both groups performing similarly to the college students. Apparently, biological motion, unlike motion coherence, continues to improve past the age of 6. Freire et al. (2006) found that 9-year-olds were more sensitive than 6-year-olds but did not differ from adults, while Pavlova et al. (2000) found differences between 14-year-olds and adults. In any case, biological motion perception appears to have a longer developmental trajectory than motion coherence, and it appears that our youngest WS group, with an average age of 14;3 years, has reached full and normal maturity on this task—and they perform better than normally developing 6-year-olds.

The third task—form-from-motion—which required the use of coherent motion to define a two- dimensional shape, showed a very different pattern of results. For the two normal groups, the pattern was similar

[7] Given the similarity between Atkinson et al.'s motion coherence task and our form-from-motion task, one might predict that WS people should be especially poor in our FFM task. This is indeed what we found.

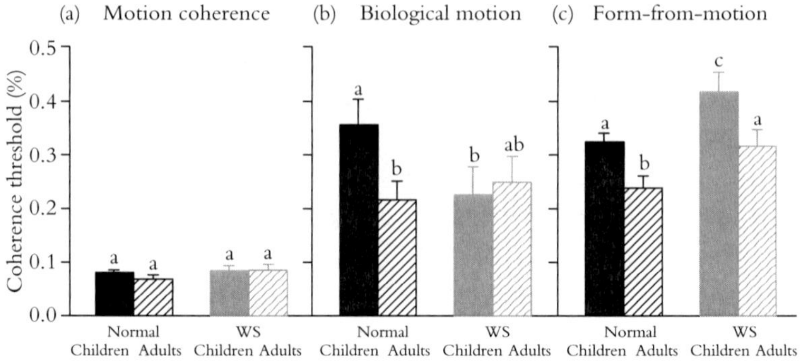

Figure 3.10. Coherence thresholds (mean coherence level from last five adaptive staircase reversals; lower values indicate greater sensitivity) for correctly reporting the target display in (a) motion coherence, (b) biological motion and (c) form-from-motion conditions across the participant groups. Within each motion task panel, means with different letters above are significantly different from one another based on planned one-tailed *t*-test. The results showed that the WS groups were no different from the normally developing children (*M* age = 6) or adults in motion coherence, suggesting that this function arises early in normal development and is intact in WS. The results for biological motion showed that the WS groups were no different from normal adults and better than normally developing 6-year-olds. In form-from-motion, the adult WS group reaches only the same threshold as 6-year-olds, and do not appear to ever reach the threshold of normal adults. These patterns indicate that the three motion systems normally develop at different rates and that children and adults with WS reach mature levels for motion coherence and biological motion, but not form-from-motion. Reprinted from Reiss et al. (2005), with permission of Elsevier.

to that obtained for biological motion: adults were superior to the 6-year-old children. In addition, the thresholds of both normal adults and 6-year-olds were similar to those observed in the biological motion condition. This is consistent with other research examining normally developing children. For example, Gunn et al. (2002) reported that sensitivity to 2D form-from-motion does not normally reach maturity until 10–11 years of age, a developmental trajectory that is similar to the case of biological motion. Adults with WS showed performance similar to the normal 6-year-olds, but children with WS showed poorer performance than either of these groups. In addition, the thresholds of both WS groups were much higher (i.e., worse performance) than those observed in the biological motion condition. These results are consistent with Atkinson et al.'s

(2006) findings that show a specific WS impairment in perceiving motion-defined 2D shapes persisting into adulthood.

These results indicate that people with WS are not impaired on grouping from motion tasks that use structures in the dorsal visual stream: Both WS children and adults had motion coherence thresholds that were like all normal groups, from age 3 onward. WS children and adults also performed better than normal 6-year-olds (mental age matches) and like normal adults on biological motion perception, which engages more ventral structures (especially the STS). WS people did, however, show a specific impairment in the ability to perceive 2D shapes that were defined by coherently moving dots. In this task, adults with WS had thresholds that were similar to those observed in normally developing 6-year-olds, and children with WS performed more poorly. Thus the WS profile for grouping from motion appears to differ, depending on which aspect of motion processing one is considering. The same is true for the normal developmental profile.[8]

[8] It would be informative if we were able to map the patterns of performance for different kinds of motion perception onto brain areas. Unfortunately, localizing the brain areas involved in perceiving 2D form-from-motion has proven to be difficult. Blanke et al. (2007) examined perception of coherent motion and 2D FfM in 32 patients with acute posterior brain damage. Using MRI-based lesion analysis, they found that patients who had normal perception of motion coherence combined with deficient perception of FfM had lesions in the ventral-occipital-temporal (VOT) cortex, which includes ventral areas that respond selectively to objects, faces, and places. Patients who were deficient in both tasks had lesions in area MT in the dorsal stream and the lateral occipital cortex (LOC), a ventral stream area that is also selective for objects. Presumably, area MT extracts global motion information, which then forms the input to areas in the ventral stream that carry out the shape recognition. Therefore, damage to area MT results in deficits on both motion coherence and FfM tasks.

A recent fMRI paper by Vachon et al. (2009) arrived at a similar conclusion. In comparing motion coherence with FfM, they found a large number of areas in common between the two tasks but noted that area LOC was activated in FfM but not motion coherence. These results are somewhat puzzling given that people with WS appear to have a selective deficit in perceiving FfM, which would implicate damage to ventral stream areas. However, their object and face perception skills are quite good, which suggests normal functioning of these ventral steam areas. This is clearly an area that would profit from additional research, particularly fMRI studies of FfM tasks with WS participants.

3.2.2.3 Summary of Evidence on Grouping

The evidence suggests that basic grouping mechanisms in older children and adults with WS are functional and are used in a variety of tasks, including visual search, perception of illusions, contour integration, and grouping from motion. This suggests that the postulated "configural deficit" in people with WS is unlikely to be the cause of the dramatic deficits seen in visuospatial construction tasks in WS.

More crucially, examination of the profiles of normally developing children suggests that many of the grouping mechanisms we have studied emerge early in development, and those that do are likely to be fully acquired by people with WS by the time they reach late childhood. For example, thresholds for static aspects of grouping, such as contour integration or illusions, are at mature levels in normally developing children by the age of 3 or 4; the WS thresholds for these functions are also at mature levels. Thresholds for grouping from motion in normally developing children vary depending on the type of motion. Motion coherence thresholds are at mature levels by age 3 or 4, whereas biological motion and form-from-motion thresholds do not reach maturity until after age 6. People with WS show mature levels of motion coherence and biological motion, but not form-from-motion. Although we do not know the exact timing of emergence of these functions in people with WS (since we tested them in late childhood, adolescence, and adulthood), we do know that both motion coherence and biological motion have reached maturity by late childhood. Thus the overall pattern suggests that those grouping mechanisms that are acquired early in development are also acquired and reach maturity in people with WS. The one exception to this rule is biological motion, which is acquired after age 6 in normal development but is mature in people with WS by late childhood.

3.2.3 High-Level Vision: Object Recognition

Given that people with WS can group elements into larger object-like chunks, do they also recognize objects following principles shown by normal individuals? In some of the earliest investigations of spatial deficits in WS, Bellugi et al. (1994) found that performance on standardized measures of object and face recognition was much better than that observed in construction tasks. In some cases, the scores of adolescents and adults with WS were on par with their chronological age. The apparent contrast between severely impaired performance on block construction task and performance on object and face perception is consistent with the idea that the spatial deficits in WS are primarily due to abnormalities in the dorsal stream, and that the ventral stream, which handles object recognition, is not impaired (see also Wang et al., 1995).

However, standardized tests of object recognition are not generally designed to examine in detail the kinds of representations people have, or what kinds of conditions—if any—might lead to special difficulties in recognizing objects. They are also unlikely to be closely connected with the scientific literature on object representation and its neural correlates. Although problems with object recognition have not been reported in the literature for WS, careful study might reveal areas of weakness. More generally, probing the detailed nature of object representation—especially the role of spatial structure within objects—is important for understanding the WS spatial deficit.

In this section, we probe the nature of object representation in people with WS by focusing on two key issues. The first, discussed in Section 2.3.1, concerns the nature of recognition of familiar common objects. Can people with WS recognize familiar common objects under relatively demanding conditions? Of special interest, we ask whether people with WS show particularly strong performance when they view objects presented from canonical viewpoints, and weaker performance when viewing objects from unusual viewpoints—consistent with the multiple views theory of object recognition, which characterizes object recognition in normal adults (see Section 3.1, this chapter). We will see that object recognition from canonical viewpoints is indeed a strength for people with WS; but that recognition from unusual viewpoints is considerably weaker.

The second issue, discussed in Section 3.2.3.2, concerns an important puzzle: If object recognition is strong, then why do people with WS have severe difficulties in the block construction task when they must select objects (blocks) that have internal patterned structure? One possibility is that accurately selecting these blocks requires the representation of "handedness"—the left/right (or top/bottom) relationship between pattern elements. As we will see, this problem is one aspect of object representation that is, indeed, severely impaired in people with WS.

3.2.3.1 Recognizing Familiar Objects

In our first set of studies, we examined object identification in children with WS (*M* age = 11;0), compared to normally developing 4-year-olds,[9] mental-age-matched controls (*M* age = 5;8), chronological-age-matched controls (*M* age = 11;11), and normal adults (college undergraduates, *M* age = 20; Landau, Hoffman, & Kurz, 2006). On each trial, observers saw a briefly presented single full-color picture of an object and were asked to name it. These were common objects that we thought would be highly familiar to our participants, including, for example, household items (cup, toothbrush), vehicles (car, airplane, bike), and foods (banana, pumpkin, pretzel).[10] Each image was presented for 500 ms, followed by a blank screen; after the observer responded, the experimenter advanced to the next image. Each person was tested on 80 different object images, drawn from a battery of 320; no single object was presented more than once to any individual participant.

We varied two factors. In order to see whether object viewpoint mattered, we varied the orientation in which the objects were presented, including both canonical and noncanonical (or "unusual") views (see Figure 3.11). In order to make sure that we could evaluate the WS pattern against normal adult performance (which we assumed would be highly accurate), we also varied whether the objects were presented in a clear or blurred format (also in Figure 3.11). The combination of these factors ensures that all groups' performance would fall below ceiling on the more difficult conditions, allowing us to examine the effects of the two factors on all groups.

---

[9] The 4-year-olds were run later, after publication of the results with the other groups. Their responses were independently rated, along with the previously collected WS responses, by a single, experienced rater. Small differences between the new ratings of the WS group and the previous rater were used to adjust the ratings of the 4-year-olds to make them comparable to the previous ratings for the MA, CA, and adult groups.

[10] The complete set can be viewed at http://hoffman.psych.udel.edu/ObjectPicturesForWeb.pps.

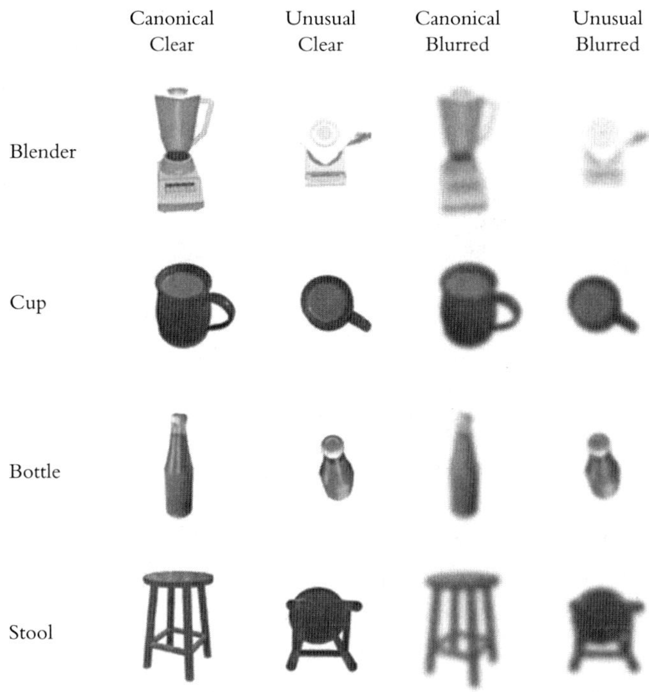

Figure 3.11. Four examples of full-color objects presented under different viewing conditions. Objects were presented from two different viewpoints (canonical and unusual), and in either clear or blurred format. Adapted from Landau et al. (2006), with permission from Elsevier. (*See* color insert.)

The two kinds of image manipulation might reveal unusual features of object identification in people with WS that would not be apparent if we had simply used clear, familiar views of common objects. Unusual views are particularly interesting because the multiple-view-with-transformation model that we reviewed earlier makes specific predictions about the effects of this transformation. Recall that this model assumes that views that have not been encountered before can be recognized only by rotating the novel view into correspondence with the nearest stored view. Mental rotation appears to be carried out in parietal cortex, predicting that recognition of objects shown in unusual views should produce more activation in parietal areas than canonical views. This appears to be the case for normal adults, as measured by fMRI (Schendan & Stern, 2007). Consistent with this, patients with right parietal damage have trouble identifying objects in unusual views (Warrington, 1982). Thus people with WS might have particular difficulty perceiving objects in unusual poses, because they are known to have deficits in parietal cortex, particularly the IPS area, which appears to be especially important for recognition of noncanonical views (Meyer-Lindenberg et al., 2006; Schendan & Stern, 2007). By contrast, the canonical views—thought to be processed by the ventral stream—should be strong, and perhaps even comparable to normally developing people of the same chronological age.

The effects of blur are also of interest. Blurring an image removes high spatial frequencies, reducing the utility of individual parts while preserving global-level image information that is carried by low spatial frequencies. The early hypothesis of "global processing deficit" (Bellugi et al., 2001) would predict severe impact of image blur, in other words, distinctly compromised performance. As we have noted, however, this hypothesis has not received support; in fact, people with WS seem to have normal perceptual grouping processes (Section 2.2). Given this, people with WS should be relatively unaffected by blur or possibly even helped by it.

The results of our study are shown in Figure 3.12 in terms of percent correct object naming as a function of age for clear images (left panel) and blurred images (right panel). Consider first the case of clear images. All groups were highly accurate for canonical views, with normal adults, WS individuals, and their mental age matches achieving accuracy above 90%. The 4-year-olds were also highly accurate, with 84% accuracy. The WS group was no different from the mental age or chronological age matches. The high levels of performance by normal 4- and 5–6-year-olds suggest that object recognition under these circumstances normally emerges quite early. The WS group is on par with both their mental age matches, who were 5–6-year-olds, and their chronological age matches, who were 12 years old.

All groups were less accurate with unusual views compared to canonical views but the WS group and normally developing MA matches showed particularly large drops in performance. The normally developing 4-year-olds also performed similarly to these two groups. These results

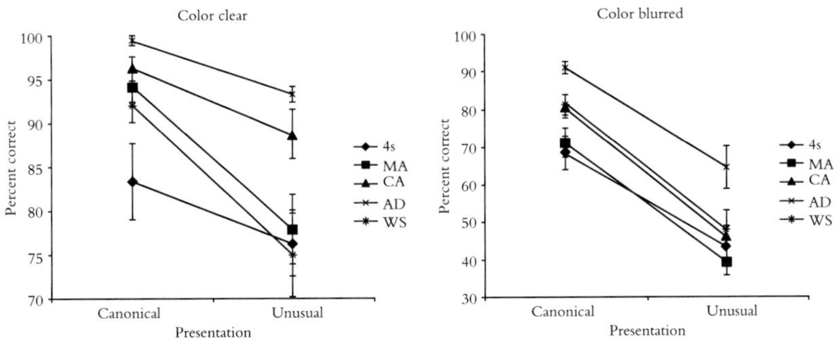

Figure 3.12. Mean percent correct as a function of viewpoint presentation (canonical versus unusual) for clear images (left panel) and blurred images (right panel). Separate lines correspond to different groups (4's: normally developing 4 year-olds; MA: mental age matches; CA: chronological age matches, AD: normal adults, WS: Williams Syndrome). Adapted from Landau et al. (2006), with permission from Elsevier.

suggest that the development of recognition of objects from unusual views is normally a rather protracted affair, with substantial growth in normally developing children between the ages of 4 and 6 (both below 80%) and the age of 11 (90%). There may be further development of this function beyond age 11, since the normal adults performed the best. In this unusual views condition, the WS group fits the profile of the normal 4- and 6-year-olds, and has not reached the level of their chronological age matches.

Now consider the blurred images. Here, all groups again fare better with canonical than unusual views, and this time the difference between conditions appears the same for all groups. Moreover, in this condition, the WS and CA groups appear to be most similar and both groups are somewhat better than the two youngest normally developing groups.

The superiority of the WS performance relative to mental age matches in the canonical blur condition is one of only two published instances that we are aware of in which people with WS have out-performed their MA matches; the other is discrimination of biological motion (see Figure 3–10). In both of these cases, people with WS performed particularly well in tasks requiring attention to global-level information relative to local details. A focus on global shape at the expense of local features is also consistent with their difficulties in the block construction task, which requires people to focus attention on the components of the global shape. Pani et al. (1999) similarly speculated that people with WS may have trouble switching from a global level to a local level of analysis to account for their finding that people with WS were particularly slow in discriminating target letters that were embedded in good global shapes.

Although the performance of WS individuals in recognizing full-color objects was quite strong—on par with their chronological age— they might depend more heavily on color or texture than normal individuals, especially if computing object shape is particularly difficult. To test this possibility, we replaced the color pictures of objects with line drawings in order to remove cues to identification based on color and/or texture (see Figure 3.13). Only clear views of canonical and unusual views were presented. Results with line

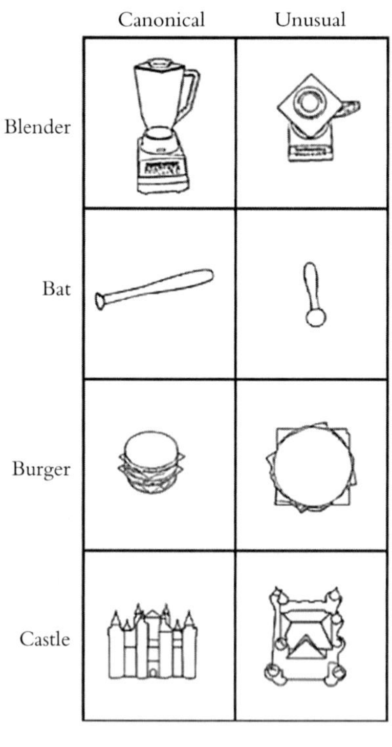

Figure 3.13. Examples of line-drawn objects presented in canonical and unusual viewpoints. These objects had no color or texture and could be identified only from overall shape information. Reprinted from Landau et al. (2006), with permission of Elsevier.

drawings were generally similar to those obtained with clear, color images (see Figure 3.14). Again, all groups performed very well, with scores above 90% for all groups except the normal 4-year-olds, who scored close to 80% correct. The WS group performed similarly to the mental-age-matched controls and this time, not as well as their chronological age matches, who performed like normal adults. Most strikingly, however, all groups again performed worse on the unusual views than the canonical views, with the WS group, the mental age matches (5–6 years old), and the normal 4-year-olds all declining to similar levels. The similarity between the unusual views profile compared to the unusual views in full color (clear view) is especially remarkable because all groups performed much more poorly in the line drawing version of this condition. Still, the relative profiles across groups were quite similar, indicating that the WS group was indeed functionally similar to both normally developing 4-year-olds and 5- to 6-year-olds.

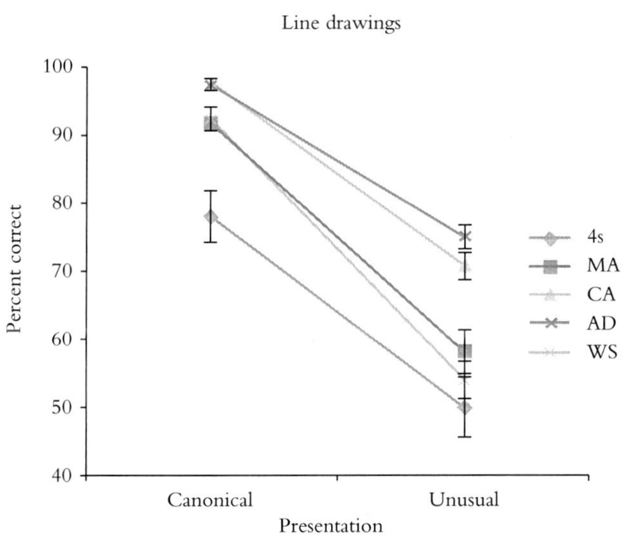

Figure 3.14. Mean percent correct as a function of view (canonical versus unusual). Separate lines correspond to different groups (4's: normally developing 4 year-olds; MA: mental age matches; CA: chronological age matches, AD: normal adults, WS: Williams Syndrome). Adapted from Landau et al. (2006), with permission from Elsevier.

Overall, it appears that there are two different profiles for object recognition—one for canonical views and the other for unusual views. For canonical views, children with WS performed at quite high levels when recognizing and identifying either full-color or line-drawn objects. Normally developing children also performed at very high levels from age 5–6 on, and 4-year-olds were not far behind. Thus there was modest development between age 4 and 6 in the ability to recognize objects from canonical viewpoint, but after that, there was little further development.

The situation for unusual views was quite different. There, children with WS showed steep declines in object recognition (relative to the canonical views), and were on par with normally developing 5- to 6-year-olds, who also showed steep declines. The absolute levels of performance for unusual views were remarkably similar for the WS children, the normal 5- to 6-year-olds, and the normal 4-year-olds. Thus, unlike the canonical views, object recognition under unusual viewpoints appears to develop rather slowly and undergoes substantial change between the ages of 6 and 12.[11]

To summarize, children with WS show a profile for recognition of familiar objects that suggests they are capable of computing object shape and category under demanding circumstances such as brief presentation and line drawings, which strip away details of surface color and texture. They have considerably more trouble identifying objects under unusual viewpoints. However, this same pattern appears in normally developing young children. Canonical object recognition appears quite strong in very normally developing young children, who nevertheless have much more difficulty recognizing objects under unusual views.

The different profiles for canonical versus unusual views are consistent with the multiple views theory of object representation that we discussed earlier. Despite the wealth of data from normal adults supporting this theory, little is known about the role of view-dependent representations of objects over development. Our results from both the WS group and from the normally developing groups suggest that there are real

---

[11] A different picture emerged when color images were blurred. The WS group performed similarly to 12-year-olds and better than their MA controls with blurred images of canonical views. We speculate that this relatively good performance with blurred images reflects an overall bias in people with WS toward processing information at a global, rather than a local, level.

differences in the mechanisms underlying canonical and unusual viewpoint recognition of objects. Recent neuroimaging studies suggest a possible neural basis for these differences. Schendan and Stern (2007) found that recognition of objects from unusual views elicits activation in dorsal, ventral, and frontal areas of the brain among adults. Some of the dorsal areas correspond to those involved in mental rotation, which is thought to play a role in rotating unusual views into correspondence with previously stored views of the object. There is evidence of slow development of both frontal and parietal areas during normal development (Casey et al., 2005), and this might account for the different developmental profiles for canonical and unusual view recognition.

3.2.3.2 A Special Problem: Handedness, or Left-Right Reflections

The strong object recognition (under canonical perspectives) shown by people with WS might be surprising on the basis of structural description accounts holding that object recognition depends on representing the spatial arrangement of parts. If people with WS suffer from a quite general impairment in representing spatial relationships, one might have expected them to be impaired in object recognition. Of course it is possible that many or all of the objects we used in our experiments were recognizable on the basis of a single part, or that the particular configuration of multiple parts was not critical for recognition and identification. This makes it important to ask how people with WS fare when accurate performance requires representing the arrangement of parts. As it turns out, we do not find any particular deficit for representing the spatial relationships of parts within objects, except when we consider one special case—the representation of objects that have undergone reflection around the vertical axis, exchanging the left for the right.

In the series of studies we used to examine these issues, we constructed a special set of stimuli. In order to avoid the problem of familiarity (which could result in matching of objects to stored images), we created novel objects composed of parts taken from actual objects. These parts were arranged using simple attachment rules. A sample object is shown in the top panel of Figure 3.15; it was created from the base of an electric drill, the handle of a hammer, and one side of a pair of eyeglasses.

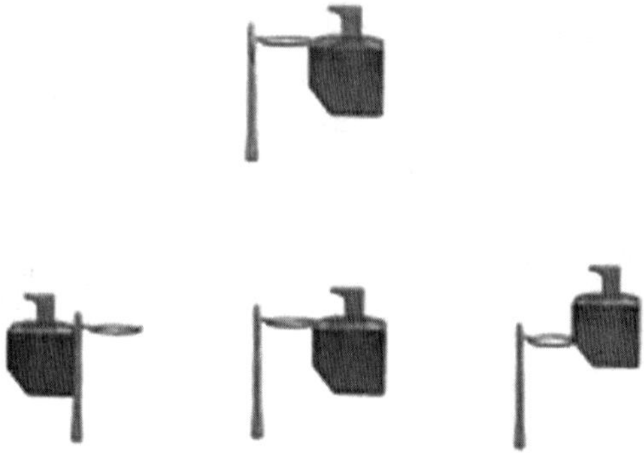

Figure 3.15. Sample novel object and three test objects, one of which matches the sample. The distractor objects have the same parts as the sample but differ in how the parts are arranged. People with WS performed no differently from normally developing children (*M* age = 6;3) who were matched for mental age when they viewed the sample as they chose the match, or when the sample was removed and they had to match after a 1- second delay.

These parts were retextured and scaled to obscure their identity and combined to form novel objects.

Observers were shown the top object (the sample) and had to choose the matching object from the three alternatives at the bottom. One of these (the object in the center, in this case) matches the target exactly, while the other alternatives have the same parts as the target object but they have been rearranged, occupying new locations relative to each other. Objects were created in a 3D object-rendering program (Carrera 3D; http://www.daz3d.com), which allowed us to use a different arrangement of lights for the sample object versus the choice objects. This should make it difficult for observers to choose the correct alternative on the basis of local cues involving reflection or shading.

People with WS (*M* age = 12;1, range = 8;11–16;3) were tested along with normally developing children (*M* age = 6;3, range = 4;3–9;7) who were matched to the WS individuals on mental age. They were asked to match the sample to the test items in two conditions. In the *immediate* condition, the sample and choice objects appeared on the screen together and remained visible until people responded by clicking on one of the choice objects. In the *delay* condition, the sample object appeared first and when the observer pressed a key on the mouse, the target object disappeared; the test alternatives appeared 1 second later. This condition obviously required the observer to hold a representation of the target object in working memory, and would be expected to be more difficult.

In both conditions, the two groups performed well above chance, with roughly 80% correct in the immediate condition, and 70% in the delay condition. There were no effects of group, with the WS group performing on par with the normally developing 6-year-old children who were mental age matches. These results indicate that people with WS are quite capable of representing the arrangement of parts in novel objects and can do so over short delays of a few seconds.

However, this raises a puzzle: If people with WS can accurately represent the spatial relationships between parts of objects, why do they perform so poorly when asked to match the individual blocks used in the block construction task? Recall that in Chapter 2, we reported that people with WS were not only severely impaired in solving block construction puzzles but they were also impaired in matching individual block in the puzzle (Hoffman et al., 2003). The most common error in the block matching task was one in which a block was confused with a *reflection* of its parts. For example, a block containing a green stripe to the left of a red stripe was confused with a block having red on the left and green on the right. This kind of confusion between reflections of the same object would not have led to errors in the present experiment because reflections were not presented as an option.

Therefore, in the next experiment, we used the same novel objects as we had used in the first experiment (see Figure 3.16a for an example) but in this case the choice objects consisted of a match (shown in the middle), a reflection of the sample object across the vertical axis (reversing left and right, far right), and a reflection across the horizontal axis (reversing the upper and lower halves, far left). The results are shown in Figure 3.17a.[12] Normally developing children (*M* age = 5;11, range = 4;11–7;5) who were matched to the WS individuals on mental age were

[12] Normal adults were uniformly good at this task, achieving virtually perfect performance across both presentation conditions.

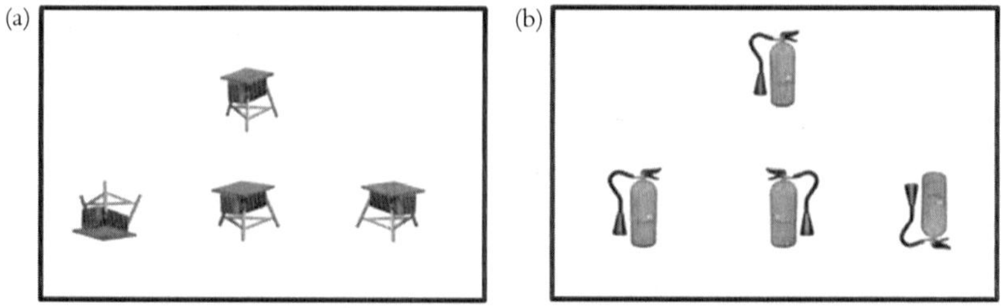

Figure 3.16. Sample object and three test objects, one of which matches the sample object. The distractor objects are mirror reflections across the vertical or horizontal axes. (a) Sample novel objects constructed from the parts of familiar objects. (b) Sample familiar objects.

very accurate in the immediate condition and, as in our previous experiment, showed a drop in accuracy of about 10% in the delay condition, when they had to hold the sample object in visual short-term memory. The WS group (*M* age = 13;10, range = 9;3–17;9) was slightly less accurate than controls in the immediate condition but showed a precipitous drop in accuracy when the choices were delayed, falling to around 65% accuracy. Notably, the errors consisted almost exclusively in choosing the vertically reflected distractor, in other words, the one that reversed the left and right. The same experiment was also carried out using real, familiar objects, with the same results (see Figure 3.16b for sample of familiar objects, and Figure 3.17b for results on familiar objects).

The results for novel and real objects suggest that the representation of object handedness may, quite generally, be a severe problem for people with WS. Their level of performance in the delay condition was reliably worse than that of mental-age-matched children who were on average 6 years old, and this pattern was the same whether the objects were completely novel or familiar. In order to test the generality—and relevance to failures in the block construction task—we carried out a third experiment, in which we used the block stimuli that we had used in the part-matching subtask of the block construction project (see Figure 2.11 for this subtask). Stimuli for this experiment are shown in Figure 3.18a. Distractors included the match, a reflection (either over the vertical or horizontal axis), and a third item that had a different geometric split from the model (e.g., a diagonal split for a target that was vertically split).

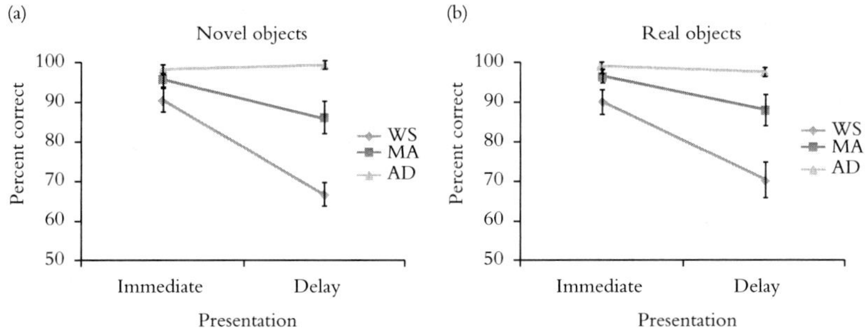

Figure 3.17. Percent correct in novel object matching task for people with WS, normally developing children (*M* age = 5;11) matched for mental age (MA), and normal adults (AD). Test choices either appeared at the same time as the sample object (immediate) or were delayed by 1 second (delay). (a) Results for the novel objects shown in Figure 3.17a. (b) Results for the familiar objects shown in Figure 3.17b.

By any measure, the block stimuli—which have exactly two parts—are considerably simpler than the objects we used in the preceding experiments, and lower object complexity might make it easier to represent the left/right or top/bottom arrangement of parts. However, as shown in Figure 3.18b, the pattern of performance is remarkably similar to that from the other two stimulus sets. All groups were at ceiling in the immediate condition. But children with WS show a much sharper drop in performance in the delay condition than do the 6-year-olds who were mental age matches. In fact, the WS group falls to about 65% accuracy, which is similar to their performance in the preceding mirror reflection experiments that used novel or familiar complex objects. Errors almost exclusively involved choosing the mirror reflection choice rather than the distractor from a different category.

The precipitous drop in accuracy under delay when the foils differed from the target by a mirror reflection raises an important question: Would this pattern of performance and error profile also hold for normally developing children who are younger than age 6? In order to see, we carried out an identical experiment using the block stimuli (Dessalegn & Landau, 2008). We tested 4-year-olds, whose data are shown in Figure 3.18b (red diamond), next to the data we have already

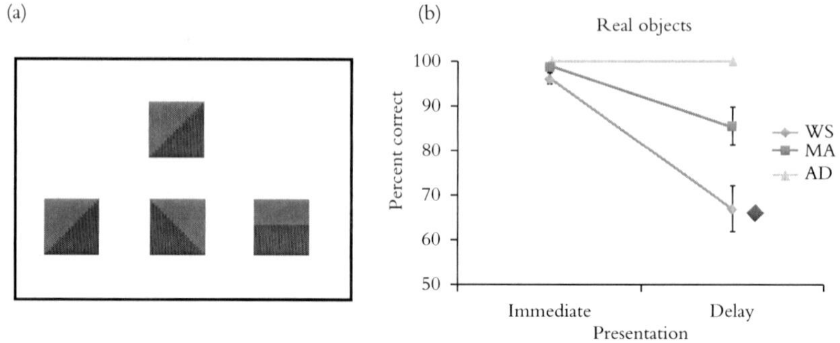

Figure 3.18. (a) Sample object and three test objects in experiment using blocks as stimuli. (b) Percent correct in block matching task for people with WS and normally developing children (*M* age = 5;11) matched for mental age (MA), and normal adults (AD). Red diamond represents performance of normally developing 4-year-olds on this task. Data taken from Dessalegn and Landau (2008).

shown for the WS group. There is clearly a striking similarity in the performance of people with WS and normally developing 4-year-old children in maintaining handedness information in working memory over a 1-second delay. Analysis of errors showed that both groups overwhelmingly selected the reflection, and not the third choice (which represented a different geometric split in the block).

Overall, these experiments show that people with WS perform considerably worse than normally developing 6-year-old children (MA controls) when they have to discriminate the handedness of objects, particularly when the sample object is held in visual short-term memory. In addition, the magnitude of this impairment appeared to be remarkably consistent across different kinds of object sets, being approximately the same for novel objects, familiar objects, and colored blocks. Given that the blocks appear to be much simpler than the novel and familiar objects, these results suggest that neither object complexity nor familiarity play an important role in the WS impairment in this aspect of object representation.

The quantitative performance and error patterns shown by people with WS were remarkably similar to normally developing 4-year-olds. Moreover, a comparison of performance between normally developing

4- and 6-year-olds suggests considerable growth in this ability during this time period. The WS group, whose members are considerably older (approximately 12 years old) than both of these normally developing groups, appears to be settled at the level of the 4-year-old group, consistent with what we observed for recognition of objects under unusual views.[13]

3.2.3.3 Summary of Evidence on Object Recognition

The early observations of normalcy in object recognition among people with WS has some validity: We observed strong performance in recognizing and identifying objects under relative demanding circumstances such as brief presentation and line drawings. However, this strength was apparent only when the objects were presented from canonical viewpoints. There, children with WS performed at quite high levels, and in a number of cases on par with their chronological age. However, object

[13] One way of thinking about the difficulty experienced with object reflections is to view the problem in terms of object orientation. The fact that people with WS are able to represent arrangement of parts within an object but are severely impaired in representing the orientation of the object itself is consistent with the idea that these two pieces of information are represented separately in the brain. As we pointed out earlier, Marr and Nishihara (1978) and Biederman (1987) proposed theories of object recognition in which the locations of the object's parts were represented in an object-based coordinate system, that is, a coordinate system centered on the object with its vertical axis oriented to match the axis of elongation of the object. As McCloskey (2009) points out, though, the orientation of the object relative to an external reference frame, such as the display monitor, the subject's body, or gravity, has to be represented as a relationship between the principal axis of the object reference frame and the external reference frame, and this may be what poses difficulty for people with WS. We discuss these issues further in Chapter 4. For most cases of object recognition, the handedness of objects is irrelevant. We need to recognize a cup regardless of whether its handle is on the left or right. However, visually controlled action, which appears to be controlled by structures in the parietal lobe, does depend on accurate representation of handedness. If we want to pick the cup up, it matters whether the handle is on the right or left side. Interestingly, several papers have reported the existence of patients with damage to parietal areas in the right hemisphere who can correctly name objects but are unable to indicate their orientation (Riddoch et al., 2004).

recognition under canonical viewpoints also appears to develop in the normal child rather early, with strong performance by normal 4-year-olds, and little development between age 4 and 6—suggesting that the strong performance of children with WS may reflect acquisition of an early developing system.

By contrast, we saw that recognition under unusual views normally undergoes more substantial development between ages 6 and 12, and for this function, people with WS appear to perform at the level of 6-year-olds (or even 4-year-olds). Similarly, representing and storing the handedness of objects appear to be quite difficult for people with WS, who perform on par with normally developing 4-year-olds, but worse than 6-year-olds who are their mental age matches. Both recognition of unusual views and representation of handedness appear to be tied to parietal functions in the brain, consistent with the abnormalities observed in the WS brain (see Chapter 2).

3.3 Face Recognition

We conclude our chapter with a review on the WS capacity to recognize faces. Like objects, recognition of faces was originally characterized as a strength in people with WS, as they were reported to score in the normal range for their age on the Benton standardized test of face recognition (Bellugi, Wang, & Jernigan, 1994) and superior to the performance of mental-age-matched controls (Bellugi et al., 1988; Udwin & Yule, 1991). Face recognition is particularly interesting as a test case for the spatial profile of WS because current evidence indicates that faces are recognized *holistically*; that is, the various internal features of the face are perceived as a single *configuration* rather than being processed as independent parts. From this perspective, the task of face recognition is highly spatial, since it requires the perception of a global spatial configuration. In addition, face recognition occurs in the fusiform face area (FFA; Kanwisher, 2010), a specialized "module" in the ventral cortex that is maximally activated by faces relative to all other objects. One might wonder, therefore, whether face recognition in people with WS conforms to normal holistic processing, and whether it activates similar areas of the brain as in normal individuals.

The evidence that faces are processed holistically generally consists of showing that face features are not processed independently. For example, Tanaka and Farah (1993) developed the *part-whole procedure* in which observers learn a set of faces, each of which have unique eyes and mouth features (see Figure 3.19). After training, they are shown one of two kinds of test stimuli. In the *whole face condition*, they are shown one of the faces from the training phase along with a foil that differs by one feature and their task is to choose the matching face. In the *part condition*, they are shown one of the features (e.g., the nose) taken from a face they saw in the training phase along with a foil and asked to indicate which is the matching feature. The logic is that if people learned the appearance of the faces in training by storing independent information about the appearance of each feature, they should be equally accurate in the whole and part conditions. On the other hand, if they have learned the configuration of the features in each face, the single feature in the part condition will not match their stored knowledge and they will have

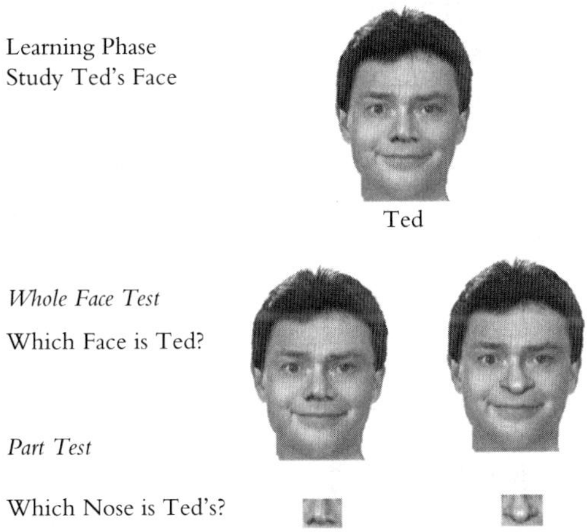

Figure 3.19. The part-whole procedure. Observers learn to identify a face and then have to discriminate that face from another differing in a single feature. Performance in this whole face test condition is usually better than a part test condition in which the discrimination is based on the nose alone.

trouble discriminating between the two isolated features at test. In general, people are more accurate in the whole face condition than in the part condition, supporting the idea of holistic processing of faces.

In the composite face effect (Carey & Diamond, 1994), observers are presented with a face in which the top and bottom halves of the face come from two different individuals (see Figure 3.20). If they are asked to name the person portrayed by the top half of the face, their recognition accuracy and latency will be impaired compared to a condition in which the two face halves are misaligned. Apparently, the appearance of the top half of the face is affected by the irrelevant bottom half, but only when they are aligned.

A final effect that is taken as evidence of configural processing of faces is the *disproportionate inversion effect*, which refers to the large deleterious effect of image inversion on face recognition compared to other objects (Yin, 1969). Inverting a face not only makes it difficult to recognize, but it also disrupts the part-whole and composite effects, which suggests that inverting the face interferes with its holistic processing. Inversion apparently disrupts configural processing, resulting in faces being processed in a feature-by-feature fashion like other objects. This is also consistent with the finding that inverted faces produce lower levels of activation in the FFA than normal faces (Mazard, Schiltz & Rossion, 2006; Yovel & Kanwisher, 2005).

We have been using the terms *holistic* and *configural* as synonymous, but some researchers draw a distinction between these terms. For example,

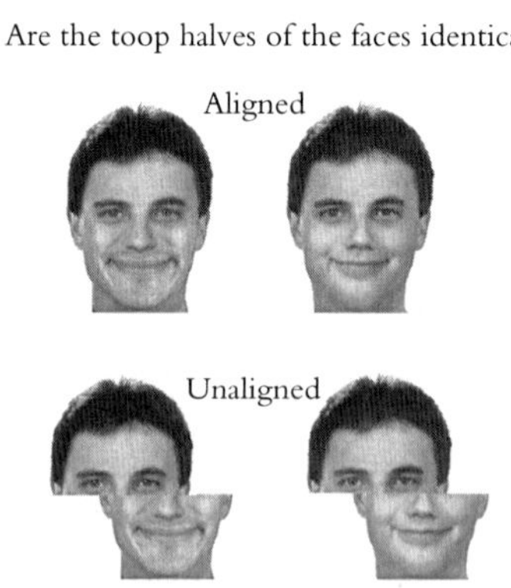

Figure 3.20. The composite face effect. Observers are presented with two faces consisting of a common top half and bottom parts from different individuals. The task is to identify the person on the basis of the upper half alone. They are more accurate when the two parts of the face are misaligned than when they are aligned.

Maurer et al. (2002) distinguish three types of configural processes in face perception: (1) *first-order relations*, that is, the eyes are always on top, the nose in the middle, and the mouth on the bottom, (2) *holistic processing*, which means that the different features are perceived as a gestalt, and (3) *second-order relations*, which refers to the metric spacing between the features. Part of their justification for separating these is that they may have different developmental trajectories (although see McKone et al., 2009, for a different view).

Maurer et al. argue that development of expertise in recognizing faces is a protracted process that extends into adolescence. Some aspects of this process, such as sensitivity to first-order relations, appear to be present in infants. Holistic processing is present in children as young as 4 years old, as shown by the presence of inversion effects, as well as part-whole and composite face effects (McKone et al., 2009). In contrast, sensitivity to second-order spatial relations appears to increase through late childhood into adolescence. Recent evidence suggests there may be prolonged development of the FFA compared to other ventral stream areas (Grill-Spector, Golarai, & Gabrieli, 2008; although see Kanwisher, 2010, for a different view). It is not clear though whether the slow development of sensitivity to second-order spatial relations in faces is really specific to face processing. In adults, limits in this sensitivity appear to correspond to the limits of hyperacuity, which is usually measured as the smallest detectable deviation in the alignment of a pair of lines, and this ability continues to improve into adolescence (Skoczenski & Norcia, 2002). So at least some of the protracted development of face recognition skills may be due to development of "general" visual abilities rather than those that are specialized for faces (McKone et al., 2009; Mondloch, Le Grand, and Maurer, 2002).

The clear role for configural processing in face recognition and the protracted developmental course of at least some aspects of face processing make it an interesting testing ground for claims about intact versus impaired visual-spatial abilities of people with WS. For example, if people with WS are impaired in configural processing, we might expect them to show a deviant processing style when recognizing faces. They should not show any of the hallmarks of holistic/configural processing such as inversion, part-whole, and composite effects because they would be processing faces as a set of nonintegrated features. In addition, they might lack an FFA, which appears to be specialized for the holistic processing of upright faces. Finally, if people with WS show spatial performances that are in some respects like those of much younger normally developing children—as we have argued is true for some aspects of object recognition—they might show lower sensitivity to the spacing of features in faces, which appears to have a prolonged developmental trajectory.

Several early papers did report that face processing in WS was aberrant and concluded that people with WS used a part-based strategy, as opposed to the holistic processing that characterizes normal face processing (Deruelle et al., 1999; Karmiloff-Smith, 1997). However, Tager-Flusberg et al. (2003) pointed out that these studies suffered from several methodological problems and reinvestigated the issue using a variant of the whole-part procedure (see Farah, Wilson, Drain, & Tanaka, 1998) along with inversion to determine whether people with WS process faces holistically. In the whole-face test procedure, observers were shown a sample face followed by two test faces, one that was identical to the sample and one that differed by a single feature (shape of the eyes, nose, or mouth). In the isolated-part test condition, the sample face was followed by only a pair of features (for example, 2 mouths), one of which matched the corresponding feature of the sample face. In both conditions, observers had to choose the matching face or part. In the inverted condition, both the sample and test stimuli were shown in an inverted orientation.

Although chronological-age-matched controls were more accurate overall than people with WS, both groups were more accurate in the whole condition compared to the part condition but only with upright faces; inversion eliminated the advantage of the whole faces. Both of these results are consistent with the claim that people with WS process faces holistically.

Karmiloff-Smith et al. (2004) investigated a different aspect of configural processing in WS: namely, sensitivity to the spatial distances between the features of the face (second-order relations). In this experiment, people with WS (*M* age = 30 years, range = 16;3–51;0) and chronological-age-matched controls viewed two sequentially presented faces in order to determine whether or not the faces were identical. In the "configural" condition, nonidentical face pairs had the same features but differed in their inter-feature spacing. In the "featural" condition, spacing was the same but the features had different shapes (e.g., the noses in the two faces were different). Faces were also presented upright or inverted as a test of holistic processing. Overall, the performance of the two groups was remarkably similar with both groups showing lower performance with inverted faces relative to upright ones.

In additional analyses, the authors divided their data into two categories, corresponding to trials in which the pair of faces was "same" or "different." For "same" trials, no significant effects of group or interactions with group were observed. For "different" trials, however, they found that people with WS were less accurate than controls in the upright, configural condition (51% versus 75%). The authors took this as evidence that processing of the configural information carried by inter-feature spacing is impaired in people with WS, and therefore face processing is not normal.

One caution in accepting this conclusion is the possibility that the results reflect a difference in decision criteria rather than a difference in sensitivity. For example, suppose that people with WS had a bias to respond "same" when faced with upright faces. One would predict that their percent correct on trials with nonidentical faces would be poor, as was observed, but this same bias would result in accurate performance when the faces actually were the same. An examination of the "same" data does indeed show that people with WS were more accurate with upright configural faces compared to controls (81% versus 74%). We converted the data for *same* and *different* trials in the upright configural condition to a d-prime measure for each group and then converted these back into percent correct ($p(c)_{max}$, the unbiased proportion correct; Macmillan & Creelman, 1991) and found that the accuracy of the two groups was now much more comparable: 74.5 % for controls versus 67.4% for the WS group. Given that the standard error was approximately 5%, this difference would not be significant.

It does not appear from these data that the WS and control groups actually differ in their *sensitivity* to configural information conveyed by inter-feature spacing. The difference that was reported may be due to differences in bias to make *same* and *different* responses. In a way, it might be surprising that people with WS are not impaired in perceiving the spacing between face features because, according to Mondloch et al. (2002), this aspect of configural processing may not be fully developed until the age of 10. However, recent work (McKone, Crookes & Kanwisher, 2009) indicates that when the difficulty levels of featural and configural processing tasks are equated, the ability to perceive inter-feature spacing is present in children as young as 4 years (McKone & Boyer, 2006). McKone et al. (2009, p. 479) summarize the evidence as follows: "Qualitatively, behavioral findings indicate establishment of *all* adult-like face recognition effects by 4 years at the latest, and in infancy wherever tested." If true, these face recognition effects would constitute early-emerging functions in *normal* development. If face processing in people with WS patterns like our results for object recognition—with much performance similar to that of normally developing 4- or 5-year-olds—then they should show "mature" performance for face functions that are normally acquired by age 4 or 5.

3.3.1 Summary of Evidence on Face Recognition

The foregoing evidence indicates that people with WS are quite good at recognizing faces and their ability does not depend on abnormal or atypical processing strategies but rather reflects the same configural and holistic processing mechanisms found in typically developing populations. Other recent papers have reported similar findings. Deruelle et al. (2003) had children match faces on the basis of low or high spatial frequencies and found that the WS group was similar to both mental-age-matched controls (*M* age = 5;5) and chronological-age-matched controls (*M* age = 10;7) in their reliance on low spatial frequencies. Because low spatial frequencies favor global configuration information over local features, these results are consistent with other studies in showing that face recognition in the WS population relies on holistic processing to the same degree as in typically developing children. Similarly, Rose et al. (2007) examined face recognition in normal children, children with WS, and children with autism. They found that all three groups were accurate at discriminating pairs of faces and that people with WS were *more impaired* by inversion than both of the other groups.

The limited neuroimaging findings that are available on how WS participants process faces are also consistent with holistic processing in people with WS. There is now strong evidence that an area in the ventral cortex called the fusiform face area (FFA) responds more to faces than to other objects (see Kanwisher, 2010, for a review). In addition, this area seems to respond to the holistic aspect of face processing as its activation level is affected by the face composite effect (Schiltz & Rossion, 2006) and inversion (Mazard, Schiltz, & Rossion, 2006; Yovel & Kanwisher, 2005). If people with WS were recognizing faces using a part-based strategy, as some have claimed, one might expect that the FFA region in WS participants would be less extensive and/or show lower levels of activation in response to face stimuli compared to control participants. However this does not appear to be the case. Sarpal et al. (2008) used fMRI to examine patterns of activation and functional connectivity in different brain regions in response to faces and houses. They found that adults with WS and a group of age- and IQ-matched controls showed greater activation for faces than houses in the FFA, confirming results of an earlier study by Meyer-Lindenberg et al. (2004).

Another recent study by O'Hearn et al. (2010) used a wider variety of objects, including houses, human faces, cat faces, and shoes, to examine ventral activation. They examined three groups: WS participants (*M* age = 18;3) and two normally developing groups, one approximately matched for mental age (*M* age = 7;4) and a second matched for chronological age (*M* age = 17;8). They reported that the FFA response to faces increased with age in the two normally developing groups, consistent with previous reports (Scherf et al., 2007). The FFA activation in WS participants was the same as that of chronological age matches, consistent with a normal FFA that has developed at approximately the same rate as typically developing children. In general, the evidence from neuroimaging studies is consistent with the behavioral data in showing that face processing is a relative strength in WS and reflects the same holistic processing of faces observed in normally developing participants.

At this point, one might wonder, how can the normal processing of configural information in objects and faces by people with WS be reconciled with their clear inability to reproduce global shape in construction tasks such as drawing and block construction?

The answer appears to be that the global deficit revealed in visuospatial construction tasks does not lie at the level of perception but rather reflects impairments in some other processing stage that is critical in construction tasks. For example, Farran et al. (2003) asked people with WS to either identify or draw the global and local letters in Navon figures, and they found impairments, relative to MA controls, in *drawing* global shapes but normal performance in *perceiving* both local and global letters. Rondan et al. (2008) reported similar results.

These behavioral results are also consistent with neuroimaging evidence reported by Ogawa and Inui (2009). They asked their participants to either trace a model or copy the model in a separate display area and found that activity in the intraparietal sulcus was greater for copying than tracing. This same area of the dorsal stream appears to be underactivated in people with WS (Meyer-Lindenberg et al., 2004). Thus the visuospatial construction impairments so clearly evident in WS do not reflect abnormal functioning of ventral stream processes that are important for recognizing faces and objects but, rather, are the result of abnormalities in areas of the parietal cortex that are important for representing space. Recall that people with WS appear to have trouble representing the "handedness of objects" so that they often mistake objects with their reflections (Section 3.2.3.2). This kind of impairment will generally not pose a problem for object recognition required for categorization and naming, which is largely designed to disregard information on the orientation of objects. And it will be even less relevant for recognizing faces, which are more or less bilaterally symmetric. However, in construction tasks, reflection errors will often lead to choosing the wrong part and placing it into an incorrect position in the copy (Hoffman et al., 2003). These kinds of errors will also propagate forward, making subsequent moves incorrect as well. Hoffman et al. showed that these two kinds of errors—choosing reflection parts and placing blocks into incorrect locations—were quite prominent in the block construction task.

3.4 Summary

In this chapter, we have shown that many of the mechanisms underlying object representation are intact in people with WS, whereas other aspects of object representation are much weaker. Grouping mechanisms for static arrays, motion coherence, biological motion, object recognition under canonical viewpoints, and face recognition are all distinct strengths, with WS performance commensurate with mental age and sometimes even on par with chronological age. Representation of objects from unusual views is considerably worse than recognition from canonical views, and representation of object handedness is considerably worse than representation of object part relationships other than handedness.

More important, we saw that the patterns of strength and weakness in the WS groups—whether adults or children—were in many ways quite similar to those of normally developing children who were much younger. For example:

- Grouping processes, such as those that underlie the perception of illusions and the integration of local elements into larger figures, are strong for people with WS, with their thresholds similar to normal adults. But these same thresholds appear for normally developing 4-year-old children, suggesting that these processes emerge quite early in normal development. The same is true for motion coherence, a form of grouping from motion.
- Recognition of familiar objects from canonical viewpoints is quite strong among people with WS, with performance at very high levels even when the objects are briefly presented, or presented as line drawings, without surface color or texture. This function also emerges early in development, with normal 6-year-olds performing at the same high levels as people with WS and 4-year-olds close to these levels.
- Recognition of familiar objects from unusual viewpoints is a weakness among people with WS, with performance much poorer than for canonical views. The same pattern is shown by normally developing 4- and 6-year-olds, and the absolute levels of performance for these unusual views are roughly similar for children with WS (age 11) and normally developing 4- and 6-year-olds. There is considerable change between 6 and 12 in normally developing children, with 12-year-olds approaching normal adult performance.
- Representation of "handedness"—for example, the difference between an object and its left/right reflection—is a weakness among people with WS. Although they do not have difficulty matching on this basis if the object is visually present, removal of the object for only 1 second leads to significant errors. The same pattern—and absolute levels of performance—is shown by normally developing 4-year-olds.

The pattern that is beginning to emerge suggests that the WS profile for object representation may be a case of strength for those functions that are normally acquired early, and weakness for those that are normally acquired over a protracted developmental timetable. If true, this hypothesis for object representation would also explain the strength in face processing, for which there is now considerable evidence.

4

Objects in Places

We have just seen that the WS spatial profile for aspects of object representation is mixed: They show strong performance in identifying common objects, even under challenging conditions such as brief presentation, and they show many normal aspects of grouping processes, including perception of illusions, motion coherence, and biological motion. At the same time, they perform more poorly when asked to identify objects that are presented from unusual viewpoints and have extreme difficulty in representing object handedness (e.g., left-right relationships between parts). These patterns of performance appear to be in line with those of normally developing children between the ages of 4 and 6, suggesting that different spatial functions have different developmental trajectories, with some reaching maturity early in life while others undergo prolonged developmental trajectories. The pattern for people with WS also begins to hint that they may show developmental arrest at the level of a normally developing 4- or 5-year-old child.

This pattern also suggests that the WS deficit may be observed most sharply in tasks engaging the parietal areas and, perhaps more generally, the dorsal stream. For example, the object functions that appear weaker—object recognition under unusual perspectives, and representation of object handedness—appear to engage the parietal regions in normally developed adults, as shown by studies of both normal and brain-damaged adults. Difficulties with handedness would certainly play a role in the observed severe deficit among people with WS in the block construction task, also consistent with impairments in a range of parietal functions.

In this chapter, we explore the profile of people with WS in a range of spatial functions that are known to engage the parietal areas and, more generally, the dorsal stream. As in Chapter 2, we will examine this profile with respect to that of normally developing children at different ages, and look to see whether the WS profile is quantitatively and qualitatively similar to that of normally developing children at some age. Our exploration will not exhaust the functions of the parietal areas: These areas are involved in many different functions, ranging from spatial attention to reaching and grasping, to perception and estimation of numerosity, to the representation of small sets of individual objects, and many other functions (for review, see Grefkes & Fink, 2005; Hubbard, Piazza, Pinel, & Dehaene, 2005; Sack, 2009). However, we will report on a range of functions that are plausibly associated with the parietal areas and, more generally, the dorsal stream, and will ask what the nature of the WS profile is across these functions, relative to normally developing children.

Our main questions will be: Do people with WS exhibit severe impairment in a variety of spatial functions that are thought to engage these areas of the brain? If so, what is the nature of the impairment? Does it reflect structure that is normal for some point in development? Or do we find structure that is different from that appearing in normal individuals? To anticipate, we find that performance among people with WS—who are children, adolescents, or adults—bears striking similarity, both quantitatively and qualitatively, to normally developing children who are on average 4 or 5 years old.

We begin by reviewing the requirements of the block construction task, which form the basis for the studies we will report. We then consider three major components of the task, probing performance among people with WS and normally developing children.

4.1 Review of the Components of the Block Construction Task and Their Relationship to Parietal Functions

As we discussed in Chapter 2, the task requires at least four steps. First, the observer must look at the model puzzle and mentally *mark* a given block in the model as the one that will serve as the starting point for reconstruction. Such mental marking—or *indexing*—can be useful during the process of block construction, for example, as an aid in checking whether a corresponding block has been correctly placed in the copy area. Second, the observer must *match* the candidate block to another in the set of available copy blocks. We have already seen that people with WS have great difficulty matching blocks that differ in handedness, even outside of the construction task. Third, the observer must be able to represent the *location* of the target block relative to the others in the model, and then to identify the "*same*" location in the copy area. Finally, the observer needs to carry out an *action*, placing the chosen block in the correct location in the copy space.

Marking, locating, and acting on objects are quite different spatial functions. Yet each of these has received attention in the extensive literature concerned with functions of the dorsal stream of the brain, in particular, functions of the parietal areas (see Culham & Kanwisher, 2001; Grefkes & Fink, 2005; Rizzolatti & Matelli, 2003; Sack, 2009, for reviews). This literature includes neurophysiological studies of the macaque, cognitive studies of human patients who have sustained brain damage, and brain imaging studies of both normal and brain-damaged adults. As a whole, results converge in suggesting that a wide variety of spatial functions—including those we just described—rely heavily on intact parietal regions of the brain, as well as their connections with more frontal areas, such as sensorimotor and frontal areas of cortex.

Key observations in this literature include examples from patient studies showing that damage to the parietal areas leads to a variety of spatial disorders. Some of the most commonly reported disorders include optic ataxia, in which patients show extreme difficulty pointing to or acting on objects; visual neglect, in which patients seem unable to attend to or adequately process certain regions of space; and apraxia, in which patients show impairment in carrying out gestures (see Rizzolatti & Matelli, 2003, for review). These clinical profiles have led to the overall conjecture that the parietal areas house major networks within the dorsal stream that support the processing of spatial information for the purposes of acting in space.

More generally, Ungerleider and Mishkin (1982) first proposed that the visual system exhibits a division of labor between the ventral and dorsal streams, corresponding to the processing of information about "what" and "where," respectively. In a more recent formulation, Milner and Goodale (1995, 2008) suggest that the division of labor is better characterized in functional terms, with the ventral stream carrying out computations relevant to the enduring properties of objects ("what") and the dorsal stream carrying out computations relevant to the on-line production of visual-manual actions ("how"). More recent formulations suggest further distinctions, with three streams connecting posterior parietal cortex to prefrontal, premotor, and medial temporal areas (Kravitz et al., 2011), each contributing to somewhat different aspects of action. Additional studies show the importance of action-oriented specialization in a number of subareas of the parietal lobe. For example, studies of the macaque have shown that the intraparietal sulcus (IPS), a key landmark dividing the superior parietal lobe (SPL) from the inferior parietal lobe (IPL), contains distinct areas responsible for encoding the locations of objects for the purposes of actions including visual saccades, reaching, and grasping (Grefkes & Fink, 2005). Evidence from patients who have sustained damage to parietal areas and human neuroimaging data are consistent with the idea that there are homologous areas in humans (Culham & Kanwisher, 2001; Grefkes & Fink, 2005).

As we saw in Chapter 2, studies of brain imaging among people with WS indicate that when adults with WS carry out a task similar to block construction, they show lower activation (hypoactivation) of the intraparietal sulcus compared to normal control participants (Meyer-Lindenberg et al., 2004). This finding, together with the many findings showing that spatial functions engage the parietal areas of normal adults, raises the possibility that the spatial impairments in people with WS may be specifically linked to dysfunction in the parietal areas of the brain. This possibility predicts that we should be able to identify a variety of quite different spatial-cognitive functions that normally activate the parietal areas and, more generally, the dorsal stream, and that these functions—regardless of how computationally distinct they are—might show a relatively consistent profile of impairment in people with WS.

We now turn to a discussion of three such functions: marking objects, locating objects, and acting on objects.

4.2 Marking Objects: More Than One at a Time, but Only Up to Two

In Chapter 2, we discussed Ballard et al.'s (1997) proposal that normal adults do not carry out the block construction tasks by looking at the whole model, remembering all parts and their locations, and then selecting the correct blocks and immediately placing each of them correctly in the copy area. Rather, Ballard et al. showed that people carry out model copying tasks in more or less piecemeal fashion, for example, first looking at a target block in the model and noting its color, then selecting a block of that color from the available set, and then returning to the original model to pick up information about the same target block's location (see Section 2.3). Indeed, in our studies of how people with WS carry out the block construction task, we found that eye movement patterns reveal a cyclical pattern reminiscent of the process that Ballard et al. described. People first looked at the model, apparently focusing on a single block. Then they picked up a matching block in the "parts area," refixated the model to get the location of the part they were holding, and placed it in the copy area. These cycles were often followed by fixations between the copy and model areas, reflecting people's checks on whether they had placed the right piece in the right place. People with WS show this entire cycle but, as we also observed, they unfortunately often end up with incorrect copies of the model.

Ballard et al.'s proposal about the process underlying copying tasks suggests a mechanism that could be crucial to success in this kind of task, namely the ability to mentally *mark* a target block in the model that could later be used during the process of selecting a copy block and placing it in the copy area. The mark could be used to return one's attention to the same target block in the model, as one tries to select an identical block from the options available, and then check on whether it was a correct selection. In Ballard's proposal, only a few markers would be required, because the copy is constructed one block at a time. This idea dovetails with another line of research from Pylyshyn (2000, 2006) arguing for the usefulness of having a small number of mental "pointers" to deploy across a variety of visual-spatial tasks.

The first proposal in this line of thinking was put forth by Pylyshyn and Storm (1988), who suggested a mechanism that would allow people to track multiple objects at a time by deploying visual "indexes," first called FINSTs, or "fingers of instantiation." These indexes were thought to be pre-attentive and limited in number, with a maximum of approximately four in normal adults. Pylyshyn and Storm showed that normal adults can, in fact, keep track of multiple objects at a time, and that they could do so under circumstances that made it unlikely that they were representing the individual locations of each object in terms of a spatial reference system.

In Pylyshyn and Storm's experiments, people were presented with 10 identical objects, and a subset of these (one to five) were cued as targets. All objects then began moving along independent trajectories for a set time, after which one of the objects flashed, and people were asked to judge whether it was one of the cued targets. People did surprisingly well at this task, as long as the number of objects to be tracked was fewer than five. Pylyshyn and Storm argued that the task of tracking multiple moving objects could not be carried out by serially moving a spotlight of attention from target to target. Because objects are moving during the time between visits to the same target, distractors would be just as likely as the target to be close to its last known location, resulting in much larger error rates than were actually observed. Instead, they argued that tracking was accomplished by a specialized mechanism that allowed individual mental markers to act like "sticky fingers," adhering to the objects and following them as they moved through space. Since the original experiments by Storm and Pylyshyn, there have been numerous replications of the phenomenon, and many extensions that have led to refinements of the theory and alternative proposals (see Scholl, 2009, for a review). What does seem to be clear, however, is that normal adults are indeed capable of tracking multiple objects at a time and that the kinds of entities that are tracked must be "object-like" (e.g., they cannot act like substances; Van Marle & Scholl, 2003). Moreover, there does seem to be an upper limit to adults' tracking capacity (although there is some debate about its cause; see, e.g., Cowan, 2000; Franconeri, Jonathan, & Scimeca, 2010). Recent evidence shows that multiple object tracking (as well as other tasks involving small numbers of objects) engages the parietal areas of the normal adult brain, and in particular, the intraparietal sulcus (Culham et al., 1998; Xu & Chun, 2006, 2009).

Multiple object tracking (MOT) thus presents itself as a candidate mechanism that could show severe impairment among people with WS. For one thing, if mentally marking multiple objects is required to successfully cycle through the steps involved in copying tasks, then it is possible that difficulty in returning gaze to a target block in the model (or its mate in the copy) might contribute to the severely impaired block construction performance that we observe even among adults with WS. Second, the fact that MOT engages parietal areas of the brain among normal adults raises the possibility that this mechanism might be impaired in people with WS.

To address this possibility, we examined the performance of people with WS on MOT as well as a control task in which they had to remember the locations of multiple *static* objects. In our first experiment (O'Hearn, Landau, & Hoffman 2005), we tested 15 people with WS (*M* age = 18;0, range = 10;5–38;11), and compared their performance to normally developing children (*M* age = 5;11, range = 4;6–7;3) who were matched for mental age. In a second experiment, we increased our control sample, adding 36 normally developing children: 12 in each age group, including 4-year-olds (*M* age = 4;6), 5-year-olds (*M* age = 5;4), and 6.5–7-year-olds (*M* age = 7;0).

In both the moving and static tasks, people viewed a computer display having eight randomly positioned red squares on a black background (see Figure 4.1, left panel). At the beginning of each trial, one, two, three, or four of the red squares "flipped over" (one at a time) to reveal identical cats on the other side. In the static condition, people were instructed to remember where the cards with cats were, while in the moving condition, they were told to track all of the cards with cats. The experimenter then clicked the computer mouse, and all cards flipped back over, with the result that all eight cards were once again red. All cards then either remained in the same spots (static condition) or moved along independent trajectories (moving) for 6 seconds. After this period, people pointed to the cards that they thought were the targets, and their responses were recorded.

Accuracy (percent error) is shown in Figure 4.1 (right panel). The top panel shows that people with WS performed more poorly than normally developing children (*M* age = 5;11) matched for mental age in the moving condition, but not the static condition. The difference became larger as the target set size increases, with reliably poorer performance among WS individuals than mental age matched children for set sizes of three and four targets.

This suggests that people with WS are more impaired in their ability to track multiple moving objects than they are in remembering the locations of multiple static objects. The bottom panel of the results compares the performance of WS participants to a larger group

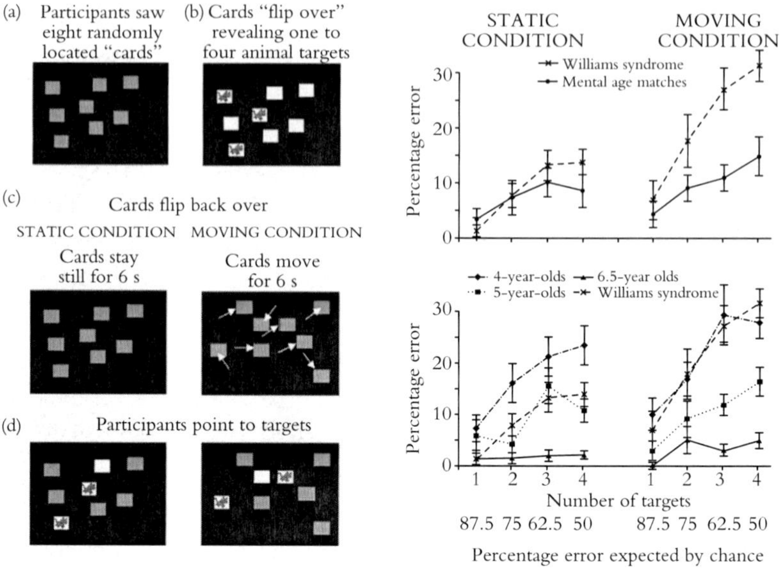

Figure 4.1. Left panel: Stimuli and method for experiment on multiple object tracking and static memory for object location. People saw a set of identical squares ("cards"), then saw several turn over to reveal animal targets. The cards then flipped back over. In the static condition, cards remained in their position for 6 seconds, and people then pointed to the ones they thought hid the animals. In the moving condition, all cards moved for 6 seconds along independent trajectories, after which people pointed to the ones they thought hid the animals. Right panel: Percent errors for all groups over target number. The upper panel shows the WS group compared to normally developing children (*M* age = 5;11) matched for mental age. The lower panel shows a larger sample of normally developing children across a broader age range. Reprinted from O'Hearn et al. (2005), with permission of Sage Publications.

of normally developing children between 4 and 6.5 years of age. This figure shows that the WS group performed like normally developing 4-year-olds in the MOT task, but like normally developing 5-year-olds in the static memory task. As this panel also shows, normally developing children improve at both tasks over age, whereas our group of WS participants—on average 18 years of age—appears to perform at the level of a normal 4-year-old in MOT, and at the level of a 5-year-old in static location memory.

One obvious question is whether people with WS make different kinds of errors in the MOT task than those made by normally developing children, either 4- or 5-year-olds. Different error patterns might reveal different underlying mechanisms for carrying out the tasks. We therefore analyzed people's error patterns, comparing two possibilities. One possibility is that people sometimes lose track of an object because its associated mental marker is lost, perhaps by a process akin to decay. If people are then probed on one of the objects that is not marked, they cannot be certain whether that object is a nontarget or corresponds to the object that lost its index. In this case, they have to guess. The second possibility is that errors occur when the mental markers "slip off" of their targets onto nearby distractors. In this case, the distractors that people erroneously identify as targets should be restricted to those that passed close to a target. In the moving condition (MOT), "nearby targets" would be those passing close to the actual targets sometime during the movement phase of the trial; in the static condition, they would be those situated fairly close to the target throughout a given trial. We evaluated the two hypotheses by asking whether distractors that were erroneously identified as targets had passed closer to a target than distractors that had not been misidentified. The results showed that this was the case for all groups of objects, suggesting that mental markers might indeed have "slipped off" of the targets and landed on a neighboring object. The same pattern occurred in an analysis of the errors for the static condition, suggesting that even when there was no motion involved, people tended to err in selecting distractors that were relatively close to the actual targets.

From these data, we know that people with WS track moving objects only at the level of normally developing 4-year-olds, but they show the same error patterns, and that these error types are similar to older children who perform better overall. Memory for static location in people with WS is somewhat better, roughly at the level of normal 5-year-old children. What underlies this specific deficit in tracking moving objects, even beyond the difficulty in remembering the locations of static objects?

Going back to Pylyshyn's view of the index, we might posit that these indexes are used in the multiple object tracking task, but that other mechanisms besides indexes are used in the static memory task. A static memory task such as ours could be carried out using other mechanisms, such as encoding the locations of individual objects in terms of a stable reference system; one possibility would be encoding the location of the objects relative to the computer screen. The MOT task is less likely to be carried out using such a reference system, since objects move along independent trajectories and would have to be simultaneously updated relative to the reference system throughout the 6-second period of motion. If indexes are used in the MOT task, but other mechanisms are available for the static task, then one might predict that people with WS simply have fewer available indexes or markers than normally developing 5-year-olds, but roughly the same number as normal 4-year-olds. More generally, it is possible that the number of available indexes grows over development, and that people with WS develop to the level of 4-year-olds but go no further.

To examine this possibility, we used our data to generate a measure of performance using Hulleman's (2005) *k* value, which is the average number of objects correctly remembered (static condition) or tracked (moving condition)—a measure used to estimate capacity among adults (Alvarez & Franconeri, 2007; Wolfe, Place, & Horowitz, 2007). We also carried out an additional study parallel to our first, in which we again tested people with WS (age range = 10;9–28;0, *M* age = 18;1) in comparison to normally developing 3- and 4-year-old children (age ranges = 3;4–3;10, *M* age = 3;7; 4;0–5;0, *M* age = 4;4, respectively; O'Hearn, Hoffman, & Landau, 2010). The combined data from the two sets of studies (O'Hearn et al., 2005, 2010) allowed us to generate an overall developmental profile for the number of objects tracked versus remembered among normally developing children between the ages of 3 and 7, and to compare this profile to that of people with WS.

The results, shown in Figure 4.2, converged clearly with those of our previous study. First, people with WS again performed better in the static condition that the moving condition; for the largest number of targets we tested (4), people with WS could remember the static locations of about 3.5 objects, but could track only 2 objects at a time. Normally developing 4-year-olds in the new study could remember the static locations of about 2.5 objects, and could track about 1.9 moving objects at a time. Thus, again, the WS group was able to track about the same number of moving objects as normal 4-year-olds, although they could remember the static locations of more objects than 4-year-olds.

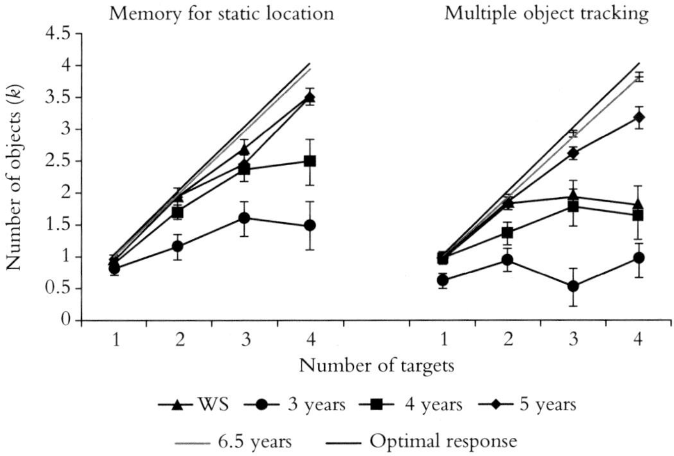

Figure 4.2. Number of objects (*k*) participants were able to represent in task requiring memory for static location of multiple objects (left panel) compared to multiple object tracking (right panel) among normally developing children from 3 to 6.5 years and people with WS. Number of objects represented was computed using Hulleman's *K* (Hulleman, 2005). Reprinted from O'Hearn, Hoffman, and Landau, 2010, with permission of John Wiley and Sons.

Looking at the profile for other age groups, normally developing 3-year-olds could remember the static locations of about 1.5 objects, and could track about 0.95 objects at a time; 5-year-olds could remember about 3.5 targets and could track about 3.2; and 6- to 7-year-olds could remember about 3.9 targets and could track about 3.8 targets. Remarkably, normally developing children within each age group could track or remember approximately the same number of objects and this number increased with increasing age In stark contrast, people with WS could remember about 3.5 objects in the static condition (roughly the same number as normal 5-year-olds) but could track only about 2, roughly the same number as normal 4-year-olds. This pattern suggests that the ability to track multiple objects is particularly impaired in people with WS, reaching the level of a 4-year-old and perhaps never moving beyond that.

Additional evidence from the literature suggests that the developmental improvement we observed among normal children probably continues for both tasks. Studies of spatial memory for static location show increases with age (see Gathercole, 1998, for review); and growth in multiple object tracking capacity also shows developmental increases from age 6 onward (Trick et al., 2005). In this context, the findings for people with WS starkly suggest developmental arrest in the number of objects that can be simultaneously tracked. The results for static memory also suggest clear limitations as well, but remembering locations of static objects may be accomplished by using external frames of reference (e.g., location relative to the side of the computer screen), and thus may take less of a "hit" than tracking of multiple objects. The limits on the number of moving objects that can be tracked by people with WS—even those who are adolescents and adults—is consistent with findings of damage in the area of the interparietal sulcus (Meyer-Lindenberg et al., 2004, 2006), since attentive tracking has been linked to this area in normal adults (Culham et al., 1998; Jovicich et al., 2001).[1]

In sum, the evidence on multiple object tracking shows that people with WS can track fewer objects than children who are mental age matches, and that their performance closely resembles that of normally developing 4-year-old children. Their somewhat better

[1] Although we have discussed the MOT results in terms of limitations in the number of objects that can be tracked, it is also possible that the results are due to relatively coarse representations of spatial location among people with WS and younger children. This possibility would explain both the apparent limitation in number of objects tracked, and the error patterns observed in O'Hearn et al. (2005). In particular, if object locations are represented rather imprecisely, this would increase the possibility that neighboring objects would be misremembered as occupying the target location. The possibility that imprecise representations of object location is at the root of errors in both kinds of tasks—tracking and static memory for location—is consistent with Franconeri et al.'s (2010) work showing that limits on object spacing plays a major role in the number of objects tracked. It is also consistent with the work of Bae and Flombaum (2012), who suggest that people's uncertainty about target location may be the central source of limitations in both MOT and working memory for objects. This possibility would predict that people with WS should have relatively coarse representations of location, perhaps at the level of a normally developing 4-year-old, and that this would be linked to the small number of objects that they can track.

performance in remembering the locations of static objects suggests that the MOT task reflects a different mechanism from that underlying memory for location per se. This mechanism undergoes development in normal children between the ages of 4 and 7; individuals with WS appear to show developmental arrest at the functional level of a normal 4-year-old.

4.3 Locating Objects: Constructing and Using Reference Frames

One of the key requirements of the block construction task is the ability to accurately represent the location of each block relative to the others. Further, in order to make a copy, the observer must then find the "same" location in a separate region of space—the copy area—and place the block in that location. Understanding how object locations are represented is, of course, crucial for understanding why people with WS have such difficulties with the block construction task. As it turns out, the more general question of how people represent object locations is a foundational issue for theories of spatial representation, its development, and its impairment in neurological disorders. At the heart of this issue is the concept of a *reference system*.

Reference systems are crucial to our representations of location because they tell us the answer to the question "*X* is located in terms of what?" Consider, for example, an observer sitting at a table on which a block has been placed (see Figure 4.3). Suppose we ask the observer the simple question, "Where is the block?" The observer has many different options, depending on how he wishes to define the location of the block. It can be described as directly *in front of him*, or *on the table*, or *in the room*, or even with specific coordinates that relate its location to the front door of the house, the neighborhood, the city, or even the country in which it is located. Each of these answers specifies a different frame of reference—in terms of which the object is located. Obviously, we do not usually choose to locate a moveable object in terms of the country in which it is located. But the point is that in order to describe the location

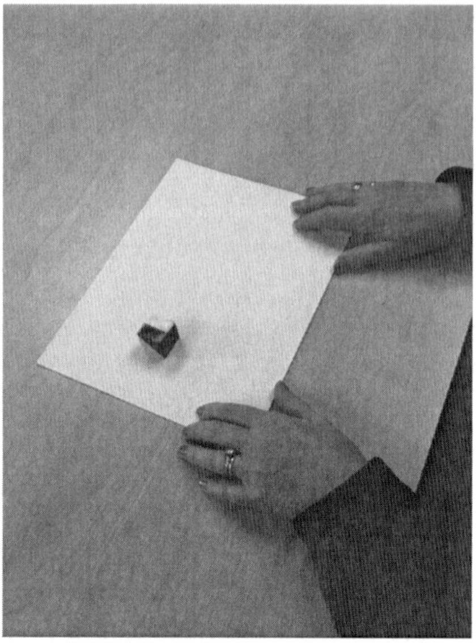

Figure 4.3. Where is the block? Many different answers are possible. It can be described as directly *in front of the observer*, or *on the table*, or *in the room*, or even with specific coordinates that relate its location to the front door of the building, the neighborhood, the city, or even the country in which it is located. Each of these answers specifies a different frame of reference—in terms of which the object is located. The particular way in which people represent and use frames of reference is a key issue for understanding how they represent location.

of an object, one must make a decision about which reference system will be used.[2]

Note that when we say that people represent location in terms of a frame of reference, we are assuming the existence of a mental structure: There is no reference system that "exists" in the world; rather, these systems are the mental representations that we naturally use to perceive and remember locations. Reference systems can then be defined in terms of their origin, the axes that intersect at the origin, and the directions within each axis (see McCloskey, 2009, for extensive discussion of the reference system and its separable components). There are several possible ways to specify the *origin* of the reference system: a *retinocentric* system has its origin at the center of the retina; a *head-centered* system has its

[2] This decision constitutes the answer to what McCloskey (2009) calls the "definition question": In relation to what are locations defined? He points out that this question is separate from what he calls the "format question": In what format are locations represented? In discussing the format question, McCloskey distinguishes between compositional and noncompositional formats, and argues for the former, with reference systems represented in terms of separable components of axes and direction within axes. Our evidence on use of reference systems by people with WS and normally developing children is consistent with this theory.

origin at the center of the head; an *egocentric* system has its origin at the center of the body (or some part thereof); an *object-centered* system has its origin at the center of some object; a *geocentric* system has its origin at the center of the earth, and so forth. Up to three sets of orthogonal axes intersect at the origin, and each axis has two distinct directions (or different "polarities" in McCloskey's terms). For example, we might consider a body-centered reference system in which one axis runs from head to toe, resulting in two different directions (let's say, + at the head and – at the feet); and a second axis that runs from one's left hand to the right, again resulting in two different directions (perhaps + for the left hand and – for the right). Conceptualized like this, one can think of the reference system rather like a Cartesian coordinate system, which includes an origin, axes, and directions. A true Cartesian system would also require that locations be defined in terms of the metric coordinates for each axis (see McCloskey, 2009).

Given the concept of a reference system, how would we represent the location of the block in our previous example? Let's simplify and assume that instead of a block, we are dealing with a flat square drawn on a sheet of paper. Figure 4.4 shows the location of the square in terms of the observer's body (an egocentric frame of reference), and in terms of the page itself.

If the page of paper is directly in front of the observer (as in Figure 4.4), then we can ask: Does the observer represent the location of the square in a reference system centered on his body, the page, or both?[3] This is an important question, because as the observer moves, the location of the object will change relative to his body but not relative to the axes defined by the page. This means that the definition of "same location" will vary, depending on what reference system we are using for a given task, as well as whether or not we move through space as we carry out the task. Because we are mobile, we must be capable of representing location in terms of different reference systems centered on parts of the body (e.g., retina, head, body, arm), and we must also be able to represent location in

[3] We could also ask whether he represents the location relative to the retinocentric or head-centered system, but for now we consider only object and body-based reference systems.

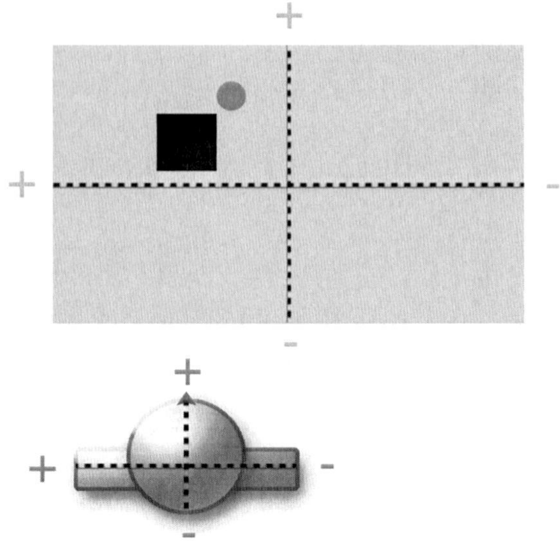

Figure 4.4. Imagine that the black square is on a gray sheet of paper positioned in front of the observer. The location of the square on the rectangular page can be defined relative to the observer's body axes, the axes of the page, or both. The dotted lines represent the axes of these two different reference systems, and the + and – represent the directions within each axis of each reference system. As one can see, the square is located *in front of* the observer, but *on the left side* of the page. These locations are defined within different reference systems—one centered on the observer, the other centered on the page itself. (*See* color insert.)

terms of different objects in the environment (e.g., the location of the square relative to the page). Solving any spatial problem will require that we encode an object's location in terms of the reference system that is appropriate for that problem.

Many spatial tasks such as block construction require that we judge the locations of corresponding parts in two different areas, such as the model and copy areas discussed earlier.

Figure 4.5 shows this problem, with one "model" page to the observer's left, and a second identical "copy" page (minus the dot to

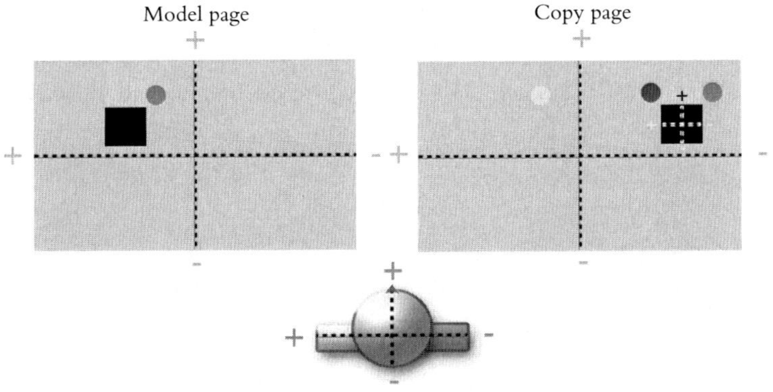

Figure 4.5. The observer can represent the location of the red dot in the model panel (left) in terms of various frames of reference. The red dot in the copy page (right) represents the "same" location using the center of the square as the origin of the reference system. The green dot represents the "same" location using the center of the page itself as the origin. The blue dot represents the "same" location using the center of the square as the origin of the reference system, but misrepresenting the direction along the horizontal axis, thereby copying the location "above and to the *left*" of the square rather than "above and to the *right*." The latter kind of error is attested in our studies of people with WS and young normally developing children. (*See* color insert.)

be copied) to his right. As we pointed out above, copying tasks require a reference system centered on the copy space, not the observer's body. In this case, we actually need two reference systems: one centered on the model located on the person's left, and another centered on the copy space, located on his right.

Using the representation of the dot in the "model" (two orthogonal axes, their direction, and the values along each axis), the observer can now transfer this representation of the dot's location relative to the square onto the second (copy) space, constructing a second reference system centered on the "copy" square, with the same axes and directional assignments. He can then place the dot at the same set of coordinates relative to this second square. If the observer has an accurate location representation, in which the dot occupies the correct coordinates for each axis, and if he can mentally hold onto this representation while he transfers it to the copy space, the copied location should be correct (as the red dot in Figure 4.5.)

Note that there are many ways that one could go wrong in this disarmingly simple copying task. First, one could represent the location of the dot relative to a reference system centered on the page, rather than the one centered on the square. If so, then even if the location representation is correct with respect to each axis, its internal directions, and the values along each axis, the dot will end up in a different location—this is shown in Figure 4.5 by the green dot. Or the observer could represent the direction within the vertical axis correctly, but misrepresent the direction within the horizontal axis. If direction is misrepresented, then the dot will end up at the opposite end of the horizontal axis, as shown by the blue dot in Figure 4.5. McCloskey's (2009) in-depth study of patient A.H. revealed a persistent pattern of this last type of error, suggesting that A.H. had some kind of misrepresentation of direction along the horizontal axis (resulting in a reflection across the vertical axis). The important point is that thinking about object location in terms of the reference system that is used—including the axes of the system and their internal directions—can often provide important information about our spatial representations. Accuracy as well as error types can illuminate how people represent location, as well as which aspects of location representation are strongest and which are most fragile.

Although we have been discussing the representation of a single dot relative to a single square on a sheet of paper, the same conceptual problems apply to the block construction task, in which a person has to copy an entire model into a second space adjacent to the first. Given this, a first and fundamental question is whether the mental structures we call reference systems are evident in people with WS. To address this question, we now report findings from two series of experiments that test for the presence of reference systems, their structure, and possible fragility in people with WS. The first series uses a matching task, and the second uses a copying task.

4.3.1 Matching Locations: Are Object Locations Defined in Terms of a Reference System?

Our first experiment was inspired by the work of Hayward and Tarr (1995), who demonstrated the powerful role of reference systems in the representation of location among normal adults. They found that if adults observed a square reference object and a dot situated close by, and were then asked to say whether a subsequent array was "same" or "different," they performed best in locations along the reference object's principal axis, in other words, the vertical and horizontal axes that run directly through the center of the square and project outward into space. Note that no visual lines were shown in Hayward and Tarr's test arrays; rather, people's patterns of responding reflected the fact that they organized locations in terms of orthogonal axes centered on the reference object. People could apparently represent the locations falling along the axis of the reference object more accurately and robustly than locations not falling on those axes. The stronger and better memory for locations along the axes suggests that people mentally represent the location of the dot in terms of the mental structure we discussed earlier—the reference system, with its origin at the center of the square, and axes projecting outward, bisecting the square both vertically and horizontally.

In our first experiment, we adapted Hayward and Tarr's method: We gave people a model display that contained a dot and square, and we asked them to *match* this model to one of two test displays also containing a dot and a square (see Figure 4.6). One test display showed a dot in the *same* location relative to the square, and the other showed a dot in a slightly *different* location. We asked people to pick the copy that looked identical to the model. We tested children with WS (ages 8–14, *M* age = 10;4) and normally developing children who were matched for mental age (ages 3–7, *M* age = 5;5).

In the study, the model displayed a single dot (0.5 in.) located in 1 of 36 target locations around a square (1.5 in. × 1.5 in., see Figure 4.6). On each trial, the two test arrays (same array, different array) were displayed in the space below the model; different arrays were identical to same arrays, except that the dot was displaced from its original location by 0.5 in. in any of four different directions.

Figure 4.7 shows proportion correct for each of the locations for children with WS (left panel) and normally developing children matched for mental age (right panel; *M* age = 5;5). The proportions correct are coded as gray scale, with the darkest regions representing the highest proportions. These data were analyzed to determine whether there was evidence of axial structure (comparing locations on-axis versus off-axis), vertical versus horizontal axis and direction within each axis, as well as

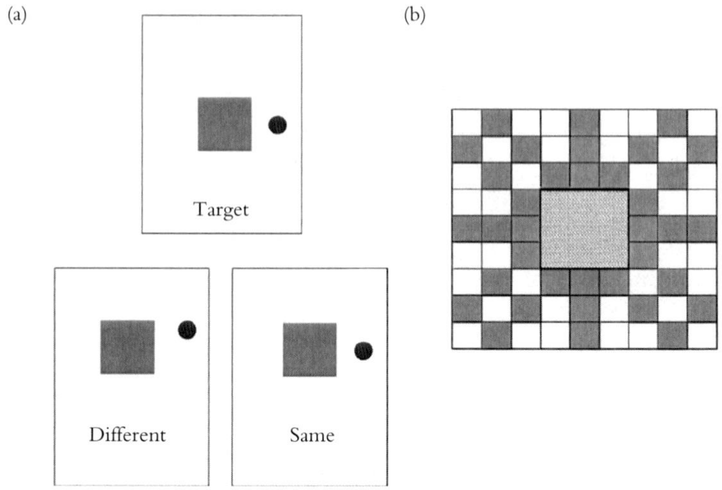

Figure 4.6. (a) Layout of model ("target") and test stimuli in matching task. People were asked to look at the model and pick the test array below that showed the dot in the "same" location relative to the square. (b) Locations tested in the matching experiment. Dark gray boxes indicate all target locations for the dot, in regions around the square. Each location was tested several times, but each trial tested just one location. Grid lines were not present in the displays used for testing. Adapted from Landau and Hoffman (2005), with permission from Elsevier.

distance from the reference object (contact, near, far from the object). These analyses confirmed what is clear from the gray-scale figures: Both children with WS and normally developing children performed better when the dot was located along the (virtual) vertical and horizontal axes extending from the square reference object than for non-axial locations. Both groups also performed better when the dot was located closer to the square than when it was farther away.

However, distance affected the two groups differently. Both groups performed at ceiling for locations in contact with the reference object, but the WS children's performance fell off more rapidly than normally developing children's as the dot's location increased in distance from the square. Moreover, analyses comparing the vertical and horizontal axes showed that both groups of children matched the dot's location better when it fell along the vertical axis than the horizontal axis; but children

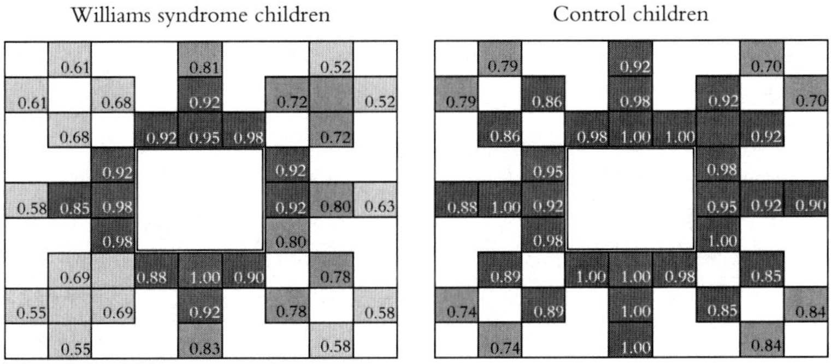

Figure 4.7. Proportions correct in the matching task for children with WS (left) and normally developing children (right; *M* age = 5;5) who were matched to the WS participants on mental age. Proportions are given for each location. Darker shades represent higher proportions correct. Adapted from Landau and Hoffman (2005), with permission from Elsevier.

with WS performed disproportionately worse along the horizontal axis, especially with greater distances.

The results suggest that both children with WS and normally developing children around 5 years of age represent the location of an object in terms of a reference system that is centered on the reference object and is composed of (at least) two distinct axes (vertical and horizontal). Locations that fall along the axes of this reference system are represented more robustly than those off the axes, but the functional structure of the reference system appears to be somewhat different for the two groups. Relative to the normally developing children who are matched for mental age, the reference system in children with WS is somehow "truncated" with respect to the distances across which location can be computed—that is, at larger distances, the WS system does not appear to function as well as the system of the normal controls. Moreover, children with WS appear to have weaker representations of the horizontal axis than do their normal mental age matches, with performance falling off more rapidly along the horizontal axis as distance increases.

The matching study asked whether children with WS represent location in terms of reference systems that are composed of two distinct axes centered on the reference object and the answer is: They do. But the design of that study did not allow us to determine whether the directions within axes—for example, "above versus below" on the vertical axis or "right versus left" on the horizontal axis—are also clearly represented as having different "polarity."

To answer this question, we carried out a second task in which people were asked to match dot locations as in the first matching task. But this time, the test items were specifically designed to probe for errors in which the directions within each axis might be confused (i.e., "above" confused with "below," "left" confused with "right").[4] In the task, people saw a model array—a dot and a square—in the upper half of a computer screen (see Figure 4.8). This target array was removed for 1 second before the appearance of the test arrays, which were shown in the lower half of the screen. On each trial, the participant was to judge which of the two test arrays displayed the dot in the "same" place relative to the model array. One of the test arrays showed the dot in the same place relative to the square. The second showed the dot situated at the same distance from the reference object, either along the same axis, but at the opposite end (e.g., "below" the square if the model dot was "above" it, "right" of the square if the target was "left" of the square), or along a different axis (e.g., "below" the square if the model dot was on the "left" or "right" of it).

We tested children with WS as before (*M* age = 11;6; range = 8;9–14;3), as well as their mental age matches (*M* age = 5;10, range = 3;11–7;2), and we added a group of adolescents and adults with WS (*M* age = 21, range = 14–30). We found that all groups performed better than chance, but more errors occurred when the dot was placed along the same axis but at the opposite end. Thus, children and adults with WS and normally developing children show fragility in the representation of direction within each axis. This result was clear when there was a brief delay (1 second), but did not appear in a control condition with no delay. This suggests that the problem more likely lies in memory for direction than in perception of direction.

[4] When we use the words "above/below" and "left/right" in the present context, we do not necessarily mean that the representation of direction that is used is linguistic. The matching task may engage language, but we cannot be sure. In Chapter 6, we review studies that focus on the linguistic understanding of these terms.

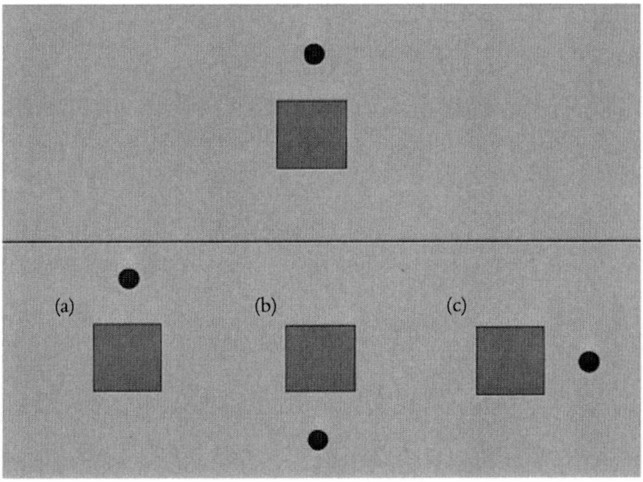

Figure 4.8. To test the representation of direction within axes, we presented people with a model (top panel), and then asked them to match it to one of two test items. The two test items included one array that was an exact match (lower panel, a), and one item that either fell along the same axis but in the opposite direction (lower panel, b) or along a different axis (lower panel, c). People with WS and normally developing children made more errors when the real match was paired with (b) than when it was paired with (c). This suggests that people find it relatively difficult to represent the particular direction (e.g., above/below) within an axis. Adapted from Landau and Hoffman (2005), with permission from Elsevier.

The findings are consistent with the evidence we presented in Chapter 3, in particular, the difficulties that children and adults with WS have in representing the unique handedness of objects (especially left-right relationships). They are also consistent with other findings from our lab showing that representation of handedness is hard for normally developing 4-year-olds to maintain even under a 1-second delay (Dessalegn & Landau, 2008). Representing handedness requires representing the relevant axis, as well as the directional asymmetry within it. By the age of 6, normally developing children become highly accurate at representing handedness under brief delays (Dessalegn & Landau, 2008). But people with WS, even adults, appear to have difficulty with handedness, in the task we just described, in object recognition tasks (see Chapter 3), and, as we will see in Chapter 6, in the use of spatial language.

4.3.2 Copying Locations: Axes, Directions, and Spatial Precision in Location Representations

The results we just described show that children and adults with WS do represent object locations in terms of reference systems—mental structures organized as sets of orthogonal axes intersecting at a common origin. Moreover, the results show that people with WS can attend to the task-relevant reference system (i.e., the one centered on the model reference object), and can convert a representation of the dot's location into a representation of the "same" location in a second reference system (the ones centered on the test array). But it is also true that the WS children's level of accuracy falls to levels just above chance for locations along the horizontal axis that are far from the reference object. Compared to normally developing 5-year-olds, they showed limits on the extent of space they can represent, fragility along the horizontal axis, and fragility in representing direction.

Two questions arise. First, does the limit in performance among WS children in the matching task extend to a "construction" task, in which they must actually *copy* the model location, rather than just select a match? Second, given their deficit relative to normally developing 5-year-olds, does the WS pattern of performance represent a pattern that is also present in even younger normally developing children? If so, this would again suggest a developing system that may be arrested at an early developmental point—rather than a system that is qualitatively different from that found in normally developing children.

To address these questions, we designed a task that was closer in requirements to the block construction task. We asked people to *copy* a dot into the "same location" relative to a square. We tested people with WS along with normally developing children who were 4, 6, and 9 years of age, to generate a normal developmental profile against which we could compare the WS group.

4.3.2.1 Copying: Task 1

The new task once again used a model containing a square reference object and a dot positioned in various locations around it (one location per trial, see Figure 4.9a). But this time, we showed people the model

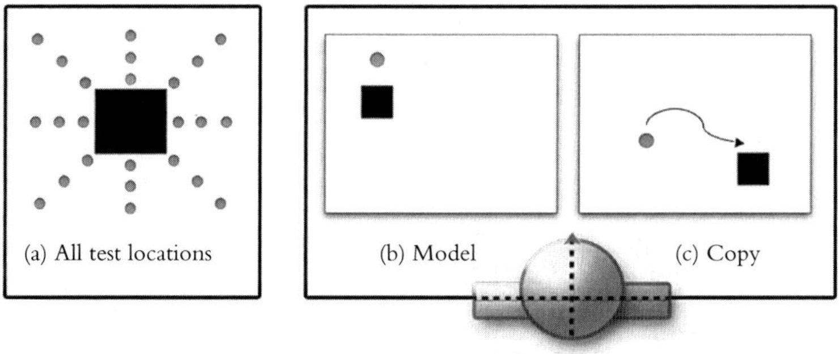

Figure 4.9. Test locations and setup for the first copying task. (a) The 24 test locations for the target dot. People saw a single dot located in one of the test locations on each trial. (Distances from center of the square to center of dot = 1.31, 3.69, 5.95 cm, respectively).[5] (b and c) The setup for the copying task. People sat midway between two computer screens. They observed a dot and a square on the model screen (b) and were then shown a second dot, placed randomly on the copy screen (c), and were asked to place it in the same location relative to the square as it was on the model screen. People moved the dot using the computer mouse.

array on a computer screen located to their left. After observing this array, people were shown a copy space (on a computer screen located to their right), containing a square, along with a dot that was to be moved into the "same" location relative to the square in the model (see Figure 4.9b, c). Half of the target locations were located along principal axes (above/below and left/right) and the rest fell along the obliques. In addition, the dots could be located at one of three distances from the reference object (contact with the square's edge, near it, and farther from it).

On half of the trials, the model and copy squares were in the same location relative to their screens, and on the other half, they were in different locations relative to the screen (see Figure 4.9b and c for an example of the latter trial type). To be accurate on both types of trials, people would have to copy the dot's location *relative to the square*, using

[5] The distances for the contact location varied slightly depending on whether they lay along the main axes or the obliques. Because we used a square, the "contact" distances for the obliques were slightly larger than those for the vertical or horizontal axes.

the square as the frame of reference, not the screen. On each trial, the dot that was to be moved into position appeared in random locations on the second screen. Participants used the computer mouse to move the dot into the "same" location relative to the square as shown on the model screen.

We tested 25 people with WS (*M* age = 21;10, range = 10;10–42;11), as well as 15 normally developing 4-year-olds (*M* age = 4;6, range = range 4;2–4;11), 12 normal 6-year-olds (*M* age = 6;7, range = 6;1–6;11), 12 normal 9-year-olds (*M* age = 9;9, range = 9;2–9;10), and 12 normal adults in order to see whether any patterns of accuracy and error in the WS group would also be shown by normally developing children and adults.

Overall, both people with WS and normally developing children did quite well on the task, with small errors of angle and distance across the trials. Average distance errors were 0.12 cm, and average angular errors were 4.25 deg. There was also very little difference depending on whether the reference object (the square) occurred in the same or different locations in the model and copy screens (differences = 0.2 deg, for angle error and 0.58 mm for location errors). For this task then, all observers used the square as the origin of the reference system, as they should have in order to accurately copy the dot's location relative to the square.

The magnitudes of errors are shown in Figure 4.10. The distance error represents how well people were able to reproduce the distance between the dot and square in the model, without regard to angle. Similarly, the angle error represents performance on matching the angle without regard to distance. These data show a striking similarity between people with WS and normally developing 4-year-olds in terms of both distance and angle errors. Four-year-olds also clearly perform worse than normal 6- and 9-year-olds, whose performance is close to normal adults. These results are consistent with our earlier findings on multiple object tracking and, more generally, with the idea that WS spatial performance appears to be arrested at the functional level of normally developing 4-year-olds for a range of spatial tasks.

In addition to these overall accuracy measures, we asked whether people made any errors that could be characterized as reflections (or

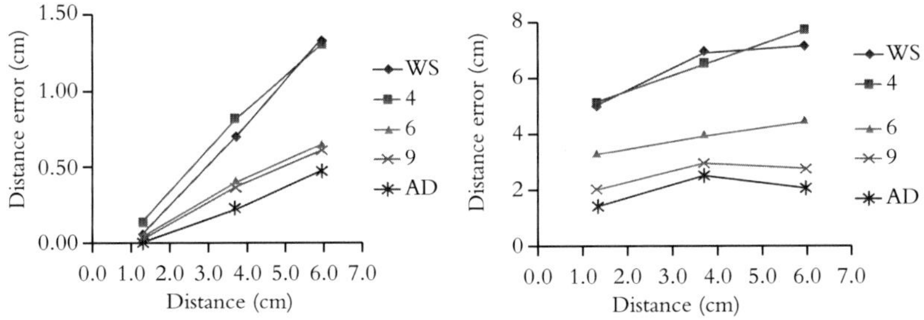

Figure 4.10. Performance on the first copying task. The left panel shows average distance errors (cm) and the right panel shows average angular errors (deg) as a function of different distances of the target dot from the square. The WS group performed virtually identically to normally developing 4-year-olds, while normal 6- and 9-year-olds showed better performance, almost at the level of normal adults.

reversal of direction) within either the vertical or horizontal axes of the square. This would mean, for example, copying a dot onto the right side of the square in the copy space, even though it was displayed on the left side of the square in the model array, or copying it below the square even though it was displayed above the model square. Although there were not many errors of this type, the patterns of performance across groups confirmed that people with WS have difficulty encoding and remembering direction: Normally developing 6-year-olds made reflection errors on half a percent of trials (0.57%), approximately the same levels as 9-year-olds (0.52%) and normal adults (0.41%). Participants with WS—whose average age was 21, made such errors on 2% of trials. Strikingly, normally developing 4-year-olds made such errors on 12.4% of trials. Thus, on this measure, people with WS fall between normal 4- and 6-year-olds.

The results of this copying task show a fair degree of absolute precision across groups; but even for the overall measures of precision, people with WS were no different from normally developing 4-year-olds, who were less precise than either 6- or 9-year-old normally developing children. These differences across groups do suggest that people with WS may represent location with as much (im)precision as normal 4-year-olds, but that WS precision does not improve beyond this point—as it does for normally developing children. But the results also fall short of illustrating the kind of severe deficit we observe in the block construction task, where very large errors are made in assembling blocks into an overall pattern. It seems likely that there are additional factors at work in copying tasks that might lead to more catastrophic failures.

4.3.2.2 Copying: Task 2

Our second copying task incorporated further complexity in order to more closely approximate the requirements of the block construction tasks and to potentially generate more errors that we could examine in detail. The task now included a reference object that had internal structure—a clear "top/bottom/right/left"—and the orientation of this reference object was varied in the model, while the copy reference object remained upright (see Figure 4.11). Including a reference object with internal structure moves the task closer to the block construction task, where individual blocks often have internal structure (e.g., a vertical split with a different color on each side). Varying the orientation of the model reference object relative to the one in the copy space also simulates a situation common in carrying out block construction tasks: Individual blocks are often set down at orientations that are slightly

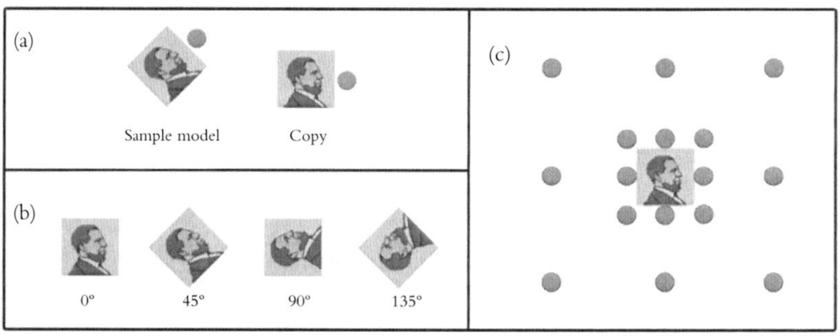

Figure 4.11. Setup and stimuli for second copying task. (a) Sample model reference object and its dot, and the corresponding copy reference object and its dot. The model and copy reference object were presented on separate sheets of paper to the participant's left and right, respectively. (b) The model reference object was presented in four different orientations. Copy reference objects were always presented upright. (c) All target dot locations presented in the models.

different from the ones in the model, possibly leading to cascading difficulties as more and more blocks are placed relative to each other.

We again presented people with a display showing a model reference object and a dot, and asked them to copy a new dot into the "same" location relative to the reference object on the copy page. The reference object in both the model and copy was a square surrounding the profile of a man's head, as in a postage stamp (see Figure 4.11a). The natural axes of the man's head—top/bottom, and right/left when upright—invited the mental imposition of a reference system within the square, with two unique orthogonal axes and two clearly different directions within these axes. We presented the model reference object at four different orientations, shown in Figure 4.11b; the copy reference object was always presented at the same, "upright" orientation.

With the model square rotated, and the man's head inside of it, the two primary axes of the reference object no longer correspond to "vertical" and "horizontal"—terms that refer to gravitational anchors. For this reason, we now refer to the axes as "primary" and "secondary," with the assumption that, when the object is upright, the primary axis is vertical and the secondary is horizontal. We designated the forehead/chin axis as "primary" and the nose/back of head axis as "secondary." Similarly, directions with each axis represent different polarities, but they do not, technically speaking, correspond to "above," "below," "left," or "right" (people generally use these terms to refer to an environmental frame of reference; Carlson-Radvansky & Irwin, 1993). We defined directions as + for the forehead and nose, and − for the chin/back of head. When we describe patterns of performance, we will refer to accuracy and error patterns for the primary and secondary (as well as oblique) axes; but for ease of exposition, we will use the terminology of above/below/left/right, while being careful to make clear that these directions are meant relative to the frame of reference centered on the man's head.

Model dots were presented in each of 16 locations around the model reference object, with a single dot presented on each trial (see Figure 4.11c). The participant's task was then to place a dot (using a pen) into the "same location" relative to the reference object in the copy space (see Figure 4.11a for a sample trial).[6] We told people that the model showed "a man" and a dot located "right here, to the man's head." We then showed people the copy page, with the upright man, and said, "This is your man. Can you make it so that there is a dot in exactly the same place to your man's head as my dot is to my man's head?" The model array was presented on a sheet of paper to the person's left, at one of four different orientations relative to the principal axes of the page (0 degrees/upright, 45, 90, and 135 degrees rotated counterclockwise from upright; see Figure 4.11b). The copy sheet was presented on an identical sheet of paper to the person's right; the man's head was always presented at 0 degrees.

The requirements of this copying task clearly build on and add to those of the previous copying task. Like the previous task, the observer still has to represent the location of the dot in the model relative to the *reference object* (i.e., the man's head), and then transfer this location to the reference object in the copy area. When both model and copy reference objects are "upright," the task remains virtually identical to the first copying task. But when the model reference object has been rotated, there is added complexity. Now, to accurately copy the location of the dot from model to copy space, people must represent the orientation of each reference object, presumably relative to the page on which it sits. McCloskey's (2009) analysis suggests that representing the orientation of each reference object entails representing the relationship between the axes of the reference object and the axes of the page on which it sits. The reference object and the page can each be represented in terms of two axes, which we can call "primary" and "secondary," and directions within each axis ("polarity"). Orientation is the mapping between the axes of the object and those of the page.

After representing each reference object's orientation, the observer would have to map each axis and direction in the model reference object onto the corresponding set of axes in the copy reference object. For

[6] The 16 locations included 4 locations along the primary axis, 4 along the secondary axis, and 8 along the oblique axes. Half of the locations for each axis contacted the square, and half were located at 4.2 cm away from the center of the man. This distance is close to the largest distance we had used in the matching task (3.2 cm) and was selected to ensure that we would be measuring spatial relationships between points distant enough to elicit substantial error.

example, a dot located along the primary axis of the model reference object, and with "positive polarity," would be copied to the location that is also along the primary axis of the copy reference object, with positive polarity.

We tested 16 people with WS (*M* age = 21;10, range 10;10–50;8), as well as 12 normally developing 4-year-olds (*M* age = 4;8), 6-year-olds (*M* age = 6;7), and 9-year-olds (*M* age = 9;6) and 12 normal adults. Analyses were carried out on the size of deviations from the correct target location in distance (cm) and in angle (degrees).

Analyses of distance showed that people were remarkably accurate, with no distance error for trials where the dot was in contact with the reference object and mean distance errors ranging from 1 cm (0.39 in) among 9-year-olds to 1.7 cm for people with WS (0.66 in) and 1.4 cm (0.55 in) for normally developing 4-year-olds for trials where the dot was "far" (4.2 cm) from the reference object. These distance effects are similar to those we observed in our first copying task. There were no effects of any variables or interactions for the measure of distance.

In contrast, there were sizeable effects for the angular deviation measures, which informed us about the strengths and weaknesses of reference systems in people with WS and normally developing children. These data are shown in Figure 4.12.

Figure 4.12 displays the mean angular deviations from the target location across all conditions for people with WS and normally developing 4-year-olds, who did not differ statistically from each other, but performed worse than normal 6- or 9-year-olds. As the figure suggests, there were clear differences in accuracy over the four orientations, especially for the WS group and the normal 4-year-olds. For these groups, the 0- and 45-degree orientations resulted in greater accuracy than the 90- or 135-degree orientations. There was clear development between the ages of 4 and 6 in the normal child groups. The 6- and 9-year-olds were extremely accurate, better than the 4-year-olds or WS group, with average angular deviations of less than 25 degrees for the most difficult (135-degree) condition. There was no difference in overall accuracy between 6- and 9-year-olds. As we had expected, the absolute angular errors in this task were much larger than in the first copying task, presumably due to the added complexity contributed by the internally structured reference object (the man's head) and its varying orientation.

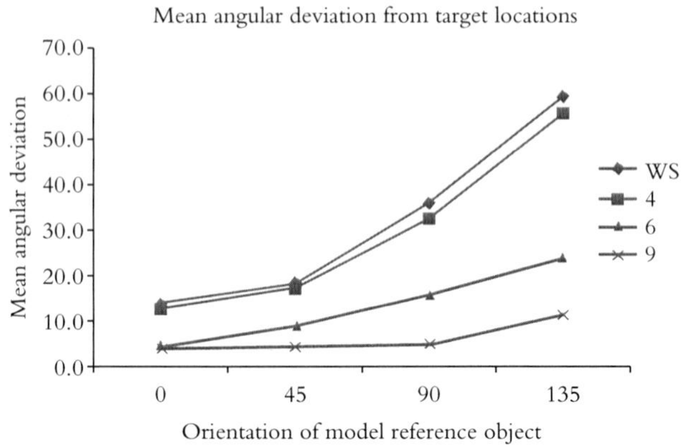

Figure 4.12. Performance on the second copying task. Mean angular deviation from target locations across the four different orientations of the model reference object (i.e., the man's head). As in the first copying task, the WS group performed virtually identically to normally developing 4-year-olds, while normal 6- and 9-year-olds showed better performance.

In addition to the effects of orientation, we observed effects of axis type, with lowest angular errors for locations along the primary axis (regardless of orientation of the object). This reinforces the idea that people with WS and normally developing children represented the reference object in terms of axes, with the primary (forehead/chin) being the most well represented. This strength for the primary axis was, however, affected by the distance from the reference object: When the dot was far from the man's head, the relative advantage for the primary axis was less obvious.

Inspection of the raw data suggested that participants at all ages—but primarily 4-year-olds and WS individuals—occasionally made errors that were grossly inaccurate, but were nevertheless systematic. These errors largely fell into three categories, two of which are shown in Figure 4.13, along with the percent of these error types for the WS group and the normally developing 4-year-olds. Six- and 9-year-old children rarely made any errors, but the few that occurred also fell in these categories.

The first category is object-based axis reversals. These are errors in which the man's head served as reference object, but the person placed the dot along the correct axis, but reversed the direction. Using our definition of axes as primary (forehead/chin) and secondary (nose/back of head), these errors occurred often enough to suggest that there were problems in representing direction along each axis. There were more errors along the secondary axis than the primary axis, consistent with our earlier findings of weakness in the "horizontal axis" of reference objects (in the matching task, see 4.3.1).

The second category is page-based errors, in which people placed the dot in the "same" location on the copy page as it appeared on the model page. That is, they used the page itself as the frame of reference, rather than the man's head. The third category was relatively rare, but reflected page-based axis reversals, in which the page itself served as reference object, but errors reflected reversal of direction along the page's primary (vertical) or secondary (horizontal) axis.

Analysis of these error types showed that all groups tended to make errors along either the primary or the secondary axis of the reference object, with errors along the secondary axis being greater than those along the primary axis. The clearest of these cases were in the 135-degree rotation condition, perhaps because this condition was the most difficult and hence produced the largest numbers of errors. Remarkably, there was qualitative similarity in the distribution of error patterns across all groups, with the exception that the WS participants made many more page-based errors than any other group, in other words, copying the dot into a location that was in the correct location relative to the page, and essentially ignoring the reference object. This solution may have been a response to the difficulty of the task, and to the fact that it is a reasonable solution to the request to copy the dot into the "same place" as in the model. Despite our attempts to emphasize that the man's head should serve as reference object, 4-year-olds and people with WS occasionally used a page-based reference system.

In sum, the error analyses showed that all groups made errors that largely reflected their use of an object-based reference system. Moreover, all groups committed directional errors, confusing direction along the secondary axis more often than the primary. These errors were reversals of direction, but they preserved the axes that organize the reference object. For example, we saw no errors in which a person copied a dot

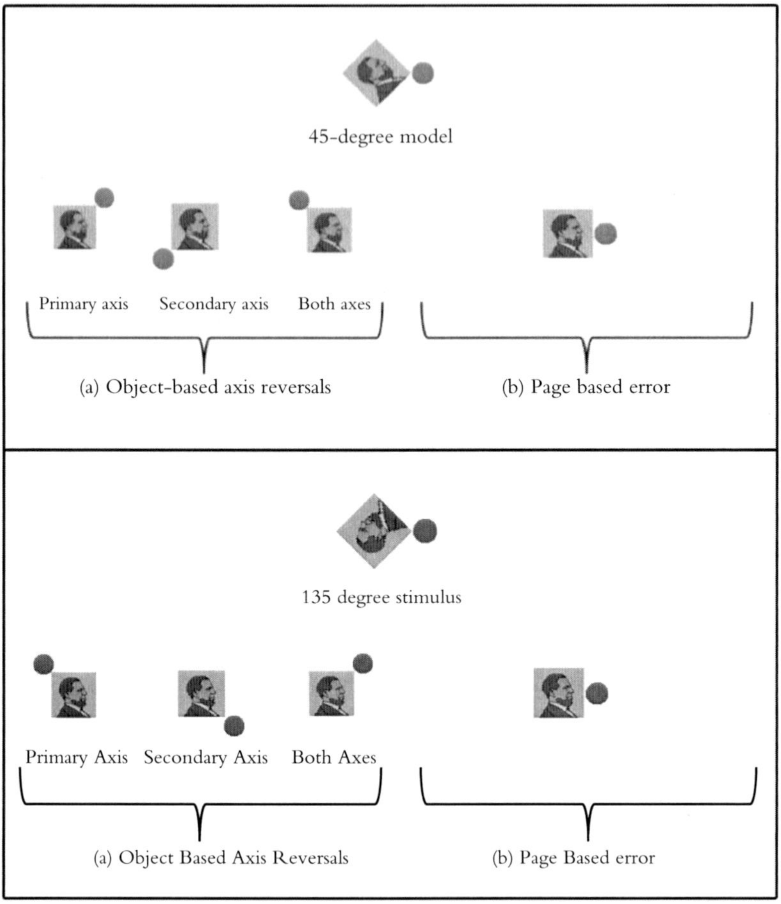

that was at the "bottom" end of the reference object's primary axis into a location that was at the "right" side of the secondary axis. The errors in this copying task are therefore quite similar to errors we have seen before: We also observed errors of direction within axes in the matching task (Section 4.3.1). We will report similar errors of direction within axes in certain spatial language tasks (reported in detail in Chapter 6). Finally, the errors we reported in our block matching task (see Chapter 3) may stem from similar difficulties. Specifically, young children and people with WS have difficulty remembering the "handedness" of objects,

◀ Figure 4.13. Examples of major error types found in the second copying task. Participants sometimes made errors in dot placement that were grossly inaccurate, but nonetheless systematic. These errors fell into two major types. Object-based axis reversals were ones in which the participant appeared to reverse the direction of the dot relative to the reference object along one of its major axes. Page-based errors were ones in which the participant appeared to place the dot in the same location relative to the page, rather than relative to the model reference object. The top panel illustrates sample errors of each type for a model that is presented at a 45-degree orientation. The bottom panel illustrates errors when the model is presented at a 135-degree orientation. Copy reference objects were always presented upright (as shown), and dots are shown in locations that represent the different error types. The total number of gross errors we considered was 208 for the WS group, and 125 for the normally developing 4-year-olds. Of these, in the WS group we observed 71 (34%) errors of Object-based axis reversals, and 113 (54%) Page-based errors. In the 4-year-olds, we observed 69 (55%) Object-based axis reversals, and 44 (35%) Page-based errors. Thus, when the WS group made gross errors, they very often did so by placing the dot in the same place relative to the page; the 4-year-olds more often placed the dot relative to the reference object's axes, but reversed the location along the axis. Still, the same qualitative types of errors occurred in all groups; we suspect that the WS tendency to use page-based solutions was due to their tendency to use the "easier" solution when the reference object was presented at extreme rotations, the most difficult condition.

which might also reflect difficulties in representing and remembering directions within axes.

4.3.3 Summary of Locating Objects: Matching and Copying

The three experiments on the representation of location suggest the following profile for people with WS. First, the data clearly show that people with WS represent locations in terms of reference systems. These reference systems are composed of at least two sets of axes, and directions within those axes. Second, there is evidence that representation of the secondary axis (or horizontal axis, for upright reference objects) is more fragile than that of the primary axis (or vertical, for upright reference objects). Third, there are clearly errors of direction within each axis, and the evidence from both the matching task and the more complex copying task suggests that representation of direction is more fragile along the secondary than the primary axis. Finally, the accuracy and error patterns among people with WS are remarkably similar to normally developing children of around age 4 or 5. This evidence coheres with the findings we presented earlier in this chapter (multiple object tracking, Section 4.2), and provides important constraints on any theory regarding the overall nature of the spatial deficit in people with WS. We now turn to the last case considered in this chapter, acting on objects.

4.4 Acting on Objects

The final component of the block construction task is action: People must pick up a target block and then place it in the "same" location in the copy area. Acting on objects is pervasive in everyday activity: We must pick up our food to eat, tilt a glass at the right angle to drink, and insert a key into a lock to get into our house. The diversity of actions on objects in our lives makes it difficult to isolate any single type of action that is most crucial or central to spatial activities. Still, the variety of actions that we carry out on objects every day places visual-manual action front and center as a capacity whose disruption or delay could play a central role in the WS profile of spatial impairment.

The literature on spatial representation in humans and other primates also gives us good theoretical reason to ask whether visual-manual actions—even of the apparently simplest sort—might be significantly damaged in people with WS. Adult patients with lesions to the parietal and sensorimotor cortex often show difficulty in grasping and manipulating common objects (Culham & Kanwisher, 2001; Grefkes & Fink, 2005; Rizzolatti & Matelli, 2003). Consistent with this, studies of macaques indicate that the parietal areas are engaged during reaching and grasping (Grefkes & Fink, 2005). Informal observations of people with WS suggest that visual-manual action may be impaired; for example, parents often report that children with WS are especially "clumsy." This general picture raises the question of whether people with WS suffer from severe impairment in visually guided action on objects, and if so, how the impairment manifests itself, both in terms of the quantitative pattern relative to normally developing children and the qualitative patterns of impairment.

Our empirical approach to these questions followed closely on the widely cited research program of Milner and Goodale (1995, 2008), who first argued that the primate visual system is divided into two streams of processing that they characterized as the "what" system and the "how" system. This theoretical division builds on a widely accepted view that beyond primary visual cortex (V1), the visual system exhibits a division of labor between the ventral and dorsal streams of the brain, often referred to as the "what" and "where" systems (Ungerleider & Mishkin, 1982). The "what" system moves from visual cortex ventrally into the temporal lobe areas supporting object and face processing. The "where" system moves from visual cortex dorsally into the parietal lobe and beyond, including the motor areas.

In Milner and Goodale's formulation of the two visual streams hypothesis, the two systems are best described by the differences in their functions, rather than the specific types of information they process. The "what" system is responsible for representing the stable and permanent properties of objects, supporting functions such as object recognition and explicit judgments of object properties. In contrast, the "how" system is designed to carry out the function of acting on objects, for example, reaching and grasping an object. Actions such as these occur in the "here and now," requiring computation of properties such as shape, size, orientation, and so forth on the fly—as needed for a present action, after which this information would no longer be required. In this formulation, the two streams carry out different functional types of processing, with the "what" system computing enduring properties of objects, but the "how" system computing properties central to the momentary execution of actions. The hypothesized different functions of the two systems led to the conjecture that whereas the "what" system should be capable of retaining object properties over time (to characterize the enduring object), the "how" system would essentially have "no memory" for object properties—which would only be computed on-line, for the immediate purposes of reaching, grasping, or otherwise manipulating an object. The latter conclusion has recently been challenged, with evidence suggesting that the parietal areas are engaged during delayed reaching, both among patients with lesions in this area and among normal adults (Himmelbach et al., 2009).

One of the most celebrated cases used to document and explore the functional distinction between the two systems was provided by evidence from Milner and Goodale's (1995) studies of patient D.F., who suffered from carbon monoxide poisoning. Observations suggested that D.F. was severely impaired in recognizing objects, but nevertheless carried out visual-manual actions on objects with little difficulty.

One critical test was a comparison of D.F.'s ability to insert an envelope into an oriented slot (as if "posting" mail) compared to her ability to match a line with the same orientation to its match. D.F. was highly accurate in posting the envelope to the oriented slot, but failed in the matching task. Milner and Goodale inferred from this striking difference in behavior that the system underlying D.F.'s visual-manual action on objects was preserved, but the system underlying her perception of oriented lines for the purposes of explicit judgments (matching) was impaired. The apparent dissociation between action and perception suggested to Milner and Goodale that the two systems are functionally separate. Additional evidence supporting the functional dissociation between the two systems comes from studies of patients with optic ataxia, who show severely impaired visual-manual action but preserved perceptual judgments (Haaxma & Kuypers, 1975; Perenin & Vighetto, 1988), and studies of normal adults under conditions of visual illusions (Bridgeman et al., 1997; but also see Franz, Hesse, & Kollath, 2009).

Given the apparent distinction between vision for perception and vision for action shown by both normal adults and neurologically impaired patients such as D.F., we asked whether the hypothetical distinction in the two functions might shed light on the WS spatial impairment. Do people with WS exhibit severe deficits in some aspects of visual-manual action, and does this differ in any way from performance on parallel tasks engaging perceptual judgments? If deficits exist in either or both task types, how do they map onto the normal developmental profile? Do they look the same, quantitatively and/or qualitatively, as normally developing children at some age? Or are the profiles of WS participants wholly different?

To address this question, we carried out a series of experiments drawing on the now-classic task used by Milner and Goodale with patient D.F. We adapted the task of "posting" versus perceiving (matching) a card to children and adults with WS (*M* ages = 12, 23;9, respectively), as well as normally developing children between the ages of 3 and 6 (Dilks, Hoffman, & Landau, 2008; see also Atkinson et al., 1997, for a similar task with WS individuals ranging from 4 to 14). The normally developing children fell into two main groups: those who were mental age matches to the WS participants (*M* age = 6;3), and those who were younger than these mental age matches (*M* age = 3;8). Under the hypothesis that functions of the dorsal stream are damaged in WS, one might expect to find severe impairment on a task requiring visually guided action, and markedly better performance on an analogous task requiring a perceptual judgment, but no directed action. As usual, the critical comparisons involve patterns of performance across the two tasks relative to normally developing children of different ages. Is the profile for people with WS the same or different across the two tasks, relative to groups of normally developing children at different ages?

Figure 4.14 illustrates a child carrying out both the action and the perceptual matching task. In the action task (right panel), we asked people to pick up a "dollar bill" and insert it into a "piggy bank" whose slot could be set at any of four different angles of orientation, including 0 degrees (vertical), 45, 90, and 135 degrees. In the perceptual matching task (left panel), we asked people to judge whether a mannequin hand holding the dollar bill was "ready to put the dollar into the slot," using the same test angles of orientation.

Overall performance is shown in Figure 4.15 as mean degrees of angular error from the target orientation for children with WS and their mental age matches (*M* age = 6;3, left panel), as well as normally developing 3- to 4-year-olds and adults with WS (right panel). The slot itself spanned 10 degrees, so any error within this range would have been a "fit" to the slot.

First consider the results of the perceptual matching task (gray bars in the figures). Both children with WS and their mental age matches could match the orientation of the dollar bill (held by the mannequin hand) quite accurately to the slot: The responses of children in both groups were within the 10-degree span that the slot occupied. That is, when the children said "Stop!" the orientation of the dollar bill was such that it would have fit through the slot. Although the children with WS showed overall larger degrees of error compared to the mental age

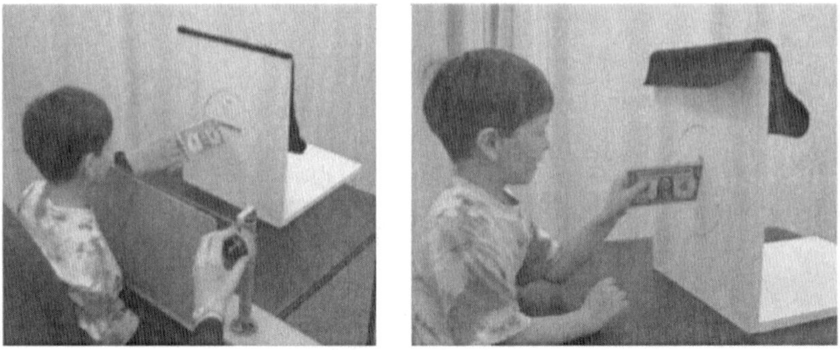

Figure 4.14. Vision-for-perception (left) and vision-for-action (right) tasks, shown with child as participant. In the perception task, people were shown a mannequin hand holding a rigid dollar bill. The experimenter rotated the hand until the subject indicated that the hand and dollar bill were ready to fit through the slot ("into the bank"). In the action task, people were asked to "put the dollar bill into the bank." They picked up the rigid dollar bill, which was lying flat on the table in front of them, and quickly inserted it into the slot. For both tasks, measurements were made of the angular deviation from the target orientation. The slot occupied one of four different orientations across trials, including 0 degrees (upright), 45 degrees, 90 degrees, and 135 degrees. The left panel shows the slot at 90 degrees orientation; the right panel shows the slot at 0 degrees orientation. Reprinted from Dilks, Hoffman, and Landau (2008), with permission of John Wiley and Sons.

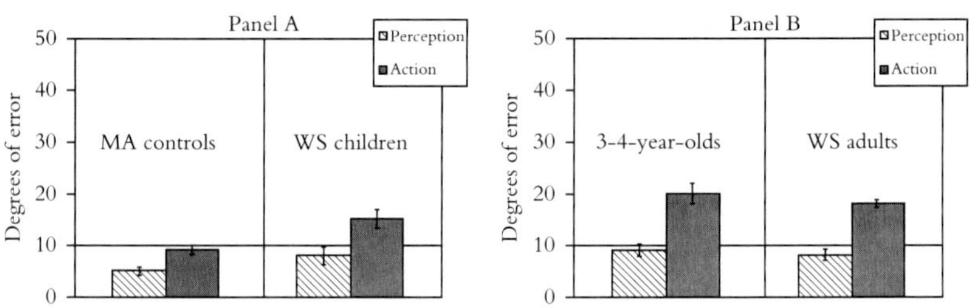

Figure 4.15. Mean degrees of angular error from the target orientation of the slot for perception task (striped bars) and action task (solid bars). We first tested children with WS and normally developing children (*M* age = 6;3) who were matched on mental age to the WS participants (left panel). We then followed up with normally developing 3–4-year-olds (*M* age = 3;8) and adults with WS (right panel). Children and adults with WS performed like normally developing 3–4-year-olds. Normal 6-year-old children matched to the WS children on mental age performed no differently from the WS children in the perception task, but performed better than them in the action task. All groups achieved higher accuracy (less error) in the perception task compared to the action task. Reprinted from Dilks, Hoffman, and Landau (2008), with permission of John Wiley and Sons.

matches, this difference did not reach significance (see Dilks et al., 2008, for details). These results fit well with the results of Atkinson et al. (1997), who used a similar method and found that children in the same age range made errors of less than 10 degrees.

Looking at the right hand panel of Figure 4.15, we can see the performance of 3–4-year-old normally developing children and adults with WS. Their performance on the perceptual matching task, too, was quite accurate, with mean degrees of error also falling within the critical 10-degree window. Again, these results are similar to those of Atkinson et al.'s (1997) results showing that normally developing children around 4 years of age showed angular errors well below 10 degrees. Statistical tests of our data showed no difference between the children with WS, the adults with WS, and the 3–4-year-old normally developing children. The normal 3–4-year-olds were less accurate, overall, than their 6-year-old peers (the mental-age-matched group), but the degree of improvement was small—both groups' means were within the 10-degree span for the slot. Children and adults with WS were less accurate than normally developing 6-year-olds, but this difference did not reach statistical significance.

We also examined the qualitative performance of individuals in each group by plotting their individual angular deviations for each orientation. These are shown in Figure 4.16. The distribution of responses across groups confirm that the perceptual judgments of when the dollar bill was "ready to put in the bank" were quite accurate, and well tuned to the four different orientations of the slot. As in the data showing mean degrees of angular error, the individual plots show that the normally developing 6-year-olds were more accurate than the other groups, with no responses falling outside the slot's borders; other groups were also very accurate, with the exception of a few stray outliers, most common among the 4-year-olds and the two groups of people with WS. It is clear that all groups were quite accurate in the perceptual matching task.

The results for the action task were quite different. As is evident from Figure 4.15 only the normally developing 6-year-olds (mental age matches, left panel) systematically inserted the dollar bill into the slot without going outside of the 10-degree boundary of its walls. The other groups were much more errorful in their action, with mean errors falling in the 15- to 20-degree range. Although some participants in each group managed to get the card into the slot on the first try, most hit the

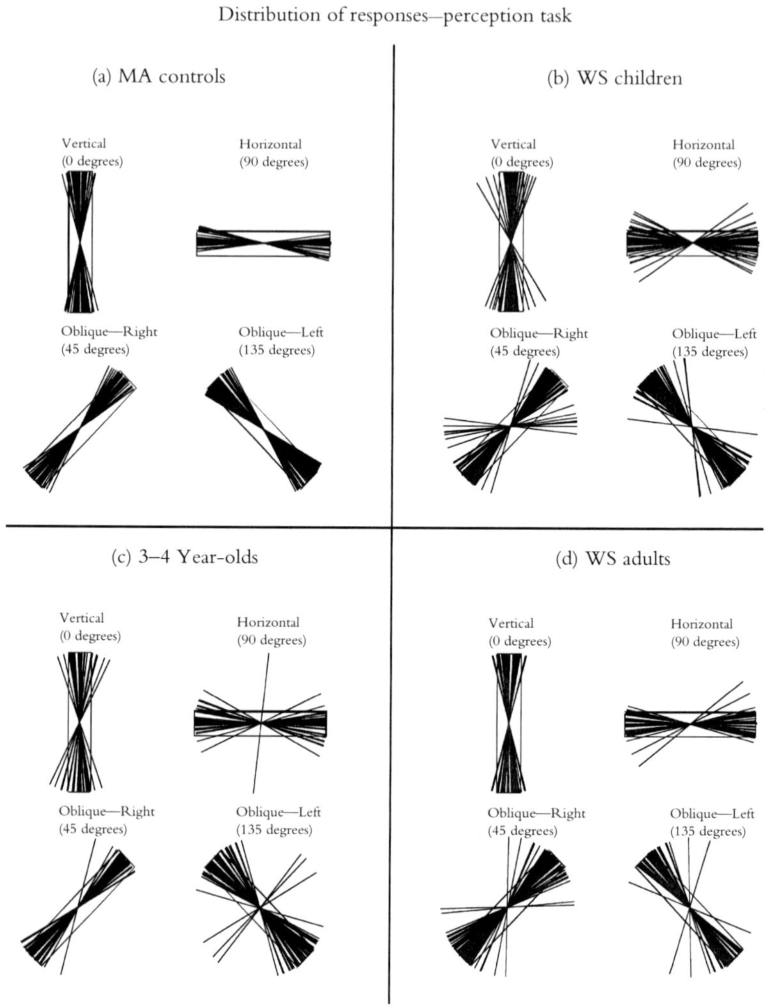

Figure 4.16. Distribution of responses in the perceptual matching task for the four groups tested: Normally developing children (*M* age = 6;3) matched to the WS participants on mental age (MA), normally developing 3- to 4-year-olds (*M* age = 3;8), WS children and WS adults. Each line represents an individual response. The spread of responses shows that the low error on this task was also accompanied by a small amount of spread around the target slot (shown as a rectangle) at each orientation. Reprinted from Dilks, Hoffman, and Landau (2008), with permission of John Wiley and Sons.

bordering surface on their way in, requiring adjustment once they had hit this wall. They did manage to insert the dollar bill, but their trajectory did not result in smoothly fitting the bill into the slot. Statistical tests showed that there were no reliable differences among the children with WS, the adults with WS, and the normally developing 3- to 4-year-old children. All three groups performed reliably worse than normally developing children whose mean age was 6, in other words, the group of mental age matches. A similar overall pattern also emerged in Atkinson et al.'s (1997) study: Children with WS between the ages of 10 and 15 made errors ranging from around 5 to 20 degrees, and younger children made larger errors. Normally developing children between ages 5 and 10 made errors of 10 degrees or less.

The distribution of responses for the action task is shown in Figure 4.17, with each panel showing the responses of a single group. The qualitative profiles are clearly very similar to each other: All groups were affected by the orientation of the slot, with most accurate performance when the slot was vertically oriented, followed by the horizontal and the obliques. However, for each orientation, the tuning was systematic, with symmetrical distributions around the slot's actual orientation. Indeed, analyses of the distribution of responses indicated that the range of actions carried out by people was quite systematic, and well-tuned to the slot's orientation.

What is also clear is that there were large quantitative differences across the groups. Looking at the two groups of normally developing children, the distribution of responses for 3–4-year-olds is much more broadly tuned than for older children (the mental age matches, average age 6). This suggests considerable change in this action task between the ages of 4 and 6 in normally developing children. More remarkable, the children and adults with WS both show a profile very similar to that of the normally developing 3–4-year-olds, and worse than normally developing mental age matches, suggesting developmental arrest at the functional level of a 3- or 4-year-old in people with Williams syndrome.

This is a strong conclusion. However, it is supported by several facts. First, the children and adults with WS performed no differently from normally developing 3–4-year-olds in the action task; that is, there was no developmental improvement between childhood and adulthood in

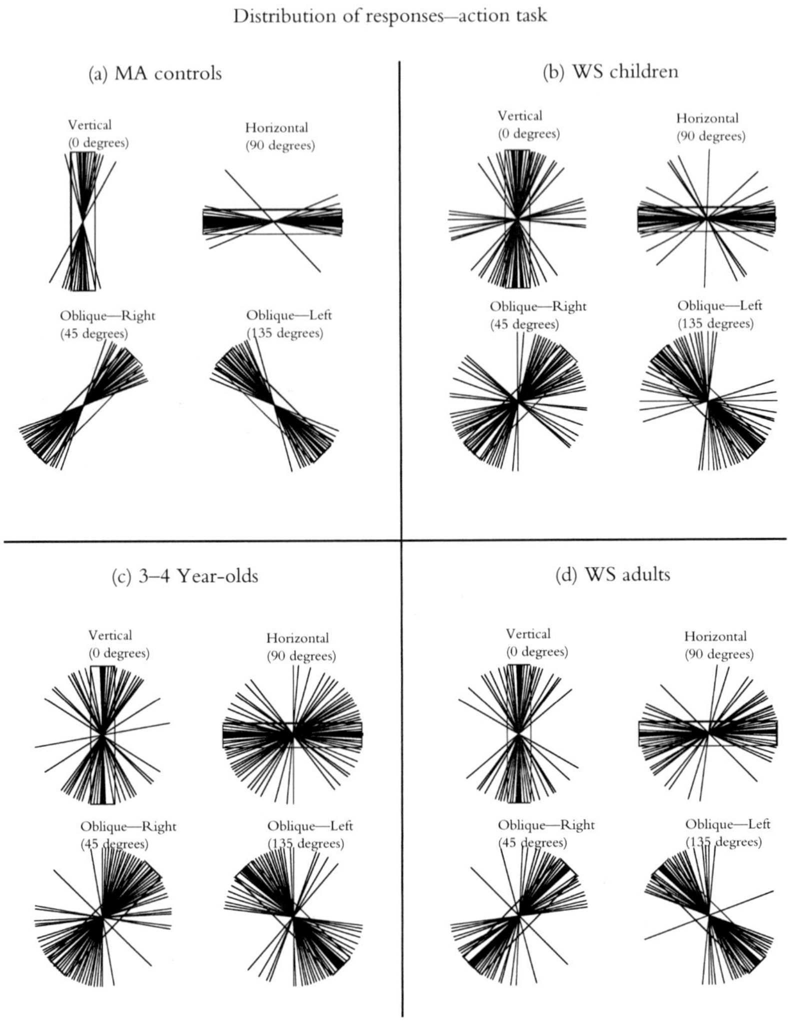

Figure 4.17. Distribution of responses in the action task for the four groups tested. Each line represents an individual response. The spread of responses shows that the errors among mental age matched controls (a) were accompanied by a small amount of spread around the target slot (shown as a rectangle) at each orientation. For the other three groups, the larger degrees of error were also accompanied by regular spread around the target slot, but the spread was much greater. Reprinted from Dilks, Hoffman, & Landau, 2008, with permission of John Wiley and Sons.

our WS participants. Second, analyses of the qualitative pattern of performance across groups show that children and adults with WS had error patterns that were highly similar to those of normally developing 4-year-olds. People with WS—and normally developing 3–4-year-olds—were also qualitatively similar to normal 6-year-olds, factoring out overall accuracy. For example, all participant groups were very accurate on trials showing vertical and horizontal target orientations, and much less accurate on trials showing oblique orientations. All groups showed error patterns of nonrandom spread around the target orientations, with the magnitude of spread larger for WS people and normal 4-year-olds relative to the normal 6-year-olds. The similarity in the qualitative nature of the spread suggests a common, underlying representation of orientation across the different groups, with differences occurring in the magnitude of the spread around the target orientation.

We should note that the particular task we used involved orientation. Other visual-manual tasks might be expected to show the same age equivalence for people with WS—that is, performance like a 4-year-old normally developing child. But the absolute level of performance might vary depending on relative difficulty. We would expect, for example, that action tasks that show highly accurate performance among young normally developing children might also show highly accurate performance among people with WS. Gregory and Landau (unpublished data) have observed this pattern in an object grasping task. In this task, people are asked to reach and grasp a wooden block varying in length, and peak grip aperture over the reaching trajectory is measured. Normally developing 4-year-olds show good tuning to the object's size in their peak grip aperture; and their performance is quite similar to normal adults (Gregory, Trzcinski, Hoffman, & Landau, 2009). Children and adults with WS also show highly accurate tuning to object size as well. This is consistent with the idea that the general level of performance among people with WS is likely to depend on when the particular spatial function emerges in the course of normal development. Visual-manual actions that become well tuned early in normal development should elicit highly accurate performance in WS, whereas actions that normally undergo a lengthy developmental trajectory should elicit relatively poor performance in people with WS. We will return to this idea in the final chapter of our book.

More generally, it is likely that not all visual-manual action tasks are equally affected in WS. Still, the important finding from the perception and posting studies is that the WS pattern is similar to the quantitative and qualitative profile of a normally developing 4-year-old child. There appears to be little or no development beyond this level for people with WS, at least as tested by our present methods.

4.5 Summary of Marking, Locating, and Acting on Objects

We organized this chapter as an inquiry into the quantitative and qualitative performance of people with WS on a broad range of tasks that are known to engage the parietal lobes and, more generally, the dorsal stream of the human brain. Evidence from other labs has already suggested that the WS spatial deficit may be best characterized as a "dorsal stream" deficit, with clear structural and functional abnormalities in the parietal regions. Cognitive performance on the range of tasks we used suggests, however, a picture of both strengths and limitations. The strengths are revealed by the fact that, in all the functions we have considered, there is a remarkable amount of preserved cognitive structure. For example:

- WS performance in the multiple object tracking task reveals the capacity to track more than one object at a time, and that errors tend to occur when the targets move by spatially neighboring items. These error patterns also appear for normally developing children.
- When we ask people with WS to match or copy the locations of simple dots, we find that the foundational cognitive structure underlying much of our spatial behavior—the reference system—is clearly a part of their representation of space.
- When we ask people with WS to carry out simple functional visual-manual actions—such as posting a rigid dollar bill into a slot—we find considerable normal structure in their oriented actions.

At the same time, the evidence shows marked limits in the levels at which people with WS carry out these tasks. Importantly:

- Comparisons with normally developing children between the ages of 4 and 9 show that the closest equivalence for people with WS places them roughly at the level of a normally developing 4- to 5-year-old for many spatial functions. Crucially, these normal young children *also* show the same remarkable cognitive structure when they carry out tasks requiring them to track, match, copy, or act. But there are limits on accuracy, and whereas the normally developing child shows considerable growth between the ages of 4 and 6 or 9, the group of people with WS—for *these tasks*—appears to remain at the level of the 4- or 5-year-old.

These facts—in conjunction with the evidence we discussed in Chapter 3, suggest that many aspects of the WS pattern of spatial representation may be better described as an overall developmental arrest than a specific impairment of the dorsal stream. Before considering how best to explain the data so far, however, we turn to two final areas of inquiry—navigation (Chapter 5) and spatial language (Chapter 6), both of which will put us in a better position to account for the WS spatial profile.

5

Finding Our Way

In the last chapter, we examined a range of spatial functions that are thought to engage the parietal areas and, more generally, the dorsal stream in normal adults. We observed that children and adults with Williams syndrome have a profile suggesting developmental arrest at the functional level of a normally developing 4- or 5-year-old child. This profile generally matches the findings for performance among people with WS on the benchmark block construction task, and suggests that many of the individual cognitive functions required for good pattern copying are severely impaired in WS. Although the block construction task itself does not reflect a single unified cognitive function, the patterns of performance across a wide range of quite different spatial tasks suggest that many spatial functions carried out by the parietal areas and, more generally, the dorsal stream, are severely impaired. At the same time, the qualitative patterns of performance in people with WS are strikingly similar to those of normally developing children who are much younger. This suggests the possibility that some aspects of spatial representation in people with WS undergo slow development followed by developmental arrest at some point. The result is a mature profile among WS people—for certain aspects of spatial representation—that is quite similar to that of a child at an early point in normal development.

In this chapter, we take up a different class of spatial functions: those that allow us to find our way through large-scale space, in other words, the spaces that we move through as we get around our home, office, or town. The study of human spatial navigation has a special status within the larger set of spatial capacities, as it is a system that is in many ways continuous with that of other species. At the core of our ability to find our way through space is the notion of a "cognitive map"—a unified representation of the spatial arrangement of objects and places in the surrounding area.

When we have a cognitive map of an area, we know the spatial relationships among different places. In this way, the cognitive map bears some similarity to real maps. For example, let's consider a real map of Keyser Quad at the Johns Hopkins Homewood campus. It includes representations of several main buildings (see Figure 5.1, left panel)—the Eisenhower Library, Krieger Hall (home of the Department of Cognitive Science), Ames Hall (home of the Department of Psychological and Brain Sciences), Gilman Hall (home of the Department of Philosophy), and Mergenthaler Hall (home of the dean's offices). Note that the real map accurately represents angles and distances between and among buildings, walkways, and various landmarks.

Our cognitive map of the same area differs from a real map. It may also represent some of the same buildings and will also likely embody the spatial relationships among the key buildings, often including relatively accurate angles and distances. But our cognitive map is not likely to be

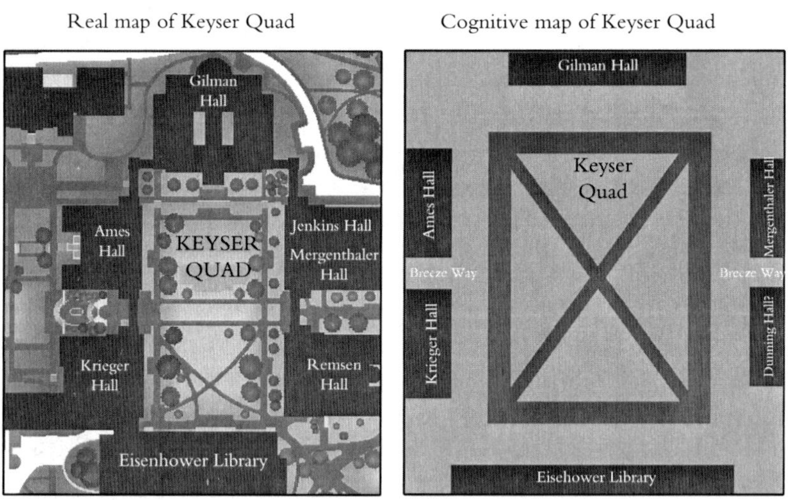

Figure 5.1. Two different representations of the Keyser Quad at Johns Hopkins University. The left panel shows a real map of the quad. The right panel shows a schematic of BL's drawing of the quad, reflecting her cognitive map of this space. Note the errors in the spatial arrangement of walkways in BL's map. These errors show that our cognitive maps represent some, but not all, of the key features of the physical spaces in which we move.

as accurate as a real map—for example, it is unlikely that our cognitive map includes the exact and complete set of walkways through the quad or the exact angles and distances among buildings. In fact, one of us (BL) drew a map of the Keyser Quad from memory; this is also shown in Figure 5.1 (right panel). This map includes several key buildings and their rough relationships, but little else. In addition, it misrepresents the walkways within the Keyser Quad as having two diagonal walkways crossing from side to side, rather than the actual set of walkways shown in the real map. This is despite having traversed the Keyser Quad almost every day for 10 years!

Despite the relatively coarse and sometimes errorful nature of the cognitive map, it crucially captures relationships among key places, allowing a person to mentally compute the relationship between individual buildings. For example, if someone phoned BL and told her that they were outside, facing the front door of Gilman Hall, she would be able to tell that person where the other buildings are, relative to his current position. In short, our cognitive map of an area is our mental representation of key places and their spatial relationships to each other, allowing us to answer the question "Where is X relative to Y?"

Our cognitive map also allows us to answer the question "Where am I relative to X or Y?" That is, we can place our own body in the cognitive map. This reflects our knowledge of where we are at present, and also allows us to track where we are in the layout as we move through it. Representing our changing position in the spatial layout is crucial in order to know where we are, relative to other objects and places at any given time.

Thus, two crucial problems for the human navigator are establishing knowledge of the relationships among places in the layout (the cognitive map) and knowing the current relationship of one's own body to various places in this map. These aspects of spatial knowledge are important for navigation when we are oriented in space, and also when we get lost and must regain our orientation.

Our scientific understanding of cognitive maps, and, more generally, their role in human navigation, has been considerably strengthened over the past several decades by behavioral and neurophysiological studies of other species. The findings, as well as those from related studies on human infants, children, and adults, show that our capacity to find our way is remarkably complex, relying on a variety of potentially dissociable mechanisms that allow us to construct cognitive maps, keep track of our own position in space (and on the map), and regain orientation when we get lost. These mechanisms may also engage different, but interconnected, areas of the human brain. Primary among these are the parietal regions of the brain and the structures in the medial temporal lobe, including the hippocampal formation and areas that are functionally connected to it, especially the parahippocampal gyrus. These regions form a network that is sensitive to different kinds of information, carrying out different kinds of computations that allow us to locate ourselves and other objects as we move through space.

There are good reasons to suspect that at least some aspects of spatial navigation are impaired in children and adults with WS: Parents report that way-finding is problematic for many children with WS (Atkinson, Anker, Braddick, Nokes, Mason, & Braddick, 2002). In fact, one might predict that people with WS should show quite widespread impairment in navigation tasks. This is because human navigation is supported by mechanisms that typically engage the parietal and hippocampal structures of the brain, and brain imaging studies of people with WS have shown structural abnormalities in both of these areas (Meyer-Lindenberg et al., 2004, 2005; see Chapter 2 for review). At the same time, the fact that multiple mechanisms are involved in human navigation raises a different possibility—that there is uneven impairment in navigation, with a profile of peaks and valleys akin to what we have observed across the range of (non-navigation) spatial functions that we have reviewed in previous chapters.

In the next sections, we first review findings from the broad navigation literature that point to several mechanisms that are candidates for any deficit in navigation among children and adults with WS. We then report several sets of studies designed to examine the navigation capabilities of people with WS. In contrast to the broader literature on spatial navigation, the literature on navigation in people with Williams syndrome is quite small, spanning only a handful of studies. Still, these studies provide a striking picture of the navigation profile in people with WS.

To foreshadow this profile, the studies that we will review suggest a possible contrast between successful navigation in tasks where people *remain oriented* in space, and significant compromise in tasks where people are disoriented and must *reorient* themselves. Mechanisms that are deployed when we remain oriented in space depend on information from our own self-movement and our representations of the locations of landmarks in a reference system centered on the surrounding space. For example, if we watch as an object is hidden in an unmarked location (A) that forms a triangular array with B and C, and we represent this location relative to B and C, we should be able to move to any new location in space, update our own location relative to B and C, and still accurately retrieve the object. Mechanisms that allow us to represent landmarks in a variety of reference systems and mechanisms that allow us to update our own location over movement both appear to be present in children and adults with Williams syndrome. However, the proficiency with which they can rely on these mechanisms to locate objects is roughly equal to that of a normally developing 4- or 5-year-old child—a pattern that is reminiscent of other spatial functions we have discussed in previous chapters.

The picture is quite different for the case of becoming disoriented and reorienting oneself in space. Disorientation can occur for a variety of reasons. Many of us have experienced disorientation when we have emerged from a subway station, facing what we assume is north, only to discover that we are completed "turned around" (mentally), and in fact are facing south. The mechanisms that we use to reorient ourselves after becoming disoriented depend on our ability to represent both "geometric" aspects of the overall spatial layout (to be discussed in detail later) and specific landmarks within that layout. Here we report initial findings indicating a striking profile in people with Williams syndrome. Evidence suggests that people with WS can use specific landmarks to reorient, but this ability may be fragile. In contrast, in at least some testing conditions, they show quite limited ability to reorient themselves using representations of the *geometry of layouts*. The contrast between navigation when one remains oriented, and navigation when one becomes disoriented and must reorient oneself, raises intriguing questions about why and how these two different aspects of navigation might be differentially compromised in people with WS.

In the next section, we discuss the different components of navigation that will be important in exploring the WS profile. These include the representation of locations in terms of egocentric (body-based) and allocentric (world-based) reference systems and the importance of representing geometric properties of layouts for navigating, both when people remain oriented and when they are disoriented. We then turn to a consideration of the evidence on WS navigation for these different aspects of navigation.

5.1 The Components of Navigation: Division of Labor

Perhaps the most basic question for understanding how we navigate through space is how we define a *place*, since places and the spatial relationships among them are the basic building blocks of the cognitive map. Cognitive maps are not, of course, physical objects; they are the mental representations that we build as we move through an area, noting and storing for later use where things are relative to each other. Like real maps, the cognitive map includes key places arranged in space; the spatial relationships between and among places can be captured using various geometric properties. For example, we might represent one building as "near" another; this kind of relationship is captured within topological geometry, which ignores properties such as exact angle or distance, or even the notion of "straight line." Or, we might represent one building as "in line with" another; this kind of relationship is captured within projective geometry, which ignores angles and distances but preserves relationships along straight lines. But navigation in the world often requires that we represent the angles and distances between places: In order to move from one place to another that is not immediately seen, for example, we need to know what angle (direction) to head out. So it is likely that when we use cognitive maps to guide our navigation, these include representations of the angles and distances between places, properties of metric geometries.

The places that we represent and the angle and distance relationships among them must be united by a common reference system, sometimes called an *allocentric*—or world-based—system (see Figure 5.2a). This kind of system is usually contrasted with *egocentric* reference systems, which are centered on our body (and discussed next). Places that we represent in our cognitive maps may be occupied by special objects, such as salient

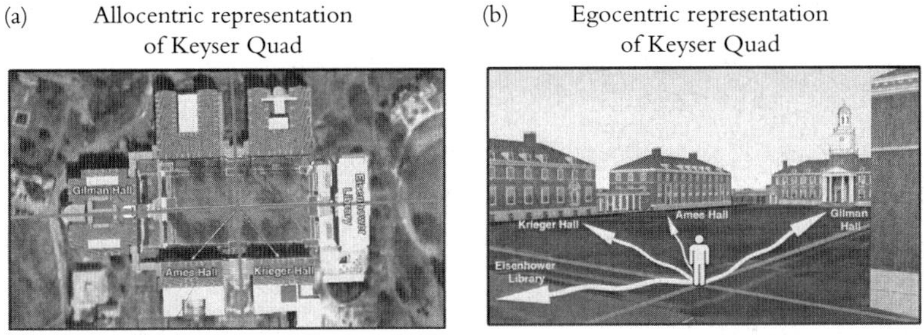

Figure 5.2. Representation of the same layout using two different reference systems. The left panel shows an allocentric (and aerial) view of Keyser Quad, in which all buildings can be represented relative to a reference system whose center is at the center of the quad. From this kind of representation, one can compute the spatial relationship of each building relative to the others; these relationships remain stable as the observer moves through space. The right panel shows an egocentric representation of the Keyser Quad, in which all buildings are represented relative to the observer's own body. This kind of representation is limited in that the direction and distance of each building relative to the observer will change as he or she moves through space. In addition, the spatial relationship of each building to every other building cannot be computed directly from the separate relationships between the observer and each building.

landmarks. But they may also be defined by general areas, such as boundaries (a garden wall, street, or hallway) or regions of space (a room, field, or parking lot). Together, our representations of the objects and the surfaces on which they rest constitute representations of the overall spatial layout of the environment. This layout is constructed as we move through space, picking up and storing information about the elements and their spatial relationships in the common, allocentric reference system.

As we already mentioned, using the cognitive map requires that we place ourselves in it, in other words, that we represent the location of our body with its own "egocentric" reference system (Figure 5.2b). The egocentric frame of reference establishes the location of objects in space relative to our body. Such a representation is crucial for action: In order to reach and grasp an object or move toward it, we need to be able to represent its location relative to our body and its effectors. Once we have placed ourselves on the map, we should be able to represent the location of places in space relative to our body—in front of us, behind us, slightly to the right and in front of us, and so forth.

Both kinds of representation can be used to direct our movement. For example, from an egocentric representation, we may know that we are facing some known building and can reach it by moving straight ahead. From an allocentric representation, we may know the relationship between two buildings. Knowing the relationship between the two buildings and our own location in the layout, we can then act, moving to the destination. We still know little about how allocentric and egocentric representations of the same place are coordinated (but see Colby & Goldberg, 1999, for coordination of retina- versus head-based systems; Soechting & Flanders, 1992, for sensorimotor transformations required for pointing).

Finally, using the cognitive map requires that we keep track of our own changing location as we move through the layout. This is necessary because as we move through space, the locations of any element in the layout will change relative to our body's position: What starts out on our right may end up on our left, and what starts out in front of us will be behind us as we move forward in space. Updating our own position in space, relative to the surrounding layout, is crucial if we are to be able to locate things and re-identify the same place after we have moved.

Thus the construction and use of a cognitive map requires at least three types of representational mechanism. It requires representations of location on the map in terms of two different frames of reference: egocentric, or "body-based," frames; and allocentric, or "world-based," frames. It also requires some mechanism that allows us to update our own location as we move through space. The latter can be accomplished by a mechanism known as path integration, or "dead reckoning," which allows us to keep track of our changed position without using any external landmarks or cues from the environment, by a process of integrating angular velocity over time (Gallistel, 1990). Dead reckoning has been shown in many species, ranging from ants to human toddlers and adults (Klatzky et al., 1998; Landau, Spelke, & Gleitman, 1984; Muller & Wehner, 1988; Newcombe, Huttenlocher, Drummey, & Wiley, 1998).

Although we might have to depend on this mechanism alone if the environment is unfamiliar and/or has few or no landmarks, dead reckoning alone has somewhat limited utility because it is subject to rapidly accumulating error as the length of the trip increases. Fortunately, in humans, dead reckoning is usually supplemented by using a cognitive map. For example, suppose we travel for some distance and direction, and then make an estimate of our current position. This estimate might not be perfect—we might have traveled farther than our estimate would suggest. By using landmarks and/or properties of the surrounding layout, we can correct our estimate and place ourselves accurately on our internal representation (cognitive map) of the environment. Thus using our cognitive map and the contents of it—including local landmarks and parts of the surrounding layout—is essential as a supplement to dead reckoning in navigation.

5.1.1 Egocentric and Allocentric Reference Systems

It is generally accepted that humans and other animals make use of these two different reference systems during navigation, and that there are mechanisms dedicated to translating between these or integrating representations of the same location over different reference systems (see, e.g., Burgess, 2008; Newcombe & Huttenlocher, 2000; Wang & Spelke, 2002).

Both kinds of reference systems appear to be functional at an early point in human development. Evidence shows that infants sometimes use an egocentric frame of reference to locate objects after they themselves have moved (Acredolo, 1978; Newcombe & Huttenlocher, 2000). But by 9 months of age, infants can also use non-egocentric frames of reference to locate objects after they themselves have been moved along paths of either rotation or translation in space (Landau & Spelke, 1988). Of particular importance is whether infants and toddlers can use external aspects of the surrounding environment, such as landmarks, to locate objects. Acredolo and Evans (1980) found that 11-month-olds who underwent movement in space relied on external landmarks to relocate an object they had seen from their original position. Newcombe and Huttenlocher (2000) reviewed several studies showing that from around 2 years of age, toddlers can use landmarks that are situated at some distance from a hidden object to locate it. For example, Newcombe et al. (1998) showed 2-year-olds a toy that was being hidden in a 5-foot sandbox. The toddlers were then walked around to the other side of the sandbox and allowed to search for the buried toy. In one condition, the toddlers could see the entire room, which held furniture—potential landmarks. In this case, toddlers were significantly more accurate than in a separate condition where the sandbox was surrounded by a curtain, concealing any external landmarks.

The evidence thus shows that by the age of about 2 years, children can make use of their own self-motion plus external landmarks to determine the location of the hidden object. The landmarks in Newcombe et al.'s (1998) studies were not solely "beacons," in other words, objects that are simple associative cues to the location of a hidden object because they are coincident with it. The use of landmarks that are not beacons suggests that toddlers can construct and use representations of the spatial relationship between the various key places in the room (including, e.g., pieces of furniture) and the hidden target object, independent of their own body's location in space. That is, they can construct and use allocentric representations of space that include specific "places." Place learning is known to engage the hippocampus in rats and other animals (e.g., O'Keefe & Nadel, 1978; see Burgess, 2008, for review), and Newcombe and Huttenlocher (2000) speculate that the use of external landmarks around age 2 in humans could be tied to maturation of the hippocampus. In addition to using external landmarks by the age of 2 years, even 18-month-old infants can use the geometric layout of surfaces in the environment to reorient themselves (Hermer & Spelke, 1996), a topic to which we return in detail in Section 5.1.3.

As a whole, the evidence suggests that infants and toddlers are not solely dependent on egocentric frames of reference, counter to the initial hypotheses of researchers who followed Piaget's theory (Acredolo, 1978; Piaget, 1954; see Newcombe & Huttenlocher, 2000, for review). Moreover, toddlers can use landmarks and the geometric properties of layouts to infer the locations of objects. Toddlers can also update their current location after moving through space using "dead reckoning" (Gallistel, 1990; Landau, Spelke, & Gleitman, 1984; Newcombe et al., 1998). Thus, by the age of 2, normally developing children are well poised to move through space purposefully, representing the locations of objects in their environment relative to each other and themselves, and updating their own location in space. These mechanisms allow toddlers to successfully locate objects (even if the objects are hidden) after they have moved through space. They clearly represent places in space, including the location of their own body.

Considerable effort has been invested in discovering the brain bases for egocentric and allocentric reference systems, and the mechanisms that allow the integration of information across these different systems. Several proposals suggest that in humans, egocentric representations of location engage the posterior parietal areas of the brain, while allocentric representations engage the hippocampus and related medial temporal areas, such as the parahippocampus (Aguirre & D'Esposito, 1999; Burgess, 2008; Epstein, 2008). Connections between the posterior parietal cortex (thought to be engaged when people use egocentric representations of space) and medial temporal areas (for allocentric representations) are thought to form a network that supports the integration of egocentric and allocentric representations, allowing us to locate objects in a stable space relative to each other, both before and after our own movement (Aguirre & D'Esposito, 1999). The general idea is that there is a division of labor in the navigation system, such that the parietal areas may be responsible for encoding locations relative to the body, whereas the hippocampus, parahippocampus, and related areas may be responsible for encoding the locations of the environment itself, in other words, the objects and places that form a layout. Connections among the different areas would effect the integration between the body-centered representations of location in the parietal area and the allocentric representations in the medial temporal lobe.

If different brain areas are involved in different aspects of navigation, one would expect different profiles of cognitive impairment to follow from damage to different areas. Evidence from human patients is consistent with the idea of selective damage, shown by specific variants of a more general "topographical disorientation." Aguirre and D'Esposito (1999) note that people who sustain damage to the posterior parietal areas of the brain tend to show egocentric disorientation, having difficulty in representing the location and orientation of objects relative to their body. In contrast, patients with damage to the lingual gyrus tend to have deficits that appear confined to landmark recognition (termed "landmark agnosia"); these people cannot remember the appearance of major salient landmarks, nor can they use them for orientation in space. Damage to the retrosplenial cortex often results in difficulty using landmarks to generate headings or orientation in space, although people with such damage do not have difficulty recognizing the landmarks. Damage to the parahippocampal cortex results in the inability to identify topographical entities, such as buildings or intersections, and difficulty learning new spatial/topographical layouts (see Epstein, 2008).

Finally, we should note that the special status of the hippocampus as the site for allocentric representations of "place" has been the subject of decades of research, originating with the proposal by O'Keefe and Nadel (1978) that the hippocampus is the neural seat of the cognitive map. In their now-classic work, O'Keefe and Nadel showed that the hippocampus of the rat contains neurons that respond vigorously when the rat occupies a particular place in its environment, irrespective of its "heading" (orientation) in that place. This suggested to O'Keefe and Nadel the existence of "place cells." Remarkably, recent research has examined the early development of place cells in the rat, as well as "head-direction" cells (which fire when the rat occupies a particular heading direction) and "grid" cells (which fire across a range of places organized as a regional grid). Wills, Cacucci, Burgess, and O'Keefe (2010) found that head direction and place cells exist in the rat in close to mature form within 2 weeks after birth; grid cells appeared slightly later and developed rapidly thereafter. The existence of each cell type—thought to be crucial in the acquisition of cognitive maps through exploration as the rat pup moves about the environment—show that at birth, the rat possesses distinct neural components of the representation of space.

The literature on spatial representation in species other than humans is important in part because one can manipulate the neural and genetic basis for navigation in ways that are impossible to do with humans. The findings from this literature are consistent with the proposed crucial role of the hippocampus in navigation. Rats undergoing lesions to this area of the brain show impaired learning of new places. For example, in the Morris water maze task, rats are trained to swim to a submerged platform; they learn the location of the platform rapidly and can then swim to it from new locations. Rats with hippocampal lesions show impaired learning of the "place" in the water maze task, as well as in other tasks involving spatial navigation (Burgess, 2008; Knierim & Hamilton, 2011; O'Keefe & Nadel, 1978). Recent studies of spatial navigation in mice bred to remove the gene LIMK1 (knockout mice) also show impaired navigation in the Morris water maze (see Chapter 2). This suggestive finding is one of the first to link the WS genetic profile—specifically, the missing gene LIMK1—to impaired navigation.

In sum, the literature points to the importance of representing spatial locations in terms of an egocentric reference system (places relative to "me") and an allocentric reference system (places relative to each other). The evidence also points to a distinct network of brain regions that appear to play an important role in navigation among humans and other species. These regions are ones already attested to show abnormalities in people with WS, raising the question of whether either or both of these representational mechanisms are impaired in WS, and if so, in what way, and to what degree. We take up these questions in Section 5.2.1.

5.1.2 The Importance of Geometry for Allocentric Representations

Although it is widely accepted that humans must have the capacity to represent places using an allocentric frame of reference, there are still many questions about the exact content of these world-based representations. Do we exclusively use individual landmarks, or do we use more global properties of the spatial layout that we have mentioned, for example, boundaries, regions, and the overall "shape"—or "geometry"—of the environment?

Recent research strongly suggests that humans and other species do use representations of the more global spatial layout, including overall environmental "shape." Some of the most striking evidence for this idea come from neurophysiological studies of the rat, which suggest that cells in the hippocampus encode spatial entities that are larger than the single landmark—entities that may reflect the more global properties of spatial layouts. Early studies provided evidence for "place" cells that fire when the animal is in a particular place in space, regardless of its heading (O'Keefe & Nadel, 1978). More recently, scientists have discovered "grid cells" that respond similarly to a range of places that occupy a grid-like structure in the rat's familiar environment (Hafting et al., 2005); these cells are present in the rat from shortly after birth (Wills et al., 2010). Place cells have also been found to encode the location of an object relative to boundaries in the environment (O'Keefe & Burgess, 1996), and recent proposals suggest that place cells may receive inputs from other cells that are tuned to barriers located at particular distances and directions in an environment ("boundary vector cells"; see Burgess, 2008).

A variety of evidence from humans also points to the importance of representations of spatial layout for human way-finding. Doeller and Burgess (2008) proposed two different learning mechanisms in humans, one that depends on the use of discrete landmarks and another that depends on information from the surface geometries of more extended layouts. They trained people to learn the locations of different sets of objects in different virtual reality environments (see Figure 5.3). One group learned to locate an object in the context of a single unique landmark and then were tested with the landmark present. A second group learned to locate an object in the context of a single unique boundary and then were tested with the boundary present. The remaining two groups learned in the context of both landmark and boundary and were then tested either with landmark or boundary. The question was whether learning in the presence of both landmark and boundary would show

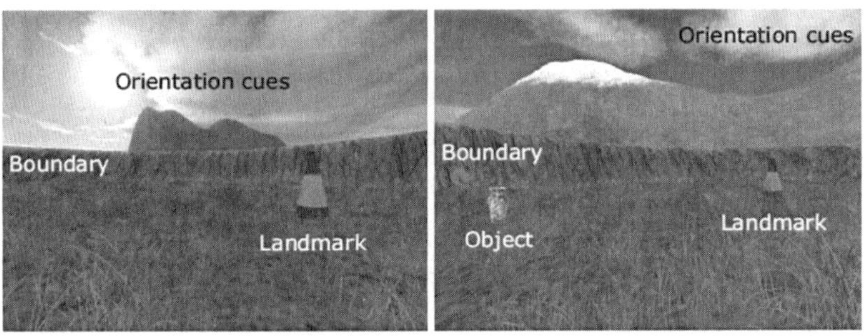

Figure 5.3. Virtual reality task from Doeller and Burgess (2008). In the task, people learned the locations of objects in the environment relative to a landmark (a traffic cone), a boundary (the circular wall), or both, and then had to replace an object (vase) relative to either the landmark or the boundary. Both panels show the virtual arena from the participant's perspective; the left panel shows the screen when people were asked to replace objects, and the right panel shows the feedback they then received. People could learn to locate objects with either the landmark or the boundary information present, but when they learned with both, boundaries were privileged. Reprinted from Doeller and Burgess, Copyright © 2008 National Academy of Sciences, U.S.A.

any asymmetry in the degree to which people learn to use the two kinds of information.

Doeller and Burgess found that people could learn to locate objects with either the landmark or the boundary information present, but they also found that when people learned with simultaneous presentation of both kinds of information, boundaries were privileged. Specifically, when people who learned with both landmark and boundary were tested with the landmark alone, they performed worse than those who learned with the landmark alone, suggesting they had not picked up information about the landmark, or could not use it as effectively when it was presented along with the boundary information. However, when people who learned with both landmark and boundary were tested with the *boundary* alone, they performed no differently from those who initially learned with the boundary alone. In other words, when people learned with both landmark and boundary, they learned the landmark worse than when they had learned it alone, but learned the boundary as well as when they learned it alone. Doeller and Burgess argued that landmark learning can be overshadowed by boundary information, but not the reverse, consistent with the idea that landmark learning and boundary learning are governed by different learning mechanisms, with landmark learning (but not boundary learning) governed by associative rules. They also cited evidence that the hippocampus in particular is more sensitive to information about boundaries than landmarks.

In humans, the neural basis of the layout-based mechanism appears to involve the hippocampus. In a brain imaging study using the task we just described, Doeller, King and Burgess (2008) observed that when people had to locate objects whose position was defined relative to the boundary, there was activity in the right hippocampal formation; but when people had to locate objects whose position was defined relative to the landmark, there was activity in the right dorsal striatum. Results of a similar behavioral (nonimaging) study in children and adults show that both groups use boundaries as well as landmarks to identify the locations of hidden objects, but that children undergo a lengthy period of development before they show the adult preference for locating objects in terms of boundaries in the environment (Bullens, Nardini, Doeller, Braddick, Postma, & Burgess, 2010). This suggests that there may be developmental changes in the weighting of different kinds of information.

The importance of layout representations, as well as their locational specificity in the human brain, has received striking support in elegant studies by Epstein and Kanwisher (1998). In their studies, adults passively viewed a variety of stimuli, including scenes, individual objects, and faces, while undergoing brain imaging (see Figure 5.4). The results showed that a specific area of the brain (the parahippocampus) responded strongly to spatial layouts (including, e.g., empty rooms), only weakly to single objects and not at all to faces (they called this area the parahippocampal place area PPA), and argued that the existence of a layout of surfaces was crucial for activation of this region.

As shown in Figure 5.4, both empty rooms and empty landscapes activated the PPA, but multiple individual objects did not. Furthermore, activation required that the surfaces cohere as a geometric layout; fractured surfaces activated the area if they were aligned to cohere geometrically, but not if they were fractured and then reassembled so as to violate geometric coherence. The activated region did not include the hippocampus itself, but only the parahippocampus, which feeds into the hippocampus proper. Epstein (2008) argued further for the important role of scene and layout perception in navigation. Patients who suffer damage to the PPA have difficulty identifying specific large topographical entities, such as streets or buildings, but know that they are large buildings or streets. These patients have difficulty learning the spatial structure of new environments, that is, developing representations of scene layout.

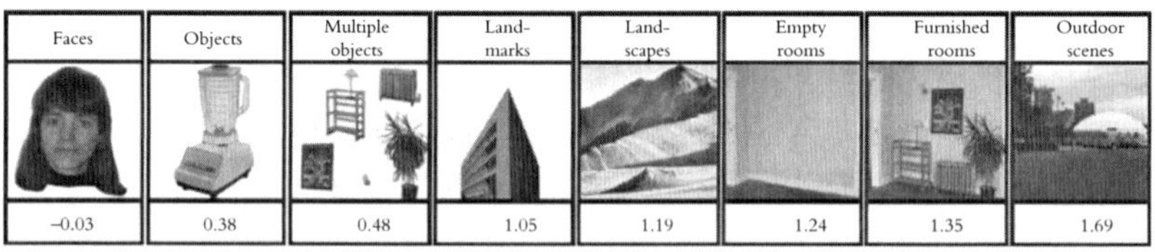

Figure 5.4. Examples of the eight different stimulus types and average percent signal change in the parahippocampal place area (PPA) when people viewed the different stimuli. The PPA appears to respond most strongly to environmental layouts, even if devoid of objects (e.g., empty room). Reprinted from Epstein and Kanwisher (1998), with permission of Nature Publishing Group.

5.1.3 The Special Importance of Geometric Layouts for Reestablishing One's Orientation After Becoming Disoriented

Most the findings we have discussed pertain to our representations of space when we remain oriented. We have seen that animals and people can use discrete landmarks and larger aspects of spatial layout to identify locations after they themselves have moved. But what happens when we are disoriented and must regain our bearings? Imagine that you have taken an underground subway and have emerged out on the street to find your destination, which is somewhat farther away. If you are like most people, you will have lost your orientation while in the subway, so you must now regain your bearings, in other words, determine what direction you are facing in the environment. How do you do this? In a common sense view, it seems like it should be equally effective to use a single discrete landmark or the geometric properties of extended layouts to do so. But a substantial body of literature over the past several decades has shown that spatial layouts—rather than individual discrete landmarks—play a privileged role as the representations we use to reorient ourselves. These representations embody the geometric structure of the layout.

The idea that the geometry of a layout—its "shape"—plays a crucial role in the mechanisms of reorientation first emerged in a set of experiments carried out by Cheng and Gallistel (Cheng, 1986; Gallistel, 1990). In these experiments, rats were introduced to a small rectangular chamber whose corners were distinguished by different kinds of information (see Figure 5.5). The chamber was baited with food. The rats were then removed from the chamber, disoriented, and returned to a separate, identical test chamber, and allowed to search for the food. Their search patterns showed an unusual signature: Rats tended to search the correct corner and the corner that was its geometrical equivalent. In the rectangular chamber, the two geometrically equivalent corners were those that preserved the overall geometric structure of the environment—that is, the two corners that preserved the sense relationship (left-right) between the two walls forming the critical corner. In other experiments, even if there were additional cues that the animal could use—for example, odors that defined the different corners—rats appeared to use this information in a very limited way, using the geometric properties of the layout to

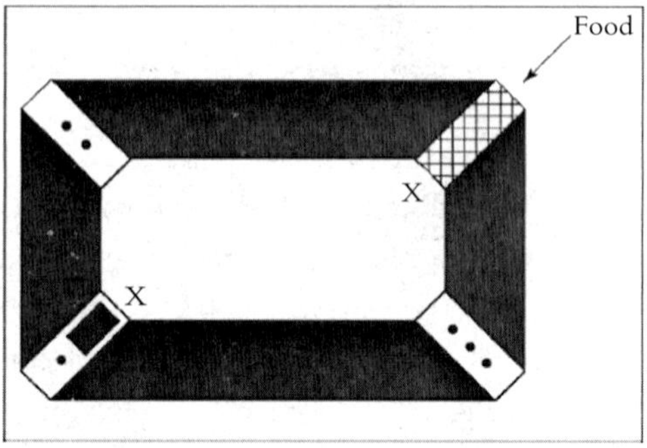

Figure 5.5. Illustration of the experimental setup and geometric pattern of search reported in Cheng (1986). In this testing environment, the location of the food is fully specified by the surfaces' salient visual features and odors (indicated by different texture elements in corners). However, after being familiarized with the testing environment, removed and disoriented, and then returned to the testing environment to search for the food, rats searched primarily the correct corner and the geometrically equivalent corner (as depicted by the "X" in the illustration), essentially ignoring the surface features of the environment. Reprinted from Landau and Lakusta (2009), with permission of Elsevier, and adapted from Cheng (1986), with permission from Elsevier.

identify the "correct" corner—that is, the one embodying the particular geometric combination of walls (one long, one short) and their sense relationship (e.g., long wall to the left of the short wall). This signature geometric pattern of search has since been documented in many different species, including chicks (Vallortigara, Zanforlin, & Pasti, 1990), fish (Sovrano, Bisazza, & Vallortigara, 2007), rhesus monkeys (Gouteux, Thinus-Blanc, & Vauclair, 2001), pigeons (Kelly, Spetch, & Heth, 1998), and human toddlers, children, and adults (Hermer & Spelke, 1996; Learmonth, Newcombe, & Huttenlocher, 2001).

Initial extension of these studies to humans showed that when human toddlers, children, or adults were tested in a small rectangular chamber that had uniformly colored walls and no landmarks, they too searched the correct corner and its geometric equivalent at roughly the same rates. However, when a single clear landmark was included—a single blue wall—adults and children age 5 years and older searched the correct corner, but not the geometric equivalent. Toddlers and younger children still searched the two geometrically equivalent corners, acting much like Cheng's rats in apparently ignoring the clear landmark (the blue wall for humans; salient visual markings and odors for rats).

These results suggested to some that the reorientation system in humans and other species is characterized by a highly specialized modular mechanism, for which geometric properties of the surface layout are, in essence, both necessary and sufficient for its operation (Gallistel, 1990; Hermer & Spelke, 1996). The claim of modularity stems primarily from the apparent failure of animals or human toddlers to use salient landmarks—objects that they are sensitive to in other tasks, but fail to use when disoriented. This "blindness" to nongeometric properties of the surface layout fits one of the principal criteria for modularity, as discussed by Fodor (1983): encapsulation, whereby the reorientation mechanism is restricted to accepting and operating on the unique property of geometric layout. The distinct ability of human adults to combine geometric properties of layouts together with individual landmarks was further hypothesized to constitute a uniquely human capacity, made possible by language (Hermer-Vazquez, Moffet, & Munkholm, 2001; Shusterman & Spelke, 2005).

More than 20 years after the first reorientation studies, a more nuanced picture has emerged (see Landau & Lakusta, 2009, for review). First, abundant evidence does suggest that geometry plays a special role in the reorienting system of humans and other species. It appears to be used by many species and in many different contexts in which the person or animal must reorient itself before finding a target. Second, the use of geometric properties of layout does not depend on experience in layouts that have particular lengths of surfaces or angles of intersection: Chicks who are raised in a rectangular environment and are then tested on a reorientation task in a circular or rectangular environment encode the geometric properties of both environments; similarly for chicks who are raised in a circular environment (Chianetti & Vallortigara, 2008). Geometric representations of surrounding layouts are more likely to be engaged when people are tested in a task that requires locomotion, compared to tasks that require reaching (Gouteux, Vauclair, & Thinus-Blanc, 2001; Hupbach & Nadel, 2005). Layouts that elicit the geometric response must be some kind of geometrically specified enclosure within which a child moves. By contrast, children do not show a geometric response if the "layout" is specified by taped boundaries on a floor, or large individual columns (Lee & Spelke, 2008).

Despite the clear evidence that geometry is special, the hypothesis that reorientation in humans and other species is modular and depends uniquely on representation of the geometry of surface layouts has been questioned (Cheng, 2008; Cheng & Newcombe, 2005). One of the main challenges has come from arguments that although geometry may be important, it is regularly combined with information from individual landmarks, and that this depends strongly on experience, which determines which kinds of information (geometry and/or other information) will most reliably lead the learner to find the target. In this alternative framework—adaptive combination of cues—the claim of modular structure, and impenetrability of the putative module, is rejected (Cheng & Newcombe, 2005; Newcombe & Ratliff, 2007).

Proponents of this alternative view point to the ability of humans and other species to use landmarks in combination with geometry. For example, human toddlers who are disoriented in a small rectangular chamber (4′ × 6′) do indeed search using the geometric properties of the layout, just as many other species do; and they do not use highly salient landmarks, such as a single clearly colored wall. However, when toddlers are disoriented in a slightly larger room (8′ × 10′), they can use landmarks as well as geometry to reorient and find the hidden toy (Learmonth, Newcombe, & Huttenlocher, 2001). In addition, a growing number of studies show that many species can use landmarks as well as geometric properties of layouts to reorient (see Cheng & Newcombe, 2005), suggesting that the reorientation system may engage a variety of solutions.

Regardless of the theoretical framework, however, one clear conclusion from this literature is that geometric properties of layouts play a special role in reorientation. There is also an additional role for individual landmarks, but it is at present unclear whether these perform a function separate from the basic mechanism of reorientation, perhaps being used as a supplement to geometry. Recall that Burgess and colleagues found that different models of learning best captured the use of unique landmarks compared to the use of boundaries to solve navigation tasks; moreover, their imaging studies revealed that the two different kinds of information engaged different brain areas in humans. It would be surprising if human reorienting used only one source of information, but the Burgess studies suggest that there may be significant differences in the kinds of mechanisms underlying use of landmarks versus more geometric properties such as boundaries and regions.

The crucial and perhaps unique role for geometry in reorientation naturally raises the question of the neural basis for this important spatial function. Although our understanding is far from complete, recent studies implicate the hippocampus, at least in some species. Rats and pigeons that have lesions to the hippocampus are impaired in using geometry for reorientation (McGregor, Hayward, Pearce, & Good, 2004; Vargas, Petruso, & Bingham, 2004). Moreover, place cells in the rat hippocampus appear to gradually and incrementally respond to the geometry of an environment during learning (Lever et al., 2002), suggesting that these cells may be important during the learning of the shapes of layouts.

In humans, it seems plausible to suggest that both the parahippocampus and its target, the hippocampus, are important supporting structures. As we discussed earlier, studies by Epstein and Kanwisher (1998; Epstein, 2008) have shown that the parahippocampus is activated when people view scenes, and that this activation is strong for empty rooms that embody only the geometry of layout, but is weak for sets of multiple objects that are not arranged in a layout. Thus this area is plausibly one of important functional sites for reorientation—possibly the region within which the brain computes information about spatial layouts that can then be integrated with our own sense of orientation (or heading), allowing us to reorient in space.

The important roles of the parahippocampus and hippocampus in reorientation is consistent with the possibility that people with WS may be impaired in reorientation, and perhaps more in navigation tasks more broadly. Recall that existing brain imaging studies of people with WS have shown structural and functional abnormalities in the parietal areas and in hippocampus (Meyer-Lindenberg et al., 2004, 2005). In addition, two separate studies using functional brain imaging have shown that people with WS have abnormally low activation in the brain during passive viewing of houses—stimuli that embody geometric layout. Sarpal et al. (2008) found that adults with WS showed reliably lower activation of the right intraparietal sulcus (IPS) than normal adult controls; this profile is consistent with previous findings implicating the IPS in the WS spatial profile (Meyer-Lindenberg et al., 2004). Sarpal et al. also found reduced connectivity between the IPS and the parahippocampal place area, compared to normal adults, again suggesting some abnormality in the areas that are important for the perception and representation of layouts. O'Hearn et al. (2010) also carried out brain imaging in people with WS during passive viewing of houses; they found reliably lower activation in the medial temporal areas of people with WS than with either chronological age- or mental-age-matched children who were normally developing. Importantly, both studies (O'Hearn et al., 2010; Sarpal et al., 2008) found that the WS group showed no differences in activation patterns for passive viewing of human faces.

To summarize, it appears that the representation of spatial layout is a crucial part of the navigation system in humans and other species. Results from brain imaging studies suggest that people with WS may have a disproportionate weakness in this aspect of spatial representation. The pattern of geometric responding in the reorientation task provides us with a clear behavioral signature that can serve as the benchmark against which to test the viability of the reorientation system. It is this signature that we will look for when we examine the reorientation system in people with Williams syndrome.

5.1.4 Summary of Behavioral and Neural Findings

The human navigation system relies on a number of different mechanisms that help us represent the stable spatial relationships among objects and surfaces as we move through space. Key among these are mechanisms that allow us to represent the places relative to our own body (in an egocentric reference system), and places relative to each other (in a world-based, or allocentric, reference system). These two kinds of representation of location play complementary roles: In order to know the location of one object relative to another regardless of our own location, we need a world-based reference system; but in order to know how to act (e.g., which way to reach or move), we need to have a representation of each object or place relative to our body.

Places can be represented relative to individual objects (landmarks) in the environment (e.g., X is 3 meters west of Y), but recent research suggests that we actually depend on somewhat richer information about the surrounding environment. In particular, our understanding of where things are depends on our representations of the larger spatial layout—the overall geometric structure or "shape" of the environment. These representations of spatial layouts play a particularly crucial role when we become disoriented and must regain our orientation.

The different kinds of mechanisms underlying navigation appear to have different neural bases. Egocentric representations of space are thought to engage the dorsal stream of the brain, especially the parietal area. Allocentric representations of space are thought to engage the medial temporal areas of the brain, including the hippocampus, which receives information from the parahippocampus, thought to be specialized for representing geometric layout. Brain imaging studies of people with WS have shown abnormalities in both the parietal areas of the brain and the hippocampus, suggesting that there may be serious impairment in one or more aspect of navigation. We now turn to the empirical facts about navigation in people with Williams syndrome.

5.2 Navigation in People with WS

Earlier, we hinted that navigation in people with WS is likely to be impaired to some extent. Parents' informal reports suggest concerns about their children losing their way (Atkinson et al., 2002), and a recent study found that children and adults with WS had difficulty learning specific routes through an environment, even when compared to a group of age-matched participants who had mild learning disabilities (Farran et al., 2010). Moreover, the known sites of abnormalities in the WS brain (parietal and hippocampal areas) make it plausible that some or all aspects of navigation might be severely impaired.

We now turn to two sets of studies that show quite different profiles. The first set focuses on the use of egocentric and allocentric reference systems in people's navigation while they remain oriented in space. The second focuses on the use of geometric layout information when people must recover from disorientation.

5.2.1 Oriented Navigation: Egocentric and Allocentric Reference Systems

The use of different frames of reference by children and adults with Williams syndrome has been tested by Nardini, Atkinson, Braddick, and Burgess (2008) and compared to the same abilities in normally developing children between age 3 and 6, reported earlier by Nardini, Atkinson, Braddick, and Burgess (2006).

Nardini et al. (2006) tested children and adults with WS between the ages of 5 and 42 years. People were fully oriented in the test space at all times, were shown an object hidden under one of a set of cups, and after a short time were asked to retrieve the hidden object. The context of the search was manipulated in such a way that one could determine whether people tended to use a reference frame centered on the body (egocentric), the larger room (allocentric), or the array itself (object-based), and whether the overall patterns of use were similar to those of normally developing children between the ages of 3 and 6.

The specifics of the task are as follows. People were shown a toy that was then hidden under one of 12 identical cups on a square board (82 cm × 82 cm; see Figure 5.6). On two sides of the board were distinct objects (e.g., a cat, a house) that could potentially serve as local landmarks for the search—that is, one could use these objects to define the location of the target cup. For example, if one observed a toy hidden under a cup immediately adjacent to the *cat* in the array, one could represent it as "target near *cat*." This type of solution might involve using the cat as a kind of "beacon," but since the locations of most of the cups could not be specified with such simple beacon descriptions, it is more likely that people would have to encode the location of a given cup in terms of more distant spatial information, either on the array or in the room. For example, the testing room had a typical structure (four walls and corners) and a variety of furniture, so observers could also make use of the room's geometric structure and its more distant fixed landmarks to represent the location of the target cup.

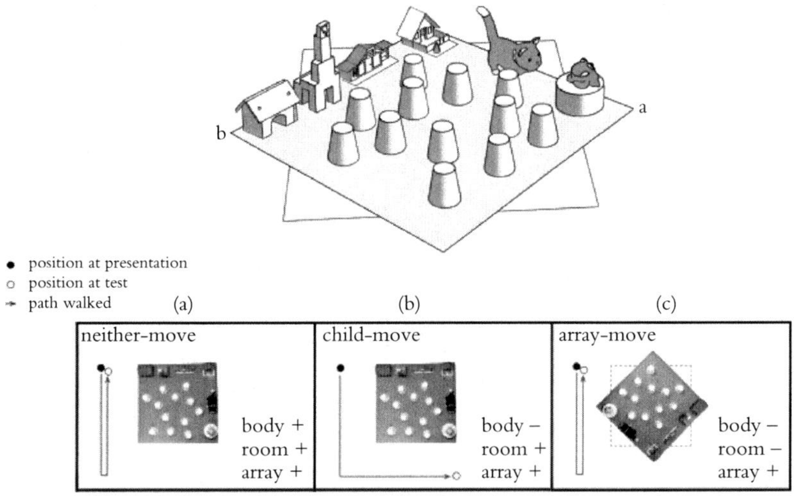

Figure 5.6. The apparatus used in Nardini et al. (2006). A toy was hidden under one of the cups. After this, one of the following changes occurred, after which the child was asked to find the hidden toy. In the baseline neither-move condition (a), the child then walked halfway to another position and back; the board was not rotated. In the child-move condition (b), the child was walked to a new position. In the array-move condition (c), the board was rotated relative to the room (while the child walked halfway to another position and back). The frame of reference provided by the array itself was always consistent between presentation and test. This frame of reference provided the only basis for correct retrieval in the array-move condition. Normally developing young children were highly successful in finding the toy in the neither-move and child-move conditions, but they found the array-move condition quite difficult. Adults with WS performed much like normally developing 3–4-year-old children. Adapted from Nardini et al. (2006), with permission from Elsevier.

In order to examine the use of different reference systems, Nardini et al. created four different conditions. For our purposes, we will consider only three, which examine the extent to which participants can retrieve a hidden object using either (a) an egocentric reference system, (b) an allocentric reference system, and/or (c) an object/array-based reference system. In the "neither-move" condition (Figure 5.6, left panel), people viewed the object being hidden, then walked along a short path and back, returning to the start position to search. The array remained stable during the trial. This condition allows people to locate the hidden object using any of three different reference frames: their body, the room, or the array itself. For example, if a person used an egocentric reference frame, he could represent the target cup relative to his own body's axes (e.g., "directly in front of me"), and retrieve it using this representation after moving.

In the "child-move" condition (Figure 5.6, middle panel), people moved along a path equal in length to the neither-move condition, but ended up at a different location relative to the room and the array. In this condition, people could locate the hidden object using a reference system centered on the room or the array. If a person had encoded the object relative to one or two objects on the array, he could use this representation after he had moved, inferring the location of the target relative to his now-moved body. If he had encoded the object relative to an object or two in the room, he could also use this representation after he moved. Information about the target cup's location relative to the room could be either specific landmarks (e.g., furniture in the room) or richer information about geometric layout of the room. In this condition, however, people could *not* effectively use the reference system centered on their own body: Because they had moved after seeing the object hidden and before searching, the object could no longer be retrieved if it had been initially encoded in a body-based reference system.

Finally, in the "array-move" condition (Figure 5.6, right panel), people walked along a short path and back, returning to the start position to search (as in neither-move), but during this time the array itself was rotated 135 degrees from its original orientation relative to the room. In this condition, people cannot locate the hidden object by solely using either their body or aspects of the room as a reference system, since the objects in the array are now in different spatial relationships relative to both body and room at search time. However, people can, of course, use the reference system based on the array itself. For example, if one encoded the location of the hidden object relative to the frog and the tree, this would allow them to reconstruct the location at their new position.

To summarize, in the neither-move condition, all reference systems were aligned between hiding and search, so people could use any of them to find the toy. In child-move, they could use the room or the array as reference system, but not their body. And in the array-move condition, they would be able to use *only* the array as the reference system (but neither their body nor the room).

The task is a complex one, and it was perhaps made more complex by testing people on each of the conditions within blocks, with one trial of each condition following one trial of the next. But it did reveal a stable pattern of responding that showed clear developmental trajectories for the normally developing children (3–6 years old) and a striking pattern of developmental arrest for people with WS.

In detail, normally developing children ages 3 years and older performed extremely well when they could solve the problem using either all reference frames (neither-move) or when they could use either the room and/or the array, but had to update their own location relative to these (child-move). There was little development between ages 3 and 6 in these conditions, showing that even very young children can update their own locations, most likely by a combination of dead reckoning and use of cues from the surrounding environment (e.g., landmarks in the room). In contrast, the youngest children performed the worst when they had to rely solely on the array's frame of reference (array-move), because the array had been rotated and was now in a new orientation relative to both the child's body and the room. In this condition, 3- and 4-year-olds hovered around chance performance,[1] and even 6-year-olds performed worse than they had when they could rely on all frames or the room's frame of reference.

The overall pattern of performance strongly suggests that young children's preferred mode of representing locations in this context is to use the cues available from self-movement and from the surrounding environment (i.e., the room). The results are consistent with other findings in the literature, showing that infants, toddlers, and young children can update their own location in space with or without room landmarks (see our earlier discussion and Newcombe & Huttenlocher, 2000, for review). The difficulty that children had in using the array as the reference object alone—when it conflicted with use of either the body

[1] Nardini et al. (2006) measured performance in terms of distance from the target location (i.e., distance error); chance was computed by comparing this to the average distances between the target and each of the 12 hiding locations, assuming that the person would search by chance at any of these locations.

(array-move) or the room (both-move)—is also consistent with well-known literature showing that children have great difficulty representing the locations of objects in an array when the array itself has undergone a change of orientation relative to the viewer (either by imagination or actual rotation; Huttenlocher & Presson, 1973; Newcombe & Huttenlocher, 1992). Nardini et al.'s results indicate that children can use the array-based reference system in this task by around age 5 or 6. But even at this age, performance was far from perfect, suggesting an even longer developmental trajectory for locating objects using the array's spatial organization independent of other information, or when it conflicts with other information. For example, if children tend to use information from the surrounding layout (i.e., room, landmarks), it might be difficult to suppress this and rely solely on the configuration internal to the array.

Given the findings on normally developing children, Nardini et al. (2008) asked how children and adults with Williams syndrome would perform on the same task. Their results show strong similarity to the performance of normally developing 3- and 4-year-old children. Their group of WS participants was split into age groups: 5–7 years, 8–11 years, 12–15 years, 16–23 years, and 26–42 years of age. Like the youngest group of normally developing children, all groups of WS people performed best in the neither-move and the child-move conditions, and the performance levels for all groups except the youngest (5–7-year-olds) were roughly in line with normally developing 3- and 4-year-old children. In the array-move condition, all groups of WS people except the oldest hovered around chance, just like the normally developing 3–4-year-olds.[2]

Although the overall profile of people with WS was quite similar to that of normally developing 3–4-year-olds, one important detail hints that there may be a qualitatively different profile across the two groups in some aspects of navigation and search. The oldest group of WS participants appeared to differ in detail from the normally developing 4-year-olds, in particular, showing less of an advantage in the

[2] Overall, the 16–23-year-olds with WS were not reliably different in overall profile from normal 4-year-olds, nor was the oldest group of 26–42-year-olds. Performance of the 12–15-year-olds with WS fell between that of 3-year-old and 4-year-old normally developing children.

child-move condition relative to array-move. Normal 4-year-olds show a large advantage for the child-move relative to array-move (which is the most difficult condition), and in absolute terms, they do very well on the child-move condition, where they must use dead reckoning (to update their location) and information from the surrounding environment. The profile for child-move and array-move was more similar among people with WS, possibly suggesting that they are not as proficient as normal 4-year-olds in using information from the surrounding environment (i.e., landmarks and/or the room's geometric layout) after they move through space. This possibility is echoed in studies of reorientation in people with WS. We now turn to these studies.

5.2.2 Reorientation and the Geometric Representation of Layouts

As we reviewed earlier, many studies have shown that human toddlers, children, and adults use geometric representations of layouts when they reorient themselves after disorientation. In the now-classic task, patterned after Cheng (1986), people are brought into an all-black rectangular chamber, shown an object being hidden in one of the corners, disoriented, and then asked to find the object (see Figure 5.7, left panel). The signature pattern shows search in the two opposing corners—those that are geometrically equivalent. This pattern appears in humans as young as 18 months and through adulthood. A second condition typically is used to test whether geometry is used by itself even when unique individual landmarks are present. To do this, a single blue wall is substituted for one of the black walls (see Figure 5.7, right panel). With a single blue wall, a person might be able to distinguish the two geometrically equivalent corners, and find the target. Alternatively, people might respond like the rats in Cheng's original studies—that is, they might ignore the landmark, and still use only the geometric properties of the layout. Adults use the blue wall, but toddlers and young children use it only under some circumstances, for example, when the room is considerably larger than the original (4 × 6 feet) size.

Given the critical importance of geometric representations in the task of reorientation by many species, including humans, we set out to test whether people with Williams syndrome use geometry to reorient

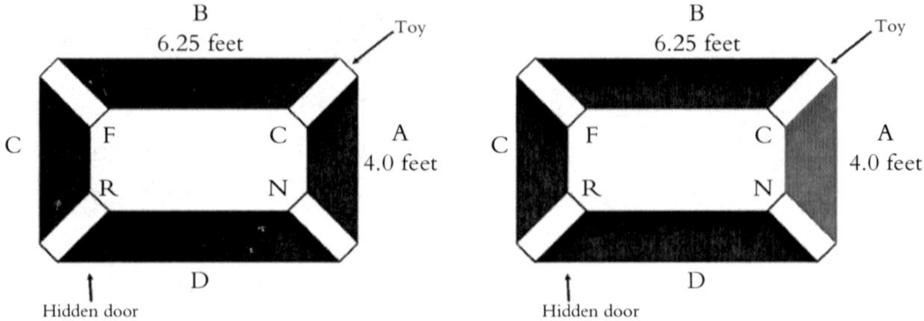

Figure 5.7. Illustration of the testing environment for reorientation experiments. A, B, C, and D denote each of the four walls. In the black wall condition (left panel), all walls were black. In the blue wall condition (right panel), wall A was blue. C, R, N, and F illustrate the four corners in which the toy was hidden (with hiding location counterbalanced across participants): C is the correct corner (i.e., corner where the toy was hidden); R, the rotationally equivalent corner (i.e., the corner that is rotationally equivalent to the correct corner); N, the near corner (i.e., the corner that is closest to the correct corner); and F, the far corner (i.e., the nonrotationally equivalent corner that is farthest from the correct corner). Adapted from Lakusta et al. (2010). (*See* color insert.)

themselves after they become disoriented (Lakusta, Dessalegn, & Landau, 2010). We carefully followed the same design and procedures used in the original studies of human toddlers, children, and adults (Hermer & Spelke, 1996; see Figure 5.7).

We tested 19 people with WS (*M* age = 17, range = 9;9–27;7). They were introduced to a small, completely enclosed chamber (4′ × 6′), and were shown a small object being hidden in one corner. They then closed their eyes and were disoriented by moving in circles for about 10 seconds, guided by the experimenter, who had linked elbows with them. They were stopped at a position facing one of the four walls, randomly determined in advance. Then they were asked to open their eyes and search for the hidden toy. This procedure—hiding, disorientation, opening of eyes, and search—was carried out four times; each time the toy was hidden in the same corner (randomly determined across participants). Other than the chamber, there was no additional information available from the surrounding environment. The chamber was placed within a larger room, but was fully enclosed by the four walls of the chamber and its ceiling; white noise was used to prevent any directional sources of information from the surround, and lighting was diffuse and evenly spread throughout the chamber.

People were tested in two conditions. In the all-black condition (Figure 5.7, left panel), the small rectangular chamber had solid black walls with no landmarks. In the blue-wall condition (Figure 5.7, right panel), the chamber was identical except that one of the short walls was solid blue. Every person was tested in both conditions, with the order counterbalanced across participants. If people with WS show the hallmark pattern of geometric responding, then they should search at the correct corner and its geometric equivalent (i.e., the corner diagonally opposite in this design) more frequently than the other two corners that are not the geometric equivalents of the correct corner. If they can use landmarks in addition to geometric representations of layout, they should search the correct corner more frequently than the geometric equivalent when the blue wall—in other words, the landmark—is present.

Analysis of performance in the all-black room showed that our participants with WS searched the four corners of the room at similar frequencies, showing no evidence of a bias to search in the correct corner and its geometrical equivalent. Figure 5.8 (panel A) shows the average proportions of search over the four test trials that each person received, normalized for the "correct" corner (C, i.e., the place where the object was hidden); its rotational equivalent (R); and the two other corners, one designated "near" (N) the correct corner; and one designated "far" (F). As can be seen, the proportions of search are distributed fairly evenly across the four corners. Statistical analyses examined how many participants searched the geometrically appropriate corners (C + R) compared to the other two corners (N + F) for each trial. Search at these pairs of corners did not differ from chance for any of the four trials. Moreover, search across the four corners did not differ from chance on three of the four trials. Analysis of individual subject data showed that 5 people showed more searches in geometric than nongeometric corners, 6 people showed the opposite pattern, and 8 people searched the two corner types equally. These results suggest that the majority of the participants with WS were not

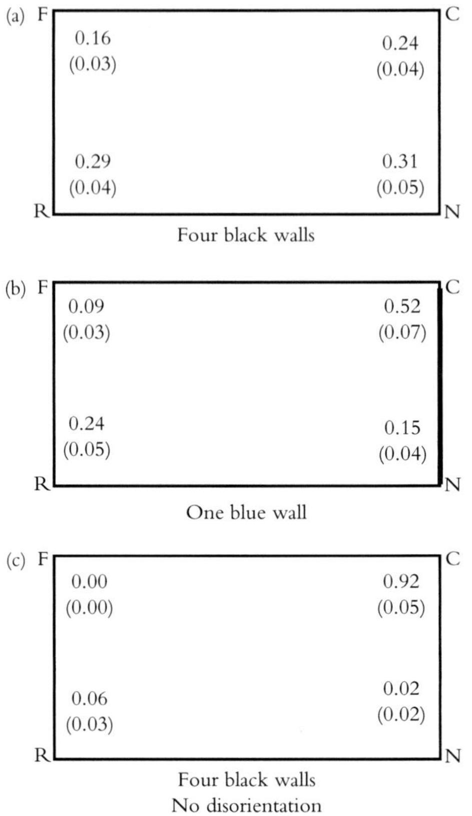

Figure 5.8. Average proportion of search (and SEs) at each corner (correct, rotationally equivalent, near, and far) for the WS participants in Experiment 1 (a, four black walls; b, one blue wall) and Experiment 2 (c, four black walls, no disorientation). Adapted from Lakusta et al. (2010). (*See* color insert.)

sensitive to the geometric layout, including the relative lengths of the walls and their left-right relationship (geometric "sense").[3]

In the room with one blue wall, the pattern was quite different, as shown in Figure 5.8 (panel b). There, the rates of search for the correct corner and its geometric equivalent exceeded the searches for the other two corners. On three out of the four trials, more participants searched at the geometrically appropriate corners (C + R) than the geometrically inappropriate corners (N + F). Moreover, of the 15 participants who showed this pattern, there was a tendency to search at the correct corner

[3] We carried out the same experiment with normal adults and normally developing 3-year-olds. Both groups showed the expected geometric response that has been demonstrated repeatedly in the literature.

more than its geometrical equivalent. Specifically, on the first two trials, search at the correct corner was greater than search at its rotationally equivalent corner. On the remaining two trials, search between the two corners was not reliably different from chance.

The pattern of results from the two conditions suggests that, although many of the people with WS who we tested were unable to use strictly geometric information about layout to guide their search, they were often able to use a clear landmark to do so. We know that people did not use the blue wall (landmark) as a "beacon"—that is, a unique object that is simply associated with the target because the two are spatially coincident. For one thing, a simple association of the blue wall with the target would predict that people search equally at both sides of the blue wall: the correct corner and the one near it. But people did not search equally across these two corners; rather, they searched at the correct corner. At minimum, people would have had to identify the landmark (blue wall) and then distinguish between the two corners, possibly by encoding them as "to my right" or "to my left" (as they face the wall). Moreover, in the experiment, the toy had been hidden for different participants in different corners, whereas the blue wall was in the same place for all participants. Thus, some people would have seen the toy hidden in a corner just adjacent to the blue wall, whereas others would have seen it hidden in a corner that was adjacent to the opposite (black) wall, also ruling out the beacon explanation. We examined whether people who saw the toy hidden adjacent to the blue wall performed better than those who saw the toy hidden near the opposite wall, and there were no differences in patterns of responding.

Thus, the results from our reorientation task strongly suggest that people with WS can take advantage of landmarks to reorient, but that many do not appear to be sensitive to overall layout geometry when that is the only source of information for reorientation. Whether the pattern of failure to reorient will turn out to be true for most people with WS, or only some, is an open question. In an ongoing replication and extension, we have found that small changes in the structure of the room layout may significantly enhance the ability of people with WS to use geometry (Ferrara & Landau, 2012).

One might wonder whether the null results for the all-black room—which meant, after all, random searching—might be a direct reflection of the deficit in visual-spatial working memory that has been observed among people with WS (Jarrold, Baddeley, & Hewes, 1999; O'Hearn, Courtney, Street & Landau, 2009; Vicari, Brizzolara, Carlesimo, Pezzini, & Volterra, 1996). A control experiment suggests this is not the case, and reinforces the idea that reorientation may depend on a highly specialized mechanism. We tested 12 people with WS, 11 of whom had participated earlier in the reorientation task, using the same overall method with the all-black room, except that people remained oriented. They entered the all-black chamber, watched while the toy was being hidden, then closed their eyes and were rotated by the experimenter to face a different wall, while she counted to 10. The 10-second delay was equivalent to the disorientation period in the original experiment, except that people remained oriented and were moved to face a different wall. When they opened eyes, they searched for the toy in the correct corner on 92% of the trials (9 participants were correct on all four trials; see Figure 5.8, panel c).

This excellent performance tells us several things. First, it rules out the idea that a general visual-spatial working memory deficit was responsible for the random reorientation performance in the all-black room. Second, the fact that these participants could easily account for their own changed position in space, with their eyes shut, suggests that they do have mechanisms responsible for updating their own location in space, even without external cues (such as were present in Nardini's study). This mechanism is likely "dead reckoning," which allows humans and many other species to keep track of their own changes in angle and distance over time as they move through space (Gallistel, 1990). It has long been known that this mechanism is present in human toddlers, even those who are blind from birth (Klatzky et al., 1998; Landau Spelke, Gleitman, 1984; Newcombe, Huttenlocher, Drummey, & Wiley, 1998), and it appears that the mechanism also operates in people with Williams syndrome.

A final set of analyses on the reorientation data sheds further light on the nature of the reorientation system in humans. One examined the possible link between reorientation performance and mastery of spatial language in people with WS. The second examined any link between reorientation performance and more general measures of intelligence. The results of both analyses are shown in Table 5.1a and Table 5.1b.

Table 5.1a Logistic Regression Analysis for Left/Right Comprehension and Production Predicting Correct Performance in the Blue Wall Chamber of Experiment 1

	Blue Wall: Correct Corner			
Predictor	*B*	SE *B*	e^B	R^2
Left/right comprehension	-1.108	0.92	0.33	0.032
Left/right production	-0.501	0.858	0.606	0.007
$e^{\mathbf{B}}$, exponentiated *B*				

Reprinted from Lakusta et al. (2010).

The first analysis was motivated by the hypothesis that the combined use of landmarks and geometry in human children and adults relies on the development of spatial language, which serves as a means of binding together information from the geometric system and other surface cues (such as the color of a wall; see Hermer-Vazquez, Spelke, & Katsnelson, 1999; Shusterman & Spelke, 2005). To see whether spatial language in people with WS had any relationship to their performance in the reorientation task, we carried out a production and comprehension task with our participants, looking for their level of competence in using terms such as "above/below" and "right/left." In principle, people who have strong control over the terms "right/left" should be better at using the landmark to identify the target's location, since they could encode that location as, for example, "to the left of the blue wall." However, we found that there was no reliable correlation between individuals' mastery of the terms "left/right" and their performance in the room with the blue wall (see Table 5.1a). Because our participants showed no evidence of using geometric information in the all-black room, it is perhaps not surprising that they did not apparently use language to combine geometry with the blue wall landmark. However, the results point to the idea that people with WS did not use language to solve the reorientation problem, even in the case of having a landmark present.

The second set of analyses was motivated by the question of whether general measures of intelligence and spatial abilities would predict performance in the reorientation task. Performance in the reorientation task was reliably predicted by IQ (see Table 5.1b), perhaps not surprisingly

Table 5.1b Logistic Regression Analysis for Measure of IQ and Block Construction Predicting Geometric Response (in the Black Chamber) and Correct Performance (in the Blue Wall Chamber) in Experiment 1 (statistically significant effects indicated by *)

	Four Black Walls: Geometric Corners (C and R)				**Blue Wall: Correct Corner**			
Predictors	*B*	SE *B*	e*B*	R^2	*B*	SE *B*	e*B*	R^2
Overall IQ	0.060	0.024	1.061*	0.158	0.053	0.022	1.054*	0.113
DAS pattern construction	0.039	0.015	1.040*	0.123	0.009	0.014	1.009	0.007

Reprinted from Lakusta et al. (2010).

since IQ is correlated with many different functions. This finding raises the question of whether the WS profile for this task is unique to other groups who have mild to moderate retardation. It also raises the question of whether people with WS who have normal IQs would show a failure to use geometry to reorient as we observed in our sample. We do not yet know the answers to these questions, but a recent replication in our lab suggests that IQ may indeed play a factor in the ability to use geometry as the sole source of information for reorientation.

We also measured the ability of our participants to carry out a standardized block construction task, as measured by the Differential Abilities Scales (DAS; Elliott, 1990, see Table 5.1b). We found that performance on this task was reliably predicted by performance in the all-black room, but not in the blue wall room, suggesting that the mechanisms underlying performance in the two rooms may be somewhat different. The correlation between failure to use geometry in the all-black room and the block construction task is intriguing, because the tasks bear little similarity to each other, at least on the surface. But the fact that performance in a block assembly task results in very low parietal area activation among people with WS (Meyer-Lindenberg et al., 2004), and that reorientation probably depends on a complex network involving both parietal and medial temporal areas, is at least suggestive: The deficits are likely not identical, but may be related, and part of an overall set of circuits that are damaged in the WS brain.

Our findings raise additional questions, which we are now pursuing. One question is whether the limited use of geometric layout in people with WS is restricted to adolescents and adults (whom we tested), or whether it appears even early in life. Another is whether the failure to use geometry as a sole source of information in reorientation is robust over testing conditions, or sensitive to small changes in procedure. As we noted, an ongoing replication and extension of the reorientation studies suggests that small changes in the room layout may enhance the ability of people with WS (including young children and adolescents) to use geometry (Ferrara & Landau, 2012). Understanding the conditions under which geometry is used and fails to be used is likely to provide important insights into basic mechanisms of reorientation in both people with WS and normally developing individuals.

5.3 Summary

Navigation in people with Williams syndrome shows a highly distinctive profile that is in some ways unlike any other aspect of spatial representation we have described. In brief, we have found the following:

- When people with WS are oriented in space, they can clearly represent the locations of objects in an egocentric reference system, and in an allocentric—or world-based—reference system, and they can use these representations to find objects after they themselves have moved through space.
- The representation and updating of spatial locations over one's own movement is also present in normally developing young children, and, in fact, the specific levels of performance of people with WS under different conditions are remarkably similar to those of normally developing 3–4-year-olds.
- When people with WS are disoriented and must regain their orientation in space, many of them fail to represent and/or use the geometric structure of the surrounding environment. In contrast, they show the ability to use landmarks in this situation. The failure to reorient using geometry among some people with WS strongly suggests qualitative abnormality in this aspect of spatial representation.

The success in representing object locations in either egocentric or allocentric reference systems, and updating these over self-movement shows that one of the most basic spatial functions required of mobile animals is preserved in people with WS. Notably, the profile for use of these systems—both separately and in combination or competition with each other—is strikingly similar to that of normally developing 3- to 4-year-old children, as shown by the results of Nardini et al. And the profile shows that some kinds of search that normally develop later than age 5 are severely impaired in people with WS. In particular, Nardini et al. found that only older children can easily use an array as a stable frame of reference when it has undergone rotation, and so is the only relevant source of information about an object's location. This ability was also found to be severely compromised in people with WS, even in adulthood. The profile of strength for early developing spatial functions is, of course, what we have seen in the last chapter, where we examined a range of spatial functions thought to be engaged when people carry out the block construction task. The representation and use of various frames of reference during object search *when people remain oriented* thus fits the overall profile we have established for a wide range of spatial functions.

By contrast, a quite different profile emerges when people with WS are disoriented and must regain their heading in space. For the people we tested, and the conditions under which we tested, the profile differs qualitatively from any pattern previously observed in normal human development or among normal adults. Specifically, for at least some people with WS, there is an indication of catastrophic failure, with failure to show the behavioral pattern that is the signature of using a geometric representation of spatial layouts to reorient themselves. At the same time, some people with WS *are* able to use geometry as a sole source of information, and many can use a landmark to find the target object.

The severe difficulties in forming and/or using geometric representations of space in the now-classic reorientation task points strongly to a unique profile for at least some individuals with WS. The impaired functional basis for forming geometric representations is uniquely situated within the spatial profile of people with WS, and contrasts starkly with their other spatial capacities, which pattern very much like normally developing children at a very early point in life. At present, the evidence from WS constitutes the only clear demonstration in humans of a specific impairment in reorientation. The neural bases of this unique profile across a broader class of navigation tasks remain to be determined. However, evidence from studies of animals and humans strongly suggest the involvement of three key regions of the human brain: the parietal areas, supporting our representation of places relative to the body; the parahippocampal areas, supporting our representation of global layout; and the hippocampus, supporting our representation of places relative to each other. Together, these regions support the development and functioning of the main cognitive structure underlying human navigation—the cognitive map.

6

Space and Language

Perhaps the most hotly debated topic in the study of people with Williams syndrome is the nature of their language. When Ursula Bellugi first brought Williams syndrome to the attention of cognitive scientists, it was with the bold suggestion that this syndrome represents a clear case of modularity, with one system of knowledge—space—severely disrupted, but another system of knowledge—language, and in particular, syntax—"spared" (Bellugi, Bihrle, Jernigan, Trauner, & Doherty, 1990; Bellugi et al., 1994). Three key pieces of evidence were reported: Adolescents with Williams syndrome could produce and judge the grammaticality of complex sentences, they had moderate mental retardation, and they had severe impairments in spatial cognition, shown especially in drawing and copying tasks. This strikingly uneven pattern across different aspects of cognition suggested to Bellugi et al. that the genetic deficit could result in widespread effects on nonlinguistic cognition with little if any effect on the complex and richly structured representations known to be part of the human capacity for language.

The implications of this conclusion are enormous: If correct, it would suggest that different systems of human knowledge could be rather directly linked to the action of a small set of genes, with the genes that are missing in WS targeting nonlinguistic cognition, but not language. Indeed, language in people with WS has been widely discussed as support for a modular view of cognition by major figures such as Jackendoff (1994) and Pinker (1999), among others, who have cited Bellugi's work as evidence that language (especially grammar) in people with WS is both "spared" and independent of other aspects of cognition. According to Jackendoff (1994, pp. 116–117), "Williams syndrome individuals almost invariably show mild to moderate mental retardation . . . Particularly severe deficits show up in tests of spatial understanding such as copying patterns of blocks. Their language, though, is if anything more fluent and advanced that that of their age-mates. . . . " Pinker

(1999, p. 262) states: "The genes of one group of children impair their grammar while sparing their intelligence; the genes of another group of children impair their intelligence while sparing their grammar."

Since that time, such claims of spared language in people with WS have come under intense fire, and the nature of language in people with WS has become a test bed for theoretical debates about the more general relationship between genes and cognition. With growing understanding of the complexities of genetics and their role in development, more and more scientists have moved away from a simplistic view in which genes directly target different cognitive systems (Fisher, 2006; Karmiloff-Smith, 1998; Landau & Hoffman, 2007; Marcus, 2004; Thomas & Karmiloff-Smith, 2005). But arguments about the nature of language in people with WS have remained contentious, especially with regard to the empirical facts and their implications for modularity (see, e.g., Musolino, Chunyo, & Landau, 2010; Musolino & Landau, 2010; Thomas, Karaminis, & Knowland, 2010).

There have been two principal arguments against the idea that language in people with WS constitutes evidence for modularity. One is that the *level of language attained* by people with WS is not commensurate with the notion that it is "spared." The idea is that language in people with WS cannot be viewed as "spared" relative to other aspects of cognition, since many aspects of language learning are initially delayed, and may reach only a level equal to what would be expected for mental age based on independent measures of cognition (Karmiloff-Smith et al., 1997; Mervis & Becerra, 2007; Thomas & Richardson, 2006). This argument is rooted in the assumption that "sparing" of language means that it should at least be significantly more advanced than would be expected for overall cognitive level (estimated by mental age) and, ideally, should be equivalent to that of normally developing chronological age-mates. In short, the argument is that if the level of a person's language is not better than that expected by mental age, then it does not qualify as "spared."

A second argument is about the *internal structure* of the language that is attained by people with WS. The argument here is that language in people with WS is not "spared" because it is structurally different from language in a normally developing person (Thomas & Karmiloff-Smith, 2005; Thomas et al., 2010). This argument is rooted in the assumption that development under abnormal conditions of development (e.g., missing genes) will inevitably result in a system that has different structural properties from the norm.

Both of these arguments have been used to conclude that language in people with WS is neither *spared*, nor does it develop *normally* (Karmiloff-Smith, 1998; Thomas & Karmiloff-Smith, 2005). Facts such as initial language delay, levels of final attainment that are at best predicted by mental age, and the putative difference in language structure between people with WS and normal controls are said to be inconsistent with the view that language in people with WS is "spared." If language in WS is not independent of other aspects of cognition and if it does not embody linguistic structures that are thought to be part of the normal human linguistic system, then one cannot argue that it provides evidence for a modular view of the language faculty, spared under genetic deficit.

These same issues can be addressed for spatial language—the language that expresses aspect of the spatial world, including objects, their motions, and the spatial relationships among them. Moreover, the study of spatial language in people with WS presents a unique opportunity to understand the relationship between the two domains—language and space—that have been at the forefront of claims for a highly distinctive cognitive profile in this syndrome. On the one hand, one might expect that people with WS should perform as poorly in spatial language tasks as in other (nonlinguistic) spatial tasks; if people cannot represent aspects of space that must be encoded in language, they should show severe abnormalities. On the other hand, one might expect people with WS to perform much better in spatial language tasks than in other (nonlinguistic) spatial tasks; if they have clear strength in language, they should show strength in spatial language.

In order to evaluate these general possibilities, we will need to know about the *internal structure* of spatial language in people with WS, and the *level of language* that is attained by them. As we will see, spatial language has rich internal structure in semantics and syntax; this allows us to ask whether people with WS can learn these aspects of linguistic structure. The question of what level is attained by people with WS resonates with issues we have discussed throughout Chapters 3, 4, and 5. As we have argued throughout the book, the best approach to understanding the nature of any deficit in people with

WS is to compare their performance against the trajectory of normally developing children who span a wide developmental range.

Using this approach in previous chapters, we have moved toward a picture that suggests a WS profile of clear peaks and valleys in spatial representation, with strong performance in a range of spatial functions, and quite weak performance in others. What we have suggested, however, is that this picture of peaks and valleys must be interpreted within the context of normal developmental trajectories, where young children normally excel in some spatial functions, and show weaknesses in others. In this context, the pattern of strengths and weaknesses in people with WS resonates remarkably with the profile of normally developing children who are on average 4 to 5 years of age. We have found only one notable exception to this rule—reorientation in space—for which at least some people with WS show a striking inability to use geometric representations of a surrounding layout to reorient themselves. In this chapter, we will ask whether spatial language in people with WS is structured like language in normally developing young children (at some age), keeping in mind our findings so far that the WS *nonlinguistic* spatial profile for a variety of spatial functions appears to mirror that of a 4- to 5-year-old normally developing child.

In the next sections, we first lay out some key notions about the nature of spatial language, focusing on the way that languages encode two central concepts: places and paths. The semantics and syntax of place and path terms captures the structure of many—if not most—of the spatial terms of English, allowing us to ask focused questions about the coding of space using those terms. Next, we use the framework we have laid out to examine the results of three different sets of studies evaluating mastery of spatial terms in people with WS. These studies focus on rather different properties of spatial terms, especially in the extent to which they map directly onto known aspects of nonlinguistic spatial representations. We conclude by putting the findings from spatial language into context by considering WS performance on a range of other nonspatial aspects of language that have been reported in the literature. As we have already hinted, we believe that the profile for spatial language in people with WS bears a telling relationship to the profile for many other aspects of their language—and an equally interesting relationship to these profiles among normally developing children.

6.1 Structure in Spatial Language: Places and Paths

What *is* spatial language? The most obvious candidates are the words that, in English, encode the spatial relationships between objects, either as they stand in a place or as they move over a path. In English, this function is largely carried out by prepositions—words like *in* and *on*, *to* and *from*, *out* and *off*, *above* and *below*, and so on. Each spatial term can be characterized in terms of the number of arguments it takes and the spatial character of these arguments. Most spatial terms require two arguments: the "figure," which represents the object to be located, and the "reference object" (or "ground"), which represents the object in terms of which the figure is located (Talmy, 1983). The spatial term itself varies further depending on its spatial meaning, which usually encodes that region of the reference object that is relevant for locating the figure.

For example, the words *above* and *below* are both *place* terms, expressing the spatial relationship between a figure X and a reference object Y. When X is *above* Y, it is in a particular region of the reference object's space; that region is defined by the term *above*. Clearly, the two terms *above* and *below* differ in the region of space that they select—*above* refers to the region of the reference object that is roughly in a "positive" direction relative to its principal (vertical) axis, whereas *below* refers to a region in the "negative" direction. Words such as *to* and *from* are both *path* terms, expressing a region of space that is traversed by the figure object, with it either ending at the reference object (X moves *to* Y) or starting at the reference object (X moves *from* Y). Thus, the meaning of spatial terms can be factored into two components: what we can call the "logical" part of the meaning (representing the number of arguments required) and the "spatial" part of the meaning (representing the region of the reference object that is relevant for locating the figure). For example, in the sentence "X is above Y," the term *above* relates the figure to the reference object (two arguments) and specifies where X can be found—that is, in a particular geometric region, "above Y."

6.1.1 Geometric Meanings of Prepositions and Reference Object Construals

For both place and path terms, the choice of a preposition establishes the spatial meaning the speaker has in mind. This choice has consequences for how the reference object is represented—specifically, its "geometric" identity, or "construal." That is, the spatial meanings of prepositions require a "match" with our geometric construal of the reference object. For example, the term *in* requires that we conceive of the reference object as affording some kind of "containment"; the term *on* requires that we conceive of the reference object as affording some kind of "support." Thus, "The apple was *in* the bowl" is typically understood to mean that the apple was contained in the space created by the contours of the bowl; "The apple was *on* the bowl" is more likely to be understood to mean that the apple was either on an overturned bowl (see Figure 6.1), or perhaps that the apple was a flat design on the surface of the bowl.

The kinds of geometric properties selected by *place* and *path* terms differ somewhat. Within the set of *place terms*, the geometries that are expressed are quite limited (Landau & Jackendoff, 1993; Talmy, 1983). Some terms require a very simple geometry. For example, terms like *near* and *far* do not constrain the geometry of the reference object—any reference object can be combined with the term *near* to produce a well-formed expression, for example, *near* my hand, *near* the door, *near* Mars. For these terms, the reference object is represented as a simple point in space—with no particular shape, size, or absolute distance constraints.

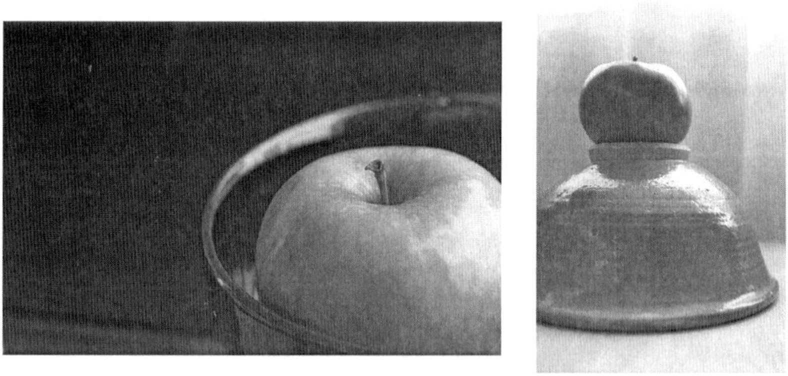

Figure 6.1. Prepositions select for different geometric "construals" of the reference object: In the left panel, the apple is *in* (but not *on*) the bowl; using the term *in* requires that we have a reference object that can be conceived as a container. In the right panel, the apple is *on* (but not *in*) the bowl; using the term *on* requires that we have a reference object that is conceived as providing support.

Other place terms require a richer geometric representation for the reference object. Terms *in* and *on* select for geometries that are (roughly speaking) "containment" and "support," requiring that the reference object be represented as a volume or a surface, respectively. Terms such as *above*, *below*, *right*, *left*, *in front of*, and *behind* require that the reference object be represented as having a set of orthogonal axes (primary, secondary, tertiary) and directions within these axes. These terms can be used with a wide variety of reference objects ranging from the body (*above* me, *left* of me) to other objects (*below* the table, to the *right* of the fork), to geographic regions (*under* the sea, *above* the Arctic pole). Another small set of terms that engages axes and directions is specialized for use with the Earth as reference system; these include *north*, *south*, *east*, and *west*.

In general, the place terms in English express a highly constrained set of geometries, resulting in just a handful of spatial meanings. These include containment (e.g., *in*), support (e.g., *on*), distance (e.g., *near*, *far*), and regions defined on the axes of an object (e.g., *above*, *below*, *right*, *left*). The meaning chosen by the speaker constrains which preposition can be used, and the selection of a preposition then constrains the geometric representation of the reference object. Knowledge of these meanings entails that speakers will produce prepositions that are appropriate for the geometric meaning they intend (*in versus on* the bowl, *above versus below* the table), and that they will be able to understand the geometric meanings intended by other speakers.

The geometries for *path terms* are also few in number in English and other languages, resulting in a small set of terms. As with the place terms, the path terms do not express the details of paths, but rather, only the coarse trajectory that an object takes—moving *to* a location, moving *from* a location, moving *past* some location, and so on. These terms are used for the path component of dynamic events, often in combination with motion verbs such as *jump*, *walk*, *swim*, *fly*, and so on. Using the terminology we mentioned earlier, in the sentence "The girl walked to the bench," the girl is the figure, the bench is the reference object, and the preposition *to* expresses a geometric path function that is defined relative to the bench. English (and many other languages) express three major types of paths: TO paths, which focus on the path's goal (endpoint), FROM paths, which focus on the path's source (starting point), and VIA paths, which focus on a point somewhere along the trajectory.

For example, "The girl walked *to* the bench" represents the bench as the goal or endpoint; "The girl walked *from* the bench" represents the bench as the source or starting point; and "The girl walked *by* the bench" represents the bench as a point somewhere along the trajectory of the path (but not its starting or ending point).

As with place meanings, the meaning of each path type (whether it focuses on goal, source, or part of the trajectory) constrains one's choice of preposition. For example, if we choose to express a TO path, we must choose from terms *to*, *into*, or *onto*; if we express a FROM path, we must choose among terms *from*, *out of*, or *off of*; if we express a VIA path, we must choose from *via*, or *by*. In other words, the particular term we use must fit the kind of path we wish to express.

6.1.2 A Basic Fact: The Small Lexicon of Place and Path Terms Results in Coarse Coding of Space by Language

As the previous discussion hints, the kinds of spatial meanings that are encoded by both place and path terms are quite limited—both in number and in kind. One estimate is that English has about 80 spatial prepositions; this number is rather large relative to other languages, which can have many fewer (Landau & Jackendoff, 1993). Moreover, the kinds of spatial relationships that the place and path terms encode are quite coarse. Although it would be possible for languages to engage very precise spatial regions of objects (hence define very precise spatial relationships between objects), spatial meanings in English and other languages do not represent such regions. For example, as Talmy (1983) pointed out, there are no individual spatial terms that describe metric regions, such as "1 cm above Y," or "3 m to the left of Y." These regions can, of course, be expressed in language; but this is usually accomplished by combining the basic spatial terms and the number system (*1 cm above Y*, *2cm above Y*, *3 cm above Y*, etc.).

One consequence of this coarse coding is that languages typically have relatively few terms that capture spatial relationships. Among languages, English has relatively many, but still only about 80 prepositions, including a number that are combinations of other terms, for example, *onto*, which combines both *on* and *to*. Many of the terms come in "pairs," for example, *above/below*, *in/out*, *on/off*, *right/left*. Given this organization—in which the meanings are in some sense opposites of each other—it becomes clear that there is a very small set of semantic "primitives"—the basic underlying features of meaning that capture the prepositional/spatial meanings. Landau and Jackendoff (1993) pointed out that this pressure to express a very small set of quite coarse spatial relationships in the set of spatial prepositions contrasts starkly with the tendency for languages to distinguish quite small geometric distinctions in the objects referred to by the set of common nouns. For example, different object categories—such as *chair* and *stool*, or *dog* and *cat*—are often differentiated by the details of their shapes, and accordingly, these differently shaped things (which belong to different categories) receive different names. The lexicon of object names is vastly larger than the small set of spatial terms in most languages, and again emphasizes the striking selectivity of the spatial term lexicon.

6.1.3 Spatial Language and Williams Syndrome

Given these key facts about spatial language, we can ask whether people with WS produce and comprehend place and path terms in a way that is consistent with the appropriate geometric meanings. We will first explore the production of *path* terms in contexts where people are asked to describe dynamic motion events. The nature of the task will also allow us to ask whether other linguistic components of the motion event (e.g., figure, reference object, motion) are also expressed properly, both syntactically and semantically. Then, we will examine the case of *places*, focusing in particular on the organization of axial terms—terms such as *above* and *below* (and related terms)—asking whether people with WS produce and comprehend these terms in a way that reflects the appropriate geometric representation of the reference object. The key structures needed to use these terms are axial reference systems, including both axes ("vertical," "horizontal") and direction within those axes (e.g., up/down, left/right). These spatial structures (axes, directions) are also required for accuracy in nonlinguistic spatial tasks (such as copying) that we discussed in Chapter 4. Therefore, the studies of axial terms will allow us to ask whether the comprehension and production of these terms reflects the same strengths and weaknesses in spatial organization that we have already observed in parallel nonlinguistic tasks (see Section 4.2).

Finally, we ask whether people with WS have control over a range of relatively abstract uses of a small set of spatial terms, *in*, *on*, *above*, *below*, *over*, and *under.* Although we have discussed geometric representations in the context of concrete physical reference objects, many of the place terms are also adapted to reference objects whose geometric meanings are quite abstract, often eluding precise description. For example, we can say "Naples is *on* the coast" but must say "Naples is *in* the state of Florida"; we can say "The classroom is *on* the third floor" but "The classroom is *in* the school." One might think that these examples reflect item-specific idiosyncrasies that must be learned one at a time; but evidence suggests that there are rules, probably culturally specific, that guide our intuitions and use of these terms. For example, although we regularly use *in* to describe our location in a small enclosed vehicle ("*in* the car," not "*on* the car" when traveling), we can also use *on* to describe our location in a larger vehicle (*on* the train/airplane/bus when traveling) and can generalize this to novel large vehicles (*on* the space shuttle, etc.; see Section 6.4.1 for further discussion).

We know little about how these more abstract senses of the place terms are learned, but previous studies tell us that they can be very difficult for second language learners (Munnich & Landau, 2010), suggesting that they may reflect complexity beyond the basic geometric uses of the place terms. Testing what people with WS know about these more abstract uses of the basic place terms may give us clues to how much of the complete adult system of place terms they have acquired. And of course, we will also ask how much of this system is acquired by the young normally developing child.

6.2 Paths

The mapping of path terms onto perceived paths has received much attention in the broader context of how people use language to encode motion events—that is, events in which an object moves from one place to another. Talmy (1978) famously proposed that the motion event as a whole is divided—for the purposes of language—into separate components, each of which is "packaged" (that is, expressed by a single term) in a somewhat different way over languages. To learn their native language, children must figure out what aspects of the entire motion event are properly encoded into different linguistic elements, including nouns, verbs, and prepositions.

More specifically, the basic components of motion events, according to Talmy (and other linguists; see, e.g., Jackendoff, 1983) include the figure, the reference object, the motion itself, its manner, and the path over which the figure moves (see Figure 6.2, for example). In an oft-cited example, "The bottle floated into the cave," the *bottle* is the figure object (that which moves) and the *cave* is the reference object (that which the figure moves with respect to). The path is expressed by the preposition *into*, which itself expresses a "path function"; this is applied to the reference object, to produce the complete path expression *into the cave*. The verb *floated* expresses the motion of the figure object, and in this example, the verb also expresses the manner of motion—the way in which the motion is executed.[1]

Because of its rich structure, the motion event has served as a good tool to explore the way that young children express space. The motion event is highly spatial: It expresses the changing spatial relationship between two objects, as one moves along a path relative to another. In addition, because the different components of the motion event are clearly distinguished in languages, there is an opportunity to determine whether any specific components of the motion event are encoded in an unusual or incorrect way, and whether there are aberrations in which different components are combined incorrectly. For example, in English, the figure and reference object are typically encoded by noun phrases,

[1] English tends to have many "manner of motion" verbs (like *float*)—including *swim*, *fly*, *run*, *walk*, *hop*, and so on. Other languages have fewer, and these languages tend to have more verbs in which the path, rather than the manner, is combined with motion in the verb. For example, Spanish has many verbs that express motion and path together: *entrar* ("go in"), *subir* ("go down"), and so on. English also has such path verbs— such as *exit* and *enter*—which express the motion and the path (motion out of or into a reference object, respectively). Talmy (1978) suggested that different languages fall into distinct typological groups characterized by which components of the motion event tend to be "packaged" into the verb, and which tend to appear as prepositions and similar elements.

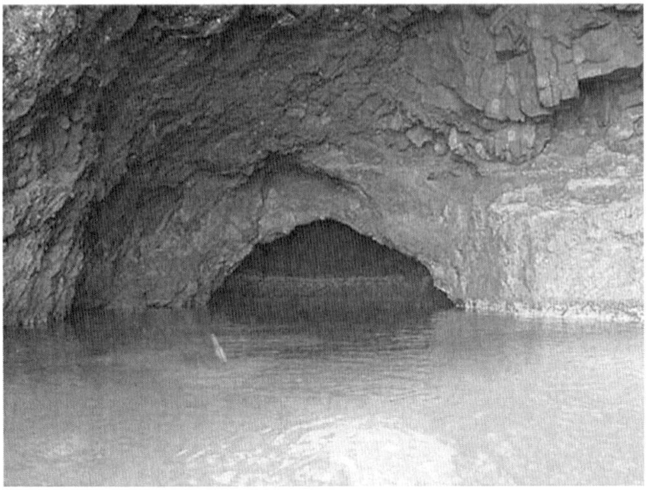

Figure 6.2. The basic linguistic encoding of motion events includes expressions for the figure, the reference object, the motion itself, its manner, and the path over which the figure moves. For example, "The bottle floated into the cave" expresses the figure with a noun phrase (*the bottle*), the motion and manner with a verb (*float*), and the path with a prepositional phrase (*into the cave*), which includes the path function term (*into*) and the reference object (*the cave*).

the motion is typically expressed by a verb (often a manner of motion verb), and the path is typically expressed by a prepositional phrase including the preposition and reference object. Finally, the mapping between the conceptual (nonlinguistic) elements of the motion event (e.g., figure, reference object, motion, path) and language are relatively clear and the rules of linguistic combination are well specified. All this means that studying the way that people with WS talk about motion events affords us the opportunity to ask whether they parse the motion event appropriately for language, and whether they then appropriately encode the distinct components.

The motion event also affords us the opportunity to look closely at a key spatial element in the sentence: path structure. Recall that English (and other languages) encodes paths in a "coarse" manner. That is, distinct path terms (prepositions) do not encode the exact metric length of a path, or its particular curvature.[2] But they *do* distinguish among three different types: *TO paths* focus on the goal or endpoint of the path, *FROM paths* focus on the source, or starting point of the path, and *VIA paths* focus on an intermediate portion of the path. As we discussed earlier, choice of these different path types constrains which path terms is used: TO paths require terms such as *to*, *into*, and *onto*; FROM paths require terms such as *out of*, *off of*, *away from*, and *from*; and VIA paths require terms such as *by* and *alongside*. Although it might seem inevitable that we *perceive* paths as being either *to* or *from* paths, a bit of reflection shows that the expression of these path types is really based on how we *choose to represent* a path.

6.2.1 The Language of Motion Events: Figure, Reference Object, Motion, and Path

To determine how people with WS encode paths within simple motion events, we first carried out an experiment in which we asked children with WS as well as normally developing children to describe to us a set of videotaped animated events (Landau & Zukowski, 2003).

We tested 12 children with Williams syndrome (*M* age = 9;7, range = 7;0–14;0), as well as 12 normally developing children (*M* age = 5;0, range = 3;6–6;9) who were matched to the WS children in terms of mental age. We also tested 12 undergraduates, in order to provide a benchmark against which the children's language could be assessed.

Participants viewed a set of 80 brief (5-second) animated video-taped segments showing simple motion events and, for each, were asked, "What happened?" Given the number of participants and the number of motion events, the procedure generated a corpus of 2880 sentences. The battery of filmed events was taken from the Verbs of Motion Production test, created and used by Ted Supalla and Elissa Newport to evaluate

[2] Of course, we *can* encode these properties in language, by using number terms or verbs and adjectives such as *zigzag* or *curvy*. But the basic path terms in English (prepositions) and in other languages do not encode these precise trajectory characteristics—these are left for other linguistic forms, and are primarily encoded by combining more basic elements.

mastery of the morphology of motion verbs in American Sign Language (Newport, 1990; Supalla, 1982).[3]

The motion events varied in the objects that moved, their motions, and their paths (see Landau & Zukowski, 2003, Appendix A, for complete set of events). In half of the events, there was only a single figure object, moving against an unmarked background; in the remaining half, the figure that moved with respect to a stationary reference object. For example, a figure-only event included a toy executing a zigzag path on a solid surface; a figure/reference object event included a girl jumping off of a platform (see Figure 6.3). Objects included toy versions of people, animals, vehicles, and common, everyday objects. Events varied in manner of motion (e.g., rolling, flying, falling, jumping) and path type. For the 40 events that included both a figure and reference object, 12 involved bounded TO paths, 16 involved bounded FROM paths, and

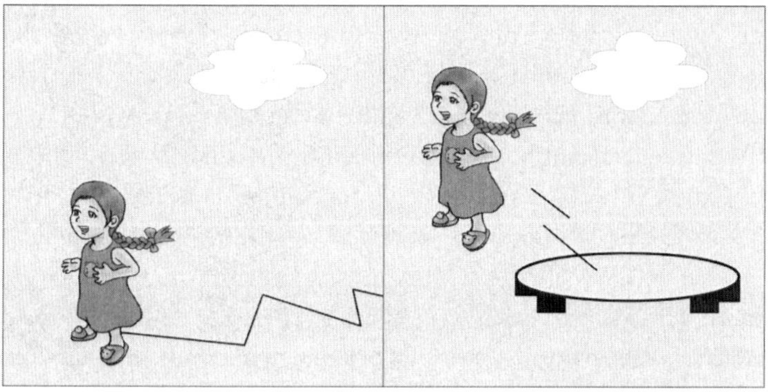

Figure 6.3. Sample of motion events used in Landau and Zukowski (2003). Animated events included a figure, motion, path, and (for half of the trials) a second object depicting the reference object. Paths included bounded-to, bounded-from, and via paths. The left panel shows an event depicting only the figure executing a zigzag path, aptly described as "The girl walked across the lawn." The right panel shows an event depicting a girl executing a bounded-from path relative to a reference object, aptly described as "The girl jumped *off* the platform."

[3] The motion events were designed to elicit contrasts relevant in ASL; many of these contrasts are also encoded in English, as discussed below; hence the battery was appropriate for use with English speakers.

12 involved VIA paths. The paths were executed in a variety of ways, including along a straight line, with a turn, or zigzagging.

6.2.2 Overall Results

We examined each of the linguistic components of the motion event, asking whether the children with WS encoded each of the elements, and if so, whether their choice of expressions was different in any significant way from the expressions produced by the normally developing children. Both of these were compared against normal adult productions, which were used as a benchmark against which to evaluate the children's encoding of the motion event structure.

In a nutshell, the descriptions produced by the children with WS showed that they encoded all of the major elements of the motion event and did so with lexically appropriate choices. The encoding of figure objects was remarkably similar across normal adults, and both groups of children. Quantitatively, people produced appropriate noun phrases for the figure object on almost every trial; these were subject noun phrases that were appropriate names for the object that underwent motion in the event, for example, *the girl* or *the man*. Similarly, participants encoded the main motion primarily using manner of motion verbs such as *jump* or *fly* and (less often) simple motion verbs such as *go* or *move*. Adults, children with WS and normally developing children produced motion verbs frequently and in correct syntactic structures (adults 92%; each group of children 89%). The particular verbs that were used were quite similar across groups, with the top seven verbs (all manner of motion) identical and identically ranked across the three groups (see Table 6.1 for the top seven verbs). Thus the children with WS encoded both figure and motion at high absolute levels and with appropriate choice of specific nouns and verbs. The overall patterns of production did not show any meaningful differences.

6.2.3 Path Expression

As we discussed earlier, the path expression is perhaps the most crucial element of the motion event. The path is composed of an expression representing the path function (the preposition) and one representing

Table 6.1 Seven Most Frequently Used Verbs, and Percentages Use Within Each Group, in Landau and Zukowski's (2003) Study

Normal Adults		Normal Child Controls		Children With Williams Syndrome	
Term	Percent	Term	Percent	Term	Percent
fall	26.6	fall	31.1	fall	28.1
jump	14.7	jump	17.2	jump	12.7
fly	9.1	fly	11.3	fly	11.5
hop	7.1	hop	7.5	hop	5.6
walk	5.6	walk	4.5	walk	7.3
roll	4.4	roll	5.5	roll	4.2
drive	4.2	drive	1.5	drive	1.9

Note: Normally developing child controls (*M* age = 5) were mental-age-matched to the children with WS (*M* age = 9;7). Adapted from Landau and Zukowski (2003).

the reference object (the noun phrase). Qualitative analysis of expressions for the reference object showed that—as with the figure objects—the WS children (as well as normally developing controls and normal adults) showed semantically appropriate choice of noun phrases to encode these objects. In addition, a qualitative analysis of the prepositions showed that people in all three groups used path function terms (prepositions) that were rich and varied, and remarkably similar across groups.

The complete corpus of path function terms over the 80 events appears in Appendix A; the corpus reveals that the bulk of the path term vocabulary that is available to normal adults is also available to children with WS by age 9 or so and normally developing children by around age 5. Moreover, when we considered the 40 events that portrayed both the figure and reference object—and where the figure's motion to, from, or via the reference object constrained their choice of preposition—we saw that children with WS used the same path terms as normally developing children and normal adults, in appropriate contexts. This is shown in Table 6.2.

There was, however, one clear difference between the use of path terms by adults and the two groups of children. Whereas adults almost always expressed the path, both groups of children tended to omit path

Table 6.2 Mean Percent Production of Five Most Frequent Path Terms for the Three Event Types

	Normal Adults		Normal Child Controls		Children With Williams Syndrome	
Path Type	Term	Percent	Term	Percent	Term	Percent
Bounded TO	into	20.5	on	31.9	on	23.3
(n = 12 events)	on top of	13.4	in	16.5	over	14.6
	up to	9.4	to	11.0	to	13.6
	toward(s)	9.4	onto	8.8	in	13.6
	on	9.4	backwards	5.5	into	12.6
	off	63.1	off	55.9	off	39.7
	out	18.2	out	10.6	over	17.3
Bounded FROM	away from	9.6	down	6.4	down	16.0
(n = 16 events)	from	4.3	over	5.3	out	5.1
	through	1.1	away from	3.7	up	2.6
					through	2.6
					backwards	2.6
					back	2.6
VIA	through	23.3	over	26.6	over	46.7
(n = 12 events)	over	22.0	through	21.9	around	5.8
	around	10.7	past	13.3	through	5.0
	past	10.0	around	7.8	to	4.2
	backwards	8.7	on	5.5	past	3.3
					off	3.3
					into	3.3
					back	3.3

expressions, and this varied systematically with the type of path that was encoded. In the events portraying the figure object only (no reference object), both children with WS and normally developing children omitted the path expression on a large proportion of trials (62% for each group). Adults did so only 12% of the time. Note that the resulting sentences were perfectly grammatical; for example, "The bunny hopped" is both syntactically well formed and semantically appropriate.

The omission of the path expression thus is not a consequence of ill-formed syntax or semantics.

The results for events that included both a figure and reference object were similar, but afforded more insight into the possible causes of the children's omissions. Again, children with WS and normally developing children omitted the complete path expression on a larger proportion of trials than adults. But this time, both groups of children showed a strong tendency to omit the path expression in two types of events. One portrayed figure objects moving away from a reference object (FROM paths), for example, a girl jumping out of a pool and landing on the ground. The second portrayed figure objects moving past a reference object (VIA paths), for example, a man moving on a path past a tree. In both cases, the figure object ended its movement at a place not occupied by a reference object.

In detail, bounded TO-path events (e.g., a bunny hopping to a tree) resulted in omissions of path expressions among WS children on 11% of the trials and among normally developing controls on 7% of the trials. Bounded FROM events resulted in omissions among WS children on 16% of the trials and among control children on 5% of the trials. VIA events resulted in omissions among WS children on 19% of the trials and control children on 12% of the trials. This pattern shows two things: First, both children with WS and normally developing children show a bias to omit path expressions more frequently in FROM and VIA events than in TO events. This suggests fragility in the expression of FROM and VIA paths, and strength in the expression of TO paths. Second, although both normally developing children around age 5 and children with WS (between 7 and 14 years) both omit these path expressions, the WS children tended to do so more often.

Does the stronger tendency of children with WS to omit path expressions stem from a difference in their *language* system per se or in the nonlinguistic representations that support language? And does the stronger tendency reflect a pattern unique to children with WS, or is it a pattern that is observed among normally developing younger children? Recall that our comparison group in the Landau and Zukowski (2003) study was a group of normally developing children who were matched for mental age and were, on average, 5 years old. Could the pattern shown by WS also be true of normally developing children who are younger than this?

6.2.4 A Follow-Up Study: Bias to Express TO Paths and Bias to Omit FROM Paths

We addressed this question by creating an entirely new set of videotaped events that portrayed a range of motion events in which a figure object was shown moving along various paths relative to two different inanimate reference objects—one a potential source (for FROM paths), and one a potential goal (for TO paths; Lakusta & Landau, 2005). For example, a bird was showing flying *out of a bucket* and *into a glass*, or a girl was shown hopping *from a lamppost to a mailbox* (see Figure 6.4, for example). The principal set of 18 events showed people or objects carrying out or undergoing motions with specific manners, including running, hopping, spinning, flying, rolling, walking, jumping, falling, and crawling; these were expected to elicit the appropriate manner of motion verbs (which they did).

We considered the manner of motion events to be good cases for testing any bias in the expression of the path, for several reasons. First, manner of motion verbs take path expressions as completely optional elements. For the flying-bird event, we can utter any of the following grammatical sentences:

a. The bird flew.
b. The bird flew out of the bucket.
c. The bird flew into a glass.
d. The bird flew out of the bucket and into a glass.

Second, the events were filmed in such a way as to show both figure and reference objects before, during, and after the event—when the participants were asked, "What happened?" Thus, TO paths and FROM paths were given equal opportunities to appear, because the potential goal and source reference objects were both present, and because the verbs we expected to be used were neutral with respect to their choices of path expressions. Grammatical and semantically coherent descriptions of these events do not require path expressions at all.

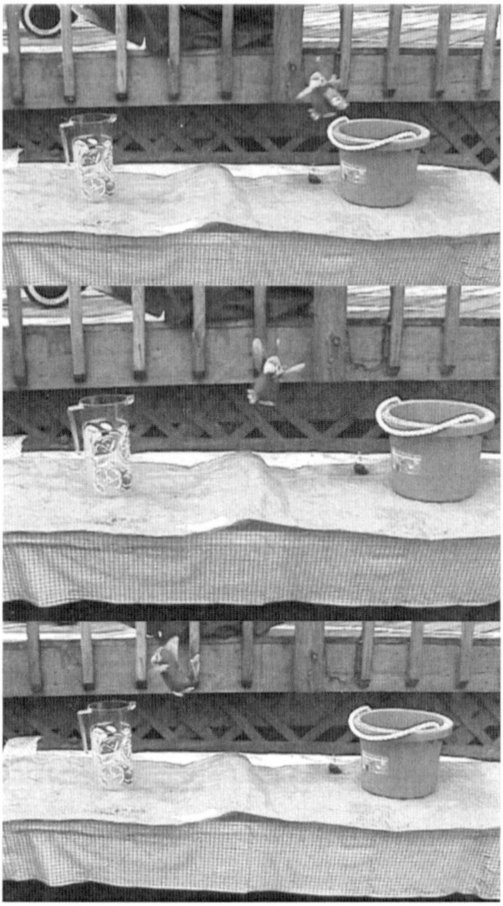

Figure 6.4. Sample motion event in Lakusta and Landau (2005). In these events, both a figure and a reference object were always visibly present during the motion. Top to bottom, the three panels show a bird flying *out of a bucket* and *into a glass*. Although both figure and reference objects were visible, there was a strong tendency for people with WS and normally developing younger children to encode the goal path but omit the source path, saying, for example, "The bird flew into a glass" rather than "The bird flew out of a bucket" or even "The bird flew out of a bucket and into a glass."

We tested 10 children with WS (*M* age = 13;7, range = 9;2–17;9) and 10 normally developing children who were matched to the WS children for mental age (*M* age = 5;9, range = 4;11–7;5). In a second study, we tested normally developing 3-year-olds. We also tested normal adults to generate a benchmark for the number and types of path expressions included in descriptions of the manner of motion events.

The verbs used for the manner of motion events were, as expected, largely the appropriate manner of motion verbs; there were no reliable differences in the proportions of these specific motion verbs, compared to more general verbs such as *come* and *go*, either between the group of children with WS and the normally developing children, or between these groups and the normal adults. Once again, children with WS used semantically appropriate verbs, and did so using appropriate syntactic structures.

The central question of interest, however, was whether we would observe the same biases in the use of path expressions as we had observed in our earlier study. The results are shown in Figure 6.5, which displays the proportions of goal path expressions and source path expressions (prepositions encoding TO paths and FROM paths, respectively).

As is evident from the graphs, both groups of children included goal path expressions more frequently than source path expressions, but

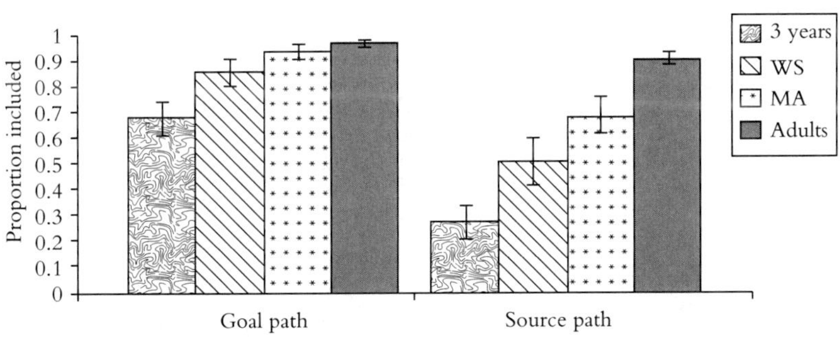

Figure 6.5. Proportions of use of goal path and source path expressions among children with WS (*M* age = 13;7), normally developing children (*M* age = 5;9) matched for mental age to the WS individuals, and normal adults. In a second study, we tested younger normally developing children (*M* age = 3;9), also shown in the figure. Adapted from Lakusta and Landau (2005), with permission from Elsevier.

adults did not. This resulted in a main effect of path type and group, and an interaction. Post-hoc comparisons showed that the goal/source path asymmetry held for both the group of children with WS and the normally developing children. The follow-up replication with normally developing 3–4-year-olds (*M* = 3;9) showed the these younger children omitted more path expressions overall than either the children with WS or the normally developing 5-year-olds. However, this younger group too showed an asymmetry in the omission of different path types, with more omissions of source path than goal path expressions. Crucially, an analysis comparing the children with WS and each group of normally developing children (*M* ages = 3;9; 5;0) showed no interaction of group with path type. In other words, the degree of asymmetry between goal and source path expressions did not differ among these groups.

We now know that the phenomenon of source path fragility—or goal path bias—is much more widespread than our earliest studies showed. We extended our studies to look at three additional classes of verbs—beyond manner of motion verbs—that nevertheless draw on the same group of path terms as we have been discussing. The influential thematic relations hypothesis (Jackendoff, 1983) states that spatial terms (such as path terms) readily encode domains other than space. For example, in the domain of possession, transfer changes are encoded in a way that is parallel to the encoding of change in space. Just as we can say "Amy gave the doll TO Beth," we can say "Amy went TO the store." In this example, there is a parallel between change of possession and change of location. Jackendoff and others have suggested that the spatial domain may serve as a kind of template that supports other domains, with the result that similar terms and structures can be used to express parallel aspects of conceptualization. This framework predicts that we should observe similar biases toward expressing Goal paths, and toward omitting source paths in other domains. Indeed, we showed that children with WS, normally developing children between the ages of 3 and 6, and normal adults all show a massive tendency to regularly encode goals and goal paths but to omit sources and source paths across a broad range of semantic domains (see Lakusta & Landau, 2005, 2012).

6.2.5 Summary: The Language of Motion Events

From the broad set of findings on how children with WS encode motion events, we can draw several conclusions about this aspect of their spatial language. First, these children can describe motion events in a way that respects the parsing of the event into components relevant for language. The children produced the correct linguistic elements for each of the major components expressed in English: noun phrases for figure and reference object, verbs for the motion itself (and specifically, manner of motion verbs for manner of motion events), and prepositions to express path functions. The children appropriately combined the path functions and the reference object into prepositional phrases that expressed the complete path. In each case, their choice of lexical items was much like that of normally developing children who were matched for mental age, and these were also similar to the choices among younger normally developing children, around 4 years old. Crucially, the different path types we portrayed (TO paths, FROM paths, VIA paths) also elicited the right set of prepositions.

The most striking pattern we observed was an asymmetry in the particular path types that were encoded or omitted: Goal paths were regularly encoded, whereas source paths were often omitted. This pattern appeared in the group of children with WS, and in normally developing children between the ages of 3 and 6. Although paths as a whole were omitted more often by younger normally developing children, the asymmetry we observed appeared in all groups. The children with WS omitted FROM paths at a rate that fell roughly between the 3-year-olds we tested and the mental-age-matched children we tested (*M* age = 5;9). But all groups showed the same patterns, suggesting that the tendency to omit FROM path expressions likely has a common cause across the three groups.

This asymmetry was even observed in the rare cases of errors of preposition choice: TO-path terms were occasionally produced for FROM paths, for example, "She hopped *to* the lamppost to the mailbox" to describe an event in which a girl hopped *from* the lamppost to the mailbox. Given the asymmetry between source and goal paths, the tendency to substitute a goal path expression for a source path expression is likely a consequence of retrieval failure, and this occurred on occasion among all child groups.[4]

Why is there fragility in the expression of FROM paths among normally developing children and people with WS? One answer is that this pattern reflects a broad-ranging bias in the way that all human represent events: Cognition is generally forward-looking, and people tend to represent events in terms of their end states rather than their start states. This idea would predict that the phenomenon of a "goal bias," or an asymmetry between goal and source paths, should be quite widespread. And it is. The same pattern has been replicated in young children learning Japanese (Lakusta, Yoshida, Landau, & Smith, 2006) and has been observed among adult agrammatics (Ihara & Fujita, 2000). It has been shown among normally developing 4-year-olds and adults in both linguistic and nonlinguistic tasks (Lakusta & Landau, 2012; Regier & Zheng, 2007). The pattern has also been shown in infants, before language is learned: Lakusta, Wagner, O'Hearn, and Landau (2007) showed that 12-month-old infants can represent both sources and goals in simple motion events; but they represent goals more robustly than sources, even when the sources are perceptually more salient than the goals.

This evidence places the site of fragility outside of language per se: Children with WS may have impairments in visual-spatial attention and/or spatial memory (as we have seen in preceding chapters), but they apparently develop a linguistic system that supports the ability to accurately

---

[4] Landau and Zukowski (2003) suggested that the tendency of WS children to omit path expressions most often in FROM- and VIA-path motion events might reflect fragile visual-spatial memory and/or attention in people with WS. In the FROM and VIA paths, the encoding of the complete path expression requires expressing both the path function and the reference object, which—in the case of these two path types—is not spatially coincident with the figure object at the time the child describes the event. For example, in an event in which a bunny hops to a carrot and rests there, the figure and reference objects are in roughly the same place at the end of the event, and thus are likely to be within the child's current attentional window; this might make it relatively easy to remember that the carrot is part of the event. By contrast, in an event in which a bunny hops *away from* the carrot, or past it on the way to his resting spot, the child with fragile visual-spatial attention and/or memory could easily fail to encode the reference object. The result is a perfectly grammatical utterance, but one that omits the path, for example, "The bunny hopped."

encode the central elements of the motion event, to make semantically appropriate lexical choices among the key elements, and, critically, to select among different spatial prepositions to accurately encode the three major categories of path types. Finally, their linguistic system supports the ability to combine these into syntactically well-formed and semantically coherent sentences. This aspect of spatial language clearly develops in such a way as to produce a richly structured system that does not appear to have significant differences from that of a normally developing child of around age 4 or 5. However, it is also notable that these complex aspects of spatial language are *normally* acquired by the age of 4 or 5—a point to which we will return.

6.3 Places

The domain of axial terms—words such as *above*, *below*, *right*, and *left*—offers perhaps the clearest case for determining whether spatial language in people with WS reflects their spatial impairment.[5] This is because understanding the spatial meanings of axial terms requires that we represent reference objects in terms of the three main sets of orthogonal axes and directions within those axes. For example, the word *above* refers to the region of a reference object that falls along its primary (often gravitationally vertical) axis and is in the "positive" region; the word *below* or *under* refers to the region that also falls along the primary axis but is

[5] This is clearly a special case of the more general question of whether language and cognition develop independently of each other. The original claim of language-cognition independence was taken to be consistent with modularity: If people with WS, who are moderately retarded and have severely impaired spatial cognition, nevertheless have spared language, this would imply that language development is independent of overall levels of cognition. The relevant evidence from Bellugi et al. (1988) concerned syntactic abilities, the paradigm case for which one might expect a modular system. The case of spatial language focuses the debate on a different question: whether the impairment in nonlinguistic representations observed among people with WS has consequences for the spatial lexicon—those terms that express spatial relationships between objects in space. The claim of modularity may not pertain to the semantics of individual spatial terms, if spatial meanings must have access to spatial systems in order to refer properly.

in the "negative" region.[6] Similarly the words *left* and *right* refer to the regions falling along the secondary (often the horizontal) axis and, again, are in the positive and negative regions, respectively. Recent research on the use of these axial terms by normal adults shows that axial terms are indeed used more densely along the reference object's axis, clear evidence for a homology between the structures used in spatial language and the structures used to represent locations without language (Hayward & Tarr, 1995), as shown in Figure 6.6 (see also Regier & Carlson, 2001).

Clearly, the structure of these regions maps closely onto the representations of reference system that we discussed in Chapter 4 (Section 4.2). There, we explained the concept of the reference system, and argued that the two central components of the reference system are axes, and the directions within them. The results of a nonlinguistic matching task showed that children with WS do represent reference systems, with clear evidence of the mental representation of two axes and direction within the axes. However, there were also weaknesses that would be relevant for using terms like *above, below, right* and *left*. First, the children with WS and normally developing 5-year-olds showed a decline in performance for locations along the horizontal axis of the reference object (compared to the vertical). The WS decline was steeper than the mental age-matched children. Second, children and adults with WS as well as normally developing controls all showed fragility in representing directions within each axis. In one task, the results for the adults with WS were no different from much younger normally developing children (*M* age = 5;10).

These findings suggest predictions for spatial language. One concerns the mapping of axial terms to *axes* of the reference object. Given that children with WS and normally developing children represent locations in terms of axes of the reference object, we would predict that both groups should use axial terms principally for locations lying along the axes of the reference object, and less often for locations lying off of these axes, consistent with the use of axial terms by normal adults (Hayward & Tarr, 1995; Munnich, Landau, & Dosher, 2001). Any differences between the groups should reflect relative difficulty for the WS children for locations that lie along the horizontal axis.

---

[6] The terms "positive" and "negative" are arbitrary, but for the vertical axis, conform to orthodox marking of units for a Cartesian coordinate system.

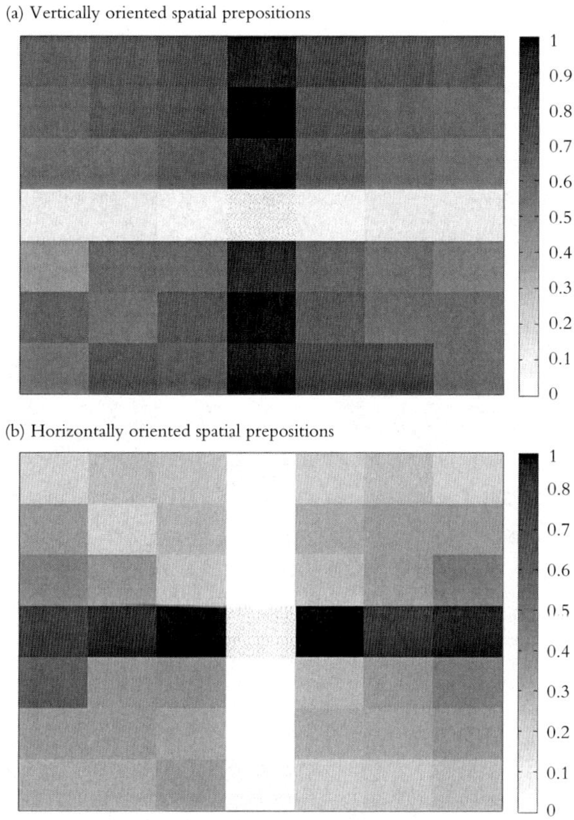

Figure 6.6. Hayward and Tarr (1995) found that normal adults' use of spatial prepositions reflects their representation and use of reference systems. People were asked to describe the location of an object that occupied various locations relative to the reference object, the square shown in the center of each panel. The figure shows the proportions of uses of "vertically oriented" spatial terms (e.g., *above, below*) and "horizontally oriented" terms (e.g., *next to, right, left*) to describe the locations of objects relative to the central square. Darker elements indicate higher usage. As can be seen, the densest use of "*above/below*" fell along the vertical axis of the square reference object, and the densest use of "*right/left*" fell along its horizontal axis. Adapted from Hayward and Tarr (1995), with permission from Elsevier.

A second prediction concerns the mapping of axial terms to *directions within axes*. Given that children with WS and normally developing children both show fragility in nonlinguistic representations of the directions within axes, we would expect similar difficulties in mapping axial terms to their proper direction within axes. For example, the terms *above* and *below* both describe locations lying along the vertical axis of the reference object (when it is upright); but *above* and *below* are distinguished by their directional component, and therefore each maps onto a different set of locations from the other. Children with WS and normally developing children should be expected to correctly map *above* and *below* to the vertical (and not horizontal) axis of the reference object; but both groups might show confusions in which term goes with which direction. The same should hold for axial terms mapping to the horizontal axis, in other words, *right* and *left*.

We examined these possibilities by testing both production and comprehension of spatial terms in a context that was designed to elicit these and other axial terms (Landau & Hoffman, 2005). The children who participated were the same as had participated in the original matching task described in Chapter 4 (Section 4.2). The 10 children with WS were between 8 and 14 years of age (*M* age = 10;4) and the 10 normally developing children were between ages of 3 and 6 (*M* age = 5;5) and were matched to the WS children for mental age. In order to see whether the axial terms undergo development in people with WS, we also tested 13 adolescents and adults with WS (henceforth "adults") ranging from 14 to 30 years (*M* age = 21). These adults had reliably higher verbal scores on the Kaufman Brief Intelligence Test (KBIT; Kaufman & Kaufman, 1990) than either normally developing young children or the children with WS.[7]

6.3.1 Production Task

Participants were shown the same displays that had been created for the matching task (see Figure 6.7a for all target locations and Figure 6.7b for

[7] The KBIT verbal means for WS adults = 47.9, range 21–64; means for WS children and normally developing 3–6-year-olds = 32 and 30.6, respectively. The WS adults' matrices (nonverbal) scores were also somewhat higher than either group (*M* = 21.7, range = 17–29; compared to 18.7, 18.5), but they were reliably higher only relative to the children with WS.

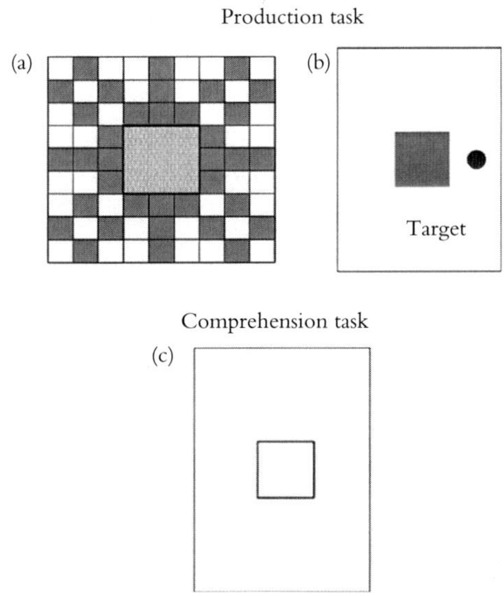

Figure 6.7. Stimulus locations and test panels for production and comprehension tasks. (a) All locations that were tested in the production task. Dark gray squares indicate individual locations. (b) A sample trial for the production task. People were shown the display and asked to complete this sentence: "The dot is ______ the square." (c) A sample trial for the comprehension task. People were shown the blank display and asked to place a dot ______ the square. See text for range of spatial terms used in the comprehension task. Adapted from Landau and Hoffman (2005), with permission from Elsevier.

sample trial), and were queried once on each of the 36 target dot locations. They were told, "See this dot? See this square? The dot is ______ to the square" using a cloze test that was expected to elicit a spatial term. In pretraining, people were instructed that they were going to talk about "where things are," and they were shown several objects being placed in locations, and were prompted with a sentence to provide a spatial term.

People's productions formed a corpus of terms and/or phrases (one per person and location), and these data were coded in terms of five categories: vertical positive terms (e.g., *above, top, up*), vertical negative terms (e.g., *below, under, down*), horizontal neutral terms (i.e., those with no directional information, such as *next to, beside*), and the two horizontal directional terms (*left* and *right*). An additional category captured the set of terms that expressed contact (e.g., *touching*) or proximity (e.g., *near, far, close to*). The six categories captured the vast majority of expressions produced (greater than 90% for each group).

6.3.1.1 Do Axial Terms Engage Axes?

Our first analyses focused on axes of the reference object. We asked whether the structured reference systems we had observed in the nonlinguistic matching location experiment would be evident when people labeled locations. We reasoned that if people represented the target locations in terms of the axes centered on the reference object, then one might expect the axial terms to be used principally for locations falling along the relevant axes (relative to locations in regions farther out from the axes), similar to the pattern found by Hayward and Tarr (1995; see Figure 6.6).

We considered all locations that were tested, and carried out two separate analyses. In the first, we grouped together four different regions that could have elicited vertical axial terms. These included locations laying in the vertical positive region on axis and off axis, and the vertical negative region on axis and off axis. For each region, we computed the proportion of locations in each region that elicited (from each person) any vertical axial term. We then did the same for the four regions that could have elicited horizontal axial terms. These included locations that lie in the region to the left of the reference object, both on axis and off axis, and in the region to the right of the reference object, again, both on axis and off axis.

Figure 6.8 shows that there was indeed an axial advantage for the axial terms. All groups produced larger proportions of axial terms for target dots that lay along the reference object's axes than for dots laying in locations off these axes. This confirms the basic pattern of axial advantage that was shown in the nonlinguistic matching task, and once again shows that children with WS represent locations in terms of reference systems. The results add to those findings by showing that mental representations of reference systems are engaged when children and adults with WS describe the locations of objects relative to a reference object. The same axial advantage was evident among normally developing children.

The data in Figure 6.8 also suggest that there are differences in the strength of the axial advantage across groups. Further analysis showed that these differences were restricted to the locations along the horizontal axis. In particular, whereas normal children and adults with WS were likely to produce more terms for on-axis locations than off-axis locations along both the horizontal and vertical axes, children with WS were only likely to do so for the vertical axis. This pattern echoes the relative weakness among children with WS in nonlinguistic matching of locations along the horizontal axis, described in Chapter 4. The fact that adults with WS did not differ from the normally developing children (*M* age = 5;5) suggests that there is some development between age 10 and adulthood among WS people in the ability to represent locations along the horizontal axis;

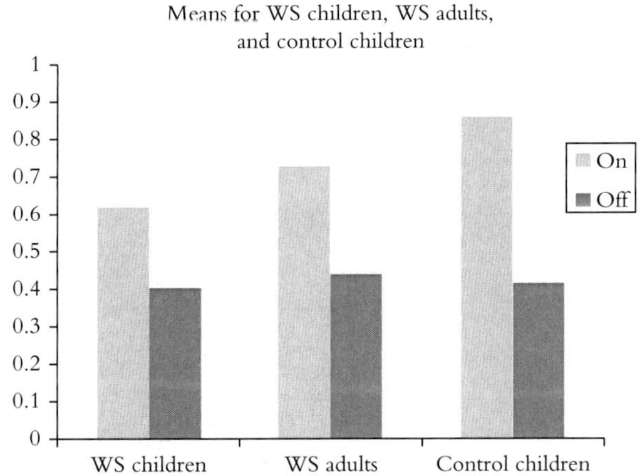

Figure 6.8. Production task: Mean proportions of target axial terms produced for locations that were on versus off axis. As can be seen, all groups showed a clear tendency to produce more target axial terms (e.g., "*above/below*" or "*next to/right/left*") for locations that were on the reference object's main vertical or horizontal axis. However, there was a sharper distinction in application for the normally developing children (*M* age = 5;5) than for the children or adults with WS. Adapted from Landau and Hoffman (2005), with permission from Elsevier.

but the gain does not exceed that of normally developing children who are on average 5;5 years old, at least in this task.

6.3.1.2 Do Axial Terms Engage Direction Within Axes?

Our second set of analyses focused on directions within axes. We again examined the proportions of target axial terms that were produced for different regions, but this time we focused only on the on-axis regions, comparing the proportions of appropriate axial terms produced in the vertical (positive, negative) and horizontal regions (left, right of the reference object). The results showed that the naming space was highly asymmetric, with all groups producing more appropriate axial terms for locations in the vertical positive (*above*) region than the vertical negative (*below*) region, but no comparable asymmetry for the two horizontal regions (*left*, *right*). Normally developing children (*M* age = 5;5) produced reliably more target terms in all of these regions than the children with WS; adults with WS were in between the two other groups, with no reliable differences. This again suggests some gains between age 10 and 20 among people with WS, but a ceiling that shows quantitatively lower production of the target terms, albeit with the same qualitative pattern.

6.3.1.3 What Else Were They Saying?

The results show that children with WS produced fewer target axial terms for on-axis locations than normally developing children who were matched for mental age, and that they produced fewer appropriate axial/directional terms for regions other than the vertical positive (*above*) region. Strikingly, the adults with WS, who were on average 21 years old, were at best no different from the normal 5-year-old children.

If the children and adults with WS produced proportionately fewer appropriate axial terms for these regions, what did they say instead? Analysis of the remaining corpus for all groups showed that the predominant response was to use a term that encoded contact or proximity without any axial information. Examples include *touching*, *near*, and *next to*, which—though less specific than the axial terms—can be used appropriately to encode many if not most of the locations that were tested. For example, *touching* was often used to describe a dot that was in contact with the square on its left side, and *near* was often used to describe a dot that was above the square but not in contact. Terms such as these comprised the bulk of the remaining corpus of the children and adults with WS, with mean proportions of .22 and .17 (WS children, adults) for the vertical negative region, and .35 and .14 (WS children, adults) for the horizontal regions. Because the normally developing children were producing more axial terms for most regions, their numbers were considerably lower, for example, .06 for the vertical negative region and .09 for the horizontal regions.

In addition to this use of terms that under-specify location, all groups also made a small number of errors in which the term they produced was incorrect with respect to either axis or direction. For example, using *beside* for a region that is above the square means that the person has engaged the wrong axis of the reference object (*beside* entails location along the horizontal axis); using *above* for a location that is below the square involves correct engagement of the reference object's axis but an error in direction. These errors were quite rare among all groups, but were more frequent among the children and adults with WS than the normally developing children, and have been observed in other reports on young normally developing children (Clark, 1980). The error of producing *above* for locations below the square was observed in children with WS on occasion, and was also observed in the youngest normally developing child we tested (3;10). Errors of direction along the horizontal axis were even rarer, likely because our participants very infrequently produced *left* or *right* at all.

The overall pattern of substitutions is noteworthy on two counts. First, the range of substitutions was common to all groups, suggesting that these productions may be the result of similar pressures. Under-specifying location is what one might expect if the individuals with WS have a fragile reference system, which might make it difficult to precisely represent a given location. Errors of axis and direction in the terms that are produced could also reflect a fragile reference system, or it could additionally reflect errors of lexical retrieval. In general, the pattern fits with the idea that while people with WS do represent locations in terms of reference systems comprised of axes and directions within axes, these systems are fragile, even relative to normally developing children who are matched for mental age. They may, however, be quite like children who are much younger than our mental age matches. This is at least suggested by the fact that similar errors of commission have been reported in studies of young children sorting out the different ends of the temporal dimension (Clark, 1971) as well as the spatial dimension (Klatzky, Clark, & Macken, 1973; Piaget & Inhelder, 1967).

6.3.2 Comprehension Task

People were shown a standard sized sheet of white paper that was blank except for a 2 × 2 inch solid square placed in the center (Figure 6.7c). They were given a marker and were asked to "Put a mark ______ the square." This was done for each of 22 spatial terms (or compound phrases including these term), including 14 that map onto locations along the vertical axis of the square (when upright), and 8 that map onto locations on the horizontal axis. The vertical terms included 7 positives and 7 negatives (*above/below, right above/right below, way above/way below, on top of/underneath, on the top of/on the bottom of, over/under*, and *higher/lower than*). The 8 horizontal terms included 4 that were neutral with respect to direction (*next to, right next to, beside, on the side of*), and 4 that encoded direction as well as axis (*on the right/left of, to the right/left of*). Terms were presented in random orders, and paired opposites were always queried on adjacent pages. Since each new page was blank, there were no constraints from previous marks on where a term's mark could be placed.

In our analysis, we asked the same questions as we had in the production task. First, we asked whether the marks for the axial terms fell along the axes of the reference object (versus off the axis) and whether they fell on the correct axis for the term (vertical versus horizontal). Second, we asked whether marks fell on the directionally appropriate segment of the axis. For both analyses, we computed the proportion of marks for each set of terms (vertical positive, vertical negative, horizontal neutral, horizontal marked) that were placed in the target axial regions. These regions were defined as extending from the appropriate edge of the square (top for vertical positive, bottom for vertical negative, right/left for horizontal neutral, right or left for horizontal marked) extending all the way to the edge of the page. These regions surrounded the axes and allowed for a small amount of extra room on each side of the axis. The entire corpus of marks for the four sets of terms is shown in Figure 6.9.

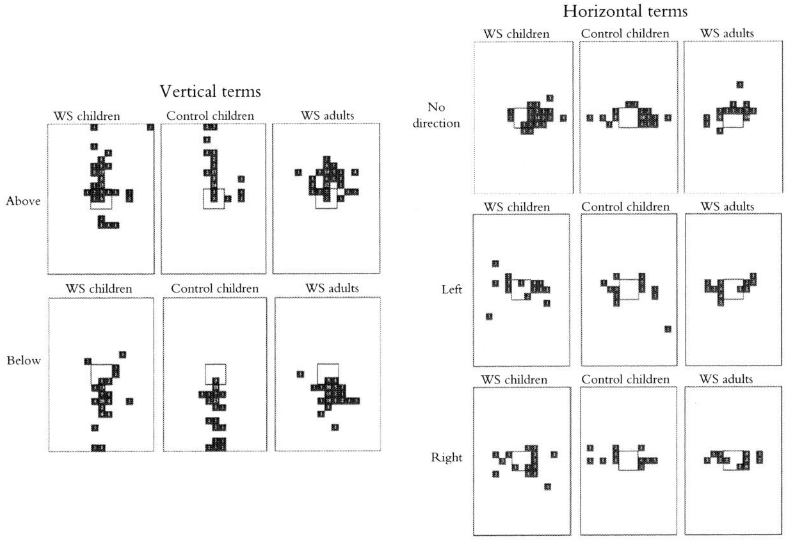

Figure 6.9. Locations of marks placed by people for different sets of terms in the comprehension task. Left upper panels: Marks produced in response to the set of vertical positive terms (e.g., *above, on top of*). Left lower panels: Marks produced in response to the set of vertical negative terms (e.g., *below, under,*). Right top panels: Marks produced in response to the set of horizontal nondirectional "neutral" terms (e.g., *next to, near*). Right middle and bottom panels: Marks produced in response to the set of horizontal directional terms, with "left" and "right" terms, respectively (e.g., *to the left, to the right*). Black squares indicate location of people's marks on the blank page. See text for complete set of terms tested. Adapted from Landau and Hoffman (2005) with permission from Elsevier.

6.3.2.1 Do Axial Terms Engage Axes?

A quick look at the figures shows that people in all groups placed their marks in the region surrounding the appropriate axis for each group of terms. Looking carefully at the numbers inside the small boxes, one can see that the vast majority of the marks were indeed placed in the appropriate region. As with the production data, this indicates that people used the main axis of the reference object and its extension as a strong organizing structure for the task. Especially with the vertical terms, people used the axis as an organizer all the way up to the top (or bottom) of the page, as appropriate. Analysis of the proportions of marks placed in appropriate regions showed only a marginal effect of group; numerically, the children with WS had the lowest proportions, the normally developing children had the highest proportions, and the adults with WS were in between the other two groups. This pattern echoes the ordering of the three groups in our production task: Normally developing children showed the sharpest asymmetry between use of axial terms for on- versus off-axis locations, children with WS the least sharp, and adults with WS were in between.

6.3.2.2 Do Axial Terms Engage Direction Within Axes?

This question can also be answered by looking at the distribution of marks for the directional terms—in other words, the vertical positive versus negative and the horizontal left versus right. (The horizontal neutrals, e.g., *next to*, can be appropriately placed to either side of the square.) Evaluating how many directional errors were made requires looking at the numbers and major types of errors committed by people in each group.

The errors fell into two types: marks that were placed along the correct axis, but in the wrong direction, or marks that were placed along the wrong axis. The overwhelming majority of errors were of the first type, and these occurred principally for the horizontal left/right terms for all groups. The children with WS and the normally developing children committed such errors roughly a third of the time (.38 each group), while the adults with WS committed them about a quarter of the time (.27). Children with WS also committed directional errors for the vertical terms on several trials (.07 of responses for V+ terms, .01 for V– terms), but neither the normal children nor the adults with WS did so. Errors in which marks were placed along the wrong axis occurred quite infrequently in each group (.06 of the time, or less often). The only remaining error type was a tendency for adults with WS to place marks for vertical terms in locations that were correct, except for falling outside the target window centered on the square's axis. Since even normal adults accept as *above* or *below* items that are placed fairly far off of the reference object's axis extension (Regier & Carlson, 2001), we do not consider these errors to be particularly meaningful.

6.3.3 Summary: Studies of Axial Term Production and Comprehension

The results of the studies of axial terms tell us several things about spatial language in people with WS. First, it is clear that representations of axes and the directions within axes are part of the knowledge that people bring to bear when they learn and use axial terms such as *above/below*. For both children and adults with WS, use of axial terms appears to respect the differences between the vertical and horizontal axes, since these people do not make errors in which they use a vertical term for a location along the horizontal axis, or vice versa. Directional differences within the axis do appear to be fragile, however, with both children and adults with WS making systematic errors for horizontal terms *left/right*, applying them fairly indiscriminately along the horizontal axis of the reference object. The relative strength in differentiating the vertical versus horizontal axes, and the relative weakness in differentiating direction within the axes, echoes the pattern we observed in the nonlinguistic matching task described in Chapter 4 (Section 4.2), showing that structure and fragility in this aspect of spatial language is linked to structure and fragility in the nonlinguistic system.

A second fact that emerges from the axial term studies is that children and adults with WS are surprisingly comparable to normally developing young children around the age of 5 years. Like the participants with WS, the normally developing children showed strength in their representations of the different axes (vertical versus horizontal), and they also showed some fragility in their representations of direction within axes. Surprisingly, even adults with WS appeared to have persistent difficulties in sorting out the directions with the horizontal axis, resulting in patterns of performance for *left/right* that look quite similar to normal children, albeit much younger. Where there were differences between the normally developing 5-year-olds and the WS participants, we saw that the children with WS looked weaker, and the adults with WS looked approximately the same as the normal children. This suggests that there is very slow development among people with WS, and that at some point in development, there is arrest. That is, somewhere between the age of the WS children (*M* age = 10) and the age of the WS adults (*M* age = 21), there is developmental arrest that results in performance roughly at the level of a normally developing 5-year-old. Since we did not carry out studies of normally developing children who were even younger—say, mean age of 3 or 4 years—we do not know whether the level of performance among WS children and/or adults is closer to the level of normal 5-year-olds or that of an even younger child. But we can say with confidence that, in our studies, the representation of axial terms in people with WS did not appear to move past a level that is approximately like a normally developing 5-year-old child. This was true both for the strengths in representation (differentiation of the vertical versus horizontal axes for the terms) and weaknesses in representation (differentiation of direction within the axes).

Finally, the studies of axial terms give us a new idea of how and why it seems that people with WS can give the appearance of having language that is highly fluent and, to an informal listener, a distinct strength. Although the directional component of the axial terms is clearly compromised in people with WS, children and adults with WS did not let this affect their willingness to describe the locations of the targets easily and freely. What they often did was use more neutral or vague terms (such as *near*), avoiding the need to use axial terms (which they might know are problematic for them). The use of these neutral terms could reflect more uncertainty about the location they are describing, or it could reflect uncertainty about the meaning of different axial terms.

We suspect it is more likely the former, since we know that the weakness in directional representation is also reflected in WS people's nonlinguistic memory for location (as seen in the matching task), as well as in some aspects of object representation and memory (see Chapter 3). But when they are required to use language to talk about locations, this weakness can be sidestepped by using more general spatial terms. This results in their "looking good," while avoiding use of terms that require that they have robust representations for axes and directions. This may be especially true for language—a domain in which one *can* describe an object's location in relatively vague terms without much of a negative consequence. This can be contrasted with the case for action, in which a poor spatial representation of location will result in missing the slot, dropping the glass, or searching in the wrong location. That is, using spatial language to talk about axial locations, you can actually do pretty well with less than perfect representation of the spatial meanings of the spatial terms. This goes back to the idea of coarse representation of spatial location in spatial language—which results in a relatively forgiving format for talking about places.

6.4 Beyond Concrete Physical Spatial Relationships

We now turn to a quite different function of spatial language—one that might provide a telling test of whether spatial language in people with WS really is qualitatively and quantitatively like that of a normal 4- or 5-year-old. This is the function that allows us to move beyond the bounds of representing concrete physical objects and their most obvious spatial relationships, to more abstract representations of entities, and the use of spatial terms to describe spatial relationships of quite abstract types. In a nutshell, not only can we talk about apples *in* bowls, we can also talk about birds *in* trees, women *in* canoes, planes *in* clouds, men *in* cages, and so on. The range of uses for place prepositions such as these—and especially their combination with appropriate reference objects—suggests that learning involves not only mapping the spatial meaning to clear and "central" types of reference objects that have obvious geometric properties, but also learning how to apply these spatial meanings in a much more abstract way, forcing us to construe reference objects in whatever way the spatial preposition demands. This learning requires what Herskovits (1986) has called our "geometric imagination."

6.4.1 Using "Geometric Imagination": Matching Spatial Prepositions and Reference Objects

The fact that the basic spatial terms—so few in number—can be used across such a diverse set of relationships suggests two things. First, as we have noted, it is likely that the basic spatial terms of a language encode only a small set of geometric and/or functional meanings pertaining to spatial relationships. Some of the most obvious and accessible meanings are acquired early in a child's life—terms such as *in*, *on*, and *under* are used by age 2 or 3. To use these terms more broadly and in combination with a range of reference objects, one must have an understanding of their spatial meanings. Although these meanings have been remarkably hard to capture in precise theoretical terms, their intuitive meanings seem clear enough: The word *in* seems to capture something about "containment," *on* captures something about "support," and so on.

As we noted earlier, these spatial meanings—the prepositions that capture place functions—combine with reference objects to produce a prepositional phrase, for example, *in the tree.* The semantics of the spatial term must "match" the geometry of the reference object, such that the reference object can, in principle, be construed as affording the right kind of geometry for the spatial term to fit. For example, "She slept *on* the bed" is fine, as is "She slept *in* the bed"; but each invites slightly different inferences. The former suggests lying on top of the bed; the latter suggests sleeping under the covers, contained somehow by the bed as enclosure. These rather delicate intuitions can become quite striking under the right circumstances: "She slept *on* the porch" is fine, but "She slept *in* the porch" sounds distinctly odd, because it requires that we think of a porch as a full-fledged containing space—not, apparently, the usual way of representing porches in English. If we change the reference object to one that more reliably invites a construal of an enclosing geometric space, we have the reverse intuition: "She slept *in* the house" is fine, but "She slept *on* the house" ensures that we call 911.[8]

The process by which preposition-reference object matches are achieved is not well understood. But what we do know is that every native speaker of English masters quite subtle distinctions in these pairings, suggesting that they represent the geometries of the spatial terms and that they can use these to select the right range of reference objects. For some preposition-noun combinations, it seems obvious how to match: Objects such as bowls naturally afford containment (hence *in* the bowl), and objects such as tables naturally afford support (hence *on* the table). But either of these construals can be shifted by shifting the spatial term: If we say that there is an apple *on the bowl*, we likely envision that the apple is a flat decoration located on the surface of the bowl; if we say that there is a groove *in the table*, we look for the groove as part of the table's material, for example, as part of the wood (see Feist & Gentner,

[8] Another example that might be compelling for speakers of American English is "She slept in the Florida room" versus "She slept on the Florida room." Florida rooms are assumed to be enclosed spaces; hence the natural use of *in* but not *on*.

1998). Moreover, many nouns represent entities that are not concrete physical objects with obvious affordances. We can describe the location of the city of Baltimore by saying that it is *in* Maryland or *on* the East Coast. Even entities that seem to have obvious affordances—vehicles—can have typical construals that vary substantially from what we might expect. We sit or ride *on* the bus or trolley, but never *on* a car (to travel); we fly *in* or *on* an airplane to a destination, but only *in* a rocket to Mars (*on* a rocket is odd to at least some native speakers, and suggests one is sitting atop it).

These surprisingly subtle cases suggest that there is a great deal for children to learn about the ways that spatial prepositions combine with reference objects, and that much of this learning goes beyond describing the physical-spatial relationships between concrete objects. Native speakers of English learn to combine prepositions with a wide range of reference objects flawlessly and with ease. By contrast, people who learn English later in life tend to make significant errors in producing and judging many combinations (Munnich & Landau, 2010). For example, describing a bird's location as *in a tree* sounds perfectly natural to native English speakers, but distinctly odd to native speakers of Korean or Japanese who learn English as a second language, later in life. The difficulty that late learners have suggests that learning how to appropriately construe reference objects is a significant challenge in acquisition. Our "geometric imagination" is likely shaped by hearing phrases like *in the tree*; these uses inform the learner that trees can be conceptualized as "containers," in other words, that they can form a good match with the preposition *in*. Our use of spatial prepositions in combination with a wide range of reference objects is flexible, but as the examples we've discussed suggest, these combinations are also significantly constrained.

Do people with WS learn to use basic spatial prepositions appropriately with a wide range of reference object types? Munnich and Landau (2010) found that adult native speakers of English show excellent agreement in their productions and judgments of a range of concrete and abstract combinations of spatial prepositions and reference objects. Using these adults' data as a benchmark, we asked whether adolescents and adults with WS also show control over the same combinations. Given our previous findings—both on nonlinguistic spatial representation and spatial language—we must also ask whether the performance of these individuals with WS looks similar to that of a normally developing very young child. Our previous findings make a striking prediction: People with WS should perform no better than normally developing children of about age 4 or 5.

This could happen in one of two ways. One possibility is that, like the recognition of objects presented from common viewpoints, learning a wide range of preposition/reference object combinations occurs quite early and effortlessly, with performance of very young children like that of adults. In this case, people with WS might be expected to perform like these very young children simply because the task of learning the combinations is one that is normally acquired quite early. A second possibility is that, like many other spatial tasks such as tracking multiple objects or representing the precise location of one object relative to another, learning the preposition/reference object combinations could undergo protracted development, with mature performance delayed until middle or even late childhood. In this case, people with WS might be expected to perform like very young children because their development in many areas of spatial language appears to be stalled at the level of a 4- or 5-year-old child. Finally, it is of course possible that our prediction will be disconfirmed, and that people with WS will perform far better than normally developing 4- or 5-year-olds, mastering many combinations of preposition and reference objects, produced by many more years of learning.

6.4.2 The Study

We adapted the stimuli and method used by Munnich and Landau (2010) to our purposes, and tested 16 adolescents and adults with WS (*M* age = 19;4, range = 12;6–28;2) as well as 12 normally developing 4-year-olds (*M* age = 4;5, range = 3;11–4;10) and 12 normal 6-year-olds (*M* age = 6;7, range = 6;2–6;10).

Munnich and Landau's stimuli included 80 different spatial scenes, which were designed to represent a range of uses of the English terms *in*, *on*, *over*, and *under*. In that study, we chose to test these terms because of specific hypotheses about performance by second language learners of English, whose native languages were Korean and Spanish (see Munnich & Landau, 2010, for details). For our present purposes, the set of terms fit three criteria. First, the terms in their most basic uses are acquired rather early by young normally developing children, and so would be expected to be in the lexicon of our WS participants. Second, the terms as a group can be used to probe people's understanding of spatial relationships intuitively understood as containment (*in*), support (*on*), and location along the vertical axis of the reference object, either with contact (*over/under*) or without contact (*above/below*). We have already seen that children and adults with WS are able to apply the latter two groups of terms to concrete physical relationships. Finally, the terms can be used with a wide range of reference object types, many of which require non-obvious and quite abstract representation, as we describe next.

6.4.2.1 Stimuli and Procedure

The structure of the stimulus set allowed us to test for the application of the target prepositions over a wide range of reference objects. To examine subtle contrasts in the applicability of the terms to different reference objects, we constructed 40 pairs of items (80 items total), consisting of contrasts between uses of *in* and *on*, and between *on*, *over*, and *under*. Two sets of figure and reference objects were used for each contrast. For example, we constructed one scene showing *pretzels in a bag*, and a paired one with very similar *pretzels on a bag*; one scene showing a *blue ball in a container* with a very similar scene showing a *blue ball on a container.* Because one of our main purposes was to examine a range of abstract uses, many of the pairs included very similar relationships between figure and reference object, but different nouns represent the reference objects, which would be likely to invite different prepositions. For example, in the set contrasting *in* and *on* (shown in Appendix B), the pairs included, for example, a scene showing an *owl in a tree* compared to *birds on a branch*; or a *classroom in a building* versus a *classroom on the second floor*; and a scene showing *two women in a canoe* versus *passengers on a ferry*. In the set contrasting *on/over/under*, we included pairs such as, for example, *a sweater on the woman* versus *a sweater over the woman's shirt*. Note that the spatial preposition in each case is conditioned to "match" the intended geometry of the reference object—for example, *in a tree* but *on a branch*—even though the stimuli being described in the two cases are physically quite similar.

The set contrasting *on/over/under* was principally designed to test contrasts between the different ends of the vertical axis (positive/negative) and their interaction with two other properties. The first was contact versus no contact (embodied by *on* versus *above* in English, which distinguishes between contact and no contact, compared to *under* in English, which can be used for locations of either kind). A sample contrast included *a lizard on a table* versus *a lizard over a table*, compared to two similar scenes involving the vertical negative direction, which could both be described with *under* (e.g., *a sticker under a table*, in other words, *stuck to the underside* versus *under a table on the floor*). The second property was that of the figure being "spread out" versus "localized" relative to the reference object (as in the blanket *on/over* the man in which the former, but not the latter, can be used for a blanket that is folded up and placed atop a man's legs, but the latter requires that the blanket be spread out atop the man). A sample contrast included a blanket folded up and sitting *on a man's legs* versus a blanket spread out *over a man*, and two similar scenes involving the vertical negative, both describable with *under*.

The 80 stimuli were photographs placed into a PowerPoint file, with one scene per slide. Each stimulus displayed two objects in some spatial relationship (see Figure 6.10 for examples).

Below each photograph, we placed a sentence including the nouns representing the figure and reference objects, and a blank space in the place where the spatial preposition would go, for example, "There is a blue ball ______ the container." On each trial, participants were given the names of the figure and reference object, and these were then put into a sentence, using the cloze technique to prompt production of a spatial term. For example, the experimenter said, "See this? Here is a blue ball (pointing), and here is a container (pointing). Where is the blue ball to the container? The blue ball is . . . " Participants readily supplied a preposition, and usually supplied the entire prepositional phrase, for example, "in the container." The spatial prepositions were immediately transcribed.

6.4.2.2 Results

The participants' responses were coded using the full corpus of terms produced by adult native English speakers (undergraduates),

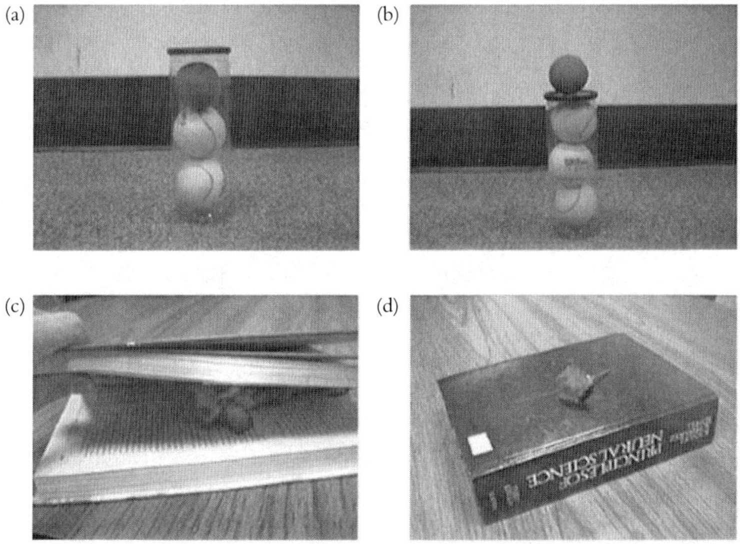

Figure 6.10. Sample of spatial semantic stimuli. Upper panel: (a) Blue ball *in* container, (b) blue ball *on* container. Lower panel: (c) Flower *in* book, (d) flower *on* book. People were given an image and were asked to complete a sentence using a spatial term. For example, they might be shown picture (a) and prompted to complete the sentence "The blue ball is ______ the container." Adapted from Munnich and Landau (2010), with permission from Taylor & Francis. (*See* color insert.)

as generated in the Munnich and Landau (2010) study. The responses of our WS participants and the normally developing child controls (4- and 6-year-olds) were coded in terms of whether they matched the modal response produced by native adult speakers, and whether they matched *any* response produced by these speakers. Although there was very high consensus on the specific preposition that was used for any given scene, adults did show some reasonable and small variation, for example, sometimes producing *under* and *below* for the same scene. For example, the terms *under/below* were appropriate for a scene in which a lizard was shown on the floor *under/below* the table, but only *under* was appropriate for a paired scene in which the lizard was situated on the underside surface of the table. Therefore, we deemed as "correct" for our participants any preposition that was also found in the native adult English corpus.[9] For each scene, we computed the proportion of subjects who produced a correct preposition.

Analyses of these proportions correct showed that the WS participants scored 82% correct, the 4-year-olds 74% correct, and the 6-year-olds 83% correct. The WS group performed reliably better than the normally developing 4-year-olds, but no differently from the 6-year-olds; there was also a reliable difference showing that the 6-year-olds performed better than the 4-year-olds.[10]

More detailed results are shown in Figure 6.11, which plots each pictured scene (i.e., stimulus) in terms of the proportion of WS participants who produced a correct preposition against the proportion of normally developing 6-year-olds who did so. This kind of plot allows us to see whether the two groups found the same scenes equally easy or difficult. As can be seen from the figure, the scenes fall roughly along the diagonal, showing that the adolescents and adults with WS found the same scenes as easy (or difficult) as normally developing 6-year-old children did. The proportions of participants in each group who produced a "correct" term were highly correlated (Spearman rho = .77).

For comparison, a similar plot of the data comparing the WS participants to normally developing 4-year-olds is also shown in the figure. Again, the performance of the WS participants was highly correlated with that of normal 4-year-olds (Spearman rho = .83). The 4- and 6-year-olds were also highly correlated (Spearman rho = .81). The high correlations between groups across the different scenes show that the pair-wise groups tended to be correct on the same sets of scenes, and tended to have difficulty on the same sets of scenes. As can be seen from the figures, many of the scenes elicited perfect or almost perfect performance by each group (witness the large number of dots clustered in the upper right-hand corner of the graph). Even after removing these items,

[9] In several cases, we found that a participant used a term that two independent raters considered acceptable but was not part of our adult English corpus. These cases were also deemed "correct."

[10] The analysis returned an $F = 6.1$, $df = 2, 37$, $p < .01$; Tamhane's post hoc tests, reliable differences, $p < .05$; no reliable difference, WS versus 6-year-olds, $p = .92$. Thus, there was significant development between 4- and 6-year-olds, and the WS group performed at the level of 6-year-olds.

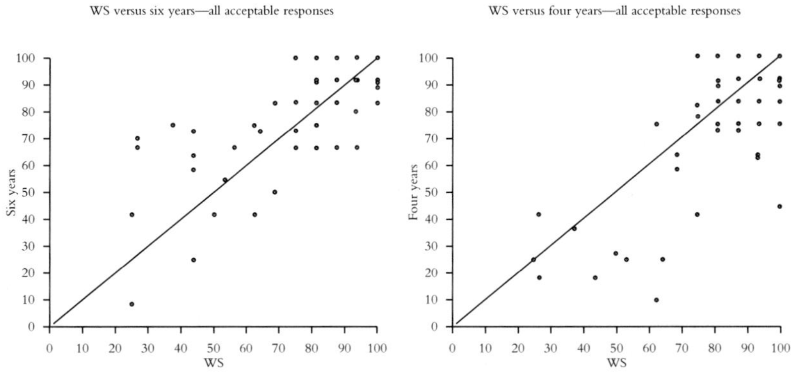

Figure 6.11. Percents of participants in each group who gave correct (i.e., adult-like) prepositions for relationships shown over individual scenes (represented by individual dots). Left panel: The WS group plotted against normally developing 6-year-olds. Right panel: The WS group plotted against normally developing 4-year-olds. In both cases, there is a high correlation between the scores of the WS group and the normally developing children for individual scenes, indicated by the close fit of the joint distribution to the diagonal (line of equality).

we found that the correlations between groups remained high (WS and 6-year-olds, r = .68, WS and 4-year-olds, r = .77, 4- and 6-year-olds, r = .69). Given the substantial variability in the types of scenes for each target preposition, the similarity across the groups is quite remarkable.

It is evident from the figure that there were a number of items for which WS participants' performance was far from perfect as well as a cluster of "easy" items (i.e., those at 100%). It is worth considering both sets of items to get a sense of what made some of the items particularly easy or difficult for people to describe using one of the target terms (*in*, *on*, *above*, *below*, *over*, *under*). The most difficult items included crack IN pavement, passengers IN seats, airport IN Paytonville, shirt IN stack, owl IN tree, dent IN can,[11] and sweater OVER shirt. The same items were most difficult for our 4-year-olds. Perhaps more remarkably, Munnich and Landau's (2010) late learners of English also found 4 of these 6 items very difficult, with less than 60% of the participants producing an acceptable adult English term.

[11] WS people were slightly better for dent IN can, with 62% of participants getting it right.

Although we do not yet fully understand the basis for the relative difficulty of these items, two things are clear. The first is that not all "easy" items are concrete uses of the prepositions: People in all groups tended to do well on items such as *passenger ON/*in ferry* and *Naples ON/*in the coast*, *birds ON/*in the branch*, and *person ON/*in the sofa*. Even normally developing 4-year-olds do rather well on these items (above 75% of participants correct). The second is that the pattern for second language learners is similar to that of the WS participants and the normally developing children. This suggests the possibility that some uses of spatial terms are acquired somewhat late in development, and so tend to be difficult for young children who are developing normally. If this is true, then people with WS may develop very slowly but stop short of the full normal developmental trajectory—resulting in permanent difficulty with some uses of spatial terms.

6.4.3 Summary of Abstract Uses of Spatial Prepositions

The results of this study are consistent with the results of the other aspects of spatial language that we have described. People with WS perform at about the same level as normally developing 4–6-year-olds on a task requiring that they produce terms like *in* and *on* in abstract usages. Like normally developing children, adolescents and adults with WS have mastered many of the uses, but have not mastered a number of other uses; they show highly similar variation in what they find easy or more difficult. Although their performance on this task admittedly places their performance at a somewhat higher age level than the tasks engaging axial terms or the elements of the motion event, they continue to show a profile that indicates their spatial language has undergone rather slow development, with arrest at the functional point of a normally developing child who is 4–6 years old. At the same time, we have shown that what people with WS know about spatial language is rather remarkable—it is structurally rich and quite abstract.

So people with WS do indeed have a rich language system. But so does the normally developing 4–6-year-old child. The system in people with WS is structurally rich and complex; and it is like that of a much younger child who does not have WS.

6.5 How Do Findings on Spatial Language Fit With Other Aspects of Language in People With WS?

In the introduction to this chapter, we promised that we would use the facts about spatial language in people with WS as a foil against which to consider more general questions about their language. Our results on spatial language indicate that children and adults with WS know a great deal about the syntax and semantics of spatial language. Still, one of the very salient facts is that the level of acquisition for children and adults with WS is roughly the same as that of a normally developing child between the ages of 4 and 6. Where errors are made, or performance differs from normal adult performance, people with WS pattern like much younger children, even showing the same patterns of errors. Even adults with WS reach only the level of normal 5- or 6-year-olds in the details of their performance. For example, WS adults perform about the same on axial terms as normally developing 5-year-olds; WS adults look about the same in their abstract uses of abstract spatial prepositions as normally developing 6-year-olds.

This pattern strongly suggests that people with WS may develop spatial language in ways that are qualitatively normal, albeit along a much more protracted (slower) timetable. The fact that the endpoint of their development looks much like that of a normal 5- or 6-year-old child further suggests that their spatial language undergoes developmental arrest at an early functional level. If so, then this invites the following key question: Do other aspects of language in people with WS also fit this pattern?

As we now describe, the findings are quite consistent with this possibility. People with WS are delayed in the onset of language milestones and in initial vocabulary growth. They also exhibit late development (relative to normally developing children) in many of the more complex aspects of language—including morphology and syntax. Finally, the findings suggest that some of the most complex aspects of language—those that normally develop after age 5 or 6—may never be completely mastered by people with WS. Despite this abnormally prolonged developmental timing, language in people with WS also shows the hallmarks of qualitative similarity to the language of normally developing children. This constrains our characterization of the profile of language in children and adults with WS.

6.5.1 Vocabulary Onset and Growth

WS children exhibit delay in the onset of vocabulary, but after initial onset, their vocabulary shows the same nonlinear growth typical of normally developing children's vocabulary (see Mervis & Becerra, 2007, for review). Using the McArthur Communicative Development Inventory (CDI), a parental report measure, Mervis and colleagues found that children with WS had expressive (production) vocabularies of 10, 50, and 100 words at ages that placed them below the 5th percentile for normally developing children. Mervis and Becerra also reported that the mean age for a 100-word vocabulary among children with WS was 40.9 months (range = 26–68 months)—a delay of almost 2 years relative to normally developing children, for whom the 50th percentile for 100 words is reached at 18 months. The 100-word milestone is significant, since it is often associated with the acquisition of verbs and the onset of syntax, after which vocabulary in normally developing children grows quite rapidly.

Despite the late onset for vocabulary, Mervis and Becerra reported that 15 of 17 children with WS in her sample showed a pattern of nonlinear growth, similar to that of normally developing children. To our knowledge, there are no reports of significant abnormalities in the qualitative nature of the early words produced by children with WS.

It is worth noting that initial reports suggesting unusual semantic organization in people with WS have recently been disproved. Bellugi, Wang, and Jernigan (1994) first reported that adolescents who were asked to name some animals produced an unusually large number of low-frequency exemplars, for example, *yak*, *ibex*, *newt*. However, a more recent study showed that the semantic organization for the domain of animal names among 9- and 10-year-old children with WS was no different from that of normally developing children matched for mental age (Mervis, Morris, Bertrand, & Robinson, 1999). Similar findings of normal semantic organization have been reported for older children with WS, and for children with WS who are native speakers of other languages, leaving no support for the proposed profile of "unusual semantic organization" in people with WS (see Mervis & Becerra, 2007, for review).

The overall picture thus suggests that although children with WS show late onset of vocabulary, they then develop vocabulary quite rapidly (like normally developing children). Standardized measures of vocabulary such as the KBIT (Kaufman & Kaufman, 1990) and the PPVT (Peabody Picture Vocabulary Test) have not shown equivalence to chronological age matches, however, possibly suggesting a permanent decrement in the maturity of the vocabulary. At the same time, vocabulary tends to grow over the lifetime, and it is likely that even if adults with WS do not obtain age-appropriate scores on standardized vocabulary measures, they likely continue to acquire new words—a point to which we return in the concluding chapter.

6.5.2 Spatial Vocabulary: Findings From Other Labs

The overall picture we've described from our own studies is consistent with those from other labs. In one study with an unusually careful approach to control subject matching, Mervis and John (2008) found that spatial language was no different for children with WS and normally developing children who were carefully matched (see below). They tested 92 children with WS between the ages of 5 and 8 years compared to 72 normally developing children between the ages of 4 and 7 years. Children were given the Test of Relational Concepts (Edmonston & Litchfield Thane, 1988), which includes items assessing knowledge of spatial concepts (e.g., *over/under*) as well as quantitative (e.g., *many/few*), temporal (e.g., *before/after*), and dimensional (e.g., *tall/short*) terms. Analyses compared performance on these relational terms to those on words for concrete objects, actions, and descriptors, as measured by the PPVT-III (Dunn & Dunn, 1997).

Mervis and John found that the children with WS had vocabulary scores that were lower than those of the typically developing children of the same ages. They also found that the WS children's scores for spatial and relational terms were lower than would be expected for their concrete vocabulary (PPVT), and that the relational language was lower relative to the PPVT in WS than it was among typically developing children. Mervis and John then asked whether the apparent deficit in WS children's language was general across all relational language, or confined to the spatial vocabulary. When the children with WS were *stringently* matched to the normally developing children for their scores on *relational* terms as a whole (using a p value > .50), there were no differences between the groups in their scores for spatial terms. This suggests that children with WS may show a profile for spatial and relational terms that resembles that of a typically developing younger child. For example, it would not be surprising if the concrete word vocabulary was more advanced than the relational vocabulary in normal children's development.

6.5.3 Morphosyntax

Morphsyntax represents one of the most contentious areas of debate about the possible "sparing" of language in people with WS. In an oft-cited paper, Karmiloff-Smith and colleagues argued that language in people with WS is not "intact," specifically that "the mechanisms by which people with WS learn language do not follow the normal path" and that "the language of WS people, although good given their level of mental retardation, will not turn out to be 'intact'" (Karmiloff-Smith, Grant, Berthoud, Davies, Howlin, & Udwin, 1997, p. 247). This paper is widely cited as evidence for impairment in language among people with WS, but we believe that there is another, more subtle and complex interpretation of the results—one that is in line with the picture we have so far painted of language in people in WS. We therefore discuss the study, its findings, and an important challenge to the findings, in some detail.

As part of the evidence for the argument against "sparing," Karmiloff-Smith et al. carried out two tests measuring knowledge of morphosyntax. They first examined overall performance on the morphosyntax items from a standardized test (the TROG; Bishop, 1983) among 20 English-speaking people with WS ranging from 8 to 34 years of age (*M* age = 18). The second examined the control of morphosyntactic rules applied to nouns and adjectives (based on gender) among French speakers with WS, using an experimental test of production.

The TROG is a test in which people listen to a word, phrase, or sentence, and pick one picture (out of four) that best corresponds to what they have just heard. The test includes a variety of items using morphosyntactic contrasts, for example, targets that include personal pronouns marked for number or gender (*She is sitting on the chair/He is sitting in the tree*), nouns marked for number (*The boy stands on the chairs/The boys pick the apples*; see Figure 6.12). It also includes items

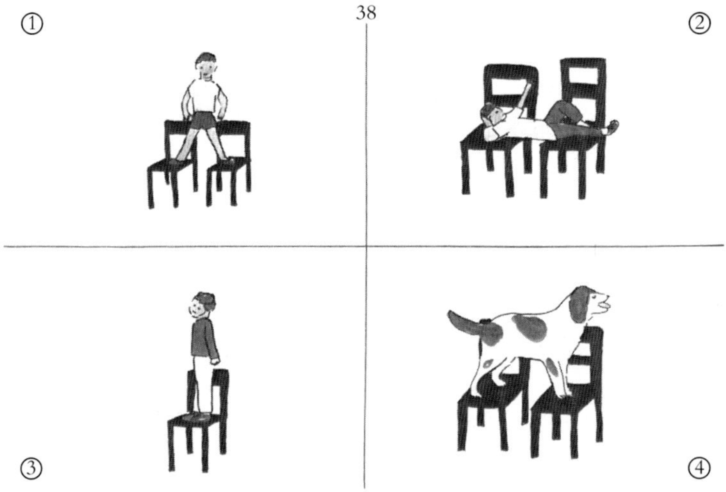

Figure 6.12. Sample item from the Test for Reception of Grammar (TROG; Bishop, 1983). The target sentence for this item is "The boy stands on the chairs," testing knowledge of number (chair/chairs). The TROG tests knowledge of a variety of morphosyntactic structures (see text for discussion) and is often used to evaluate linguistic knowledge in people with WS. Reprinted from TROG (Bishop, 1983), with permission of the Medical Research Council.

representing comparatives, passives, prepositional phrases, relative clauses, and negation. The test is normed, and so can yield an age equivalent for a given score—the age at which a normally developing child might be expected to attain that score. Karmiloff-Smith's results from the TROG showed that the WS participants (*M* age = 18) had a mean test age of 6 years, 3 months—clearly much lower than their chronological age, indicating impaired morphosyntax.

Karmiloff-Smith et al. then devised an experimental test of production to examine in detail people's control over the morphosyntax of gender in French. The rule they examined concerned the requirement in French to match the gender of the article, noun, and adjective in a noun phrase (*une chaise/la chaise/une chaise verte* versus *un tapis/le tapis vert*). Previous work by Karmiloff-Smith had shown that young normally developing children between 4 and 5 years of age have control of the grammatical gender of known words. In addition, the system of gender in French is probabilistically linked to the sounds of corresponding word endings; children of this age can also generalize the morphology to correct articles and adjectives for novel nouns (see Karmiloff-Smith et al., 1997).

Karmiloff-Smith et al. tested 14 native French speakers with WS (*M* age = 15;9, range = 9–22;6), and compared their performance to 18 native French-speaking children (*M* age = 5;1, range = 4;6–5;11). People were shown pictures of known items and novel items, named by noun phrases that represented either concord between the article and the noun's ending (e.g., feminine, *une flute*) or discord (e.g., feminine article, noun that ends in "masculine" ending, such as *une fourmi*). The novel words were constructed to fit these patterns as well.

People saw pairs of pictures for each item, and were either asked its name (known items) or given the name (for novel items, e.g., *une podine*). The two pictures in each pair were identical except for color. The experimenter put her ring under one of the pictures, and the person was then asked to tell the experimenter where the ring had been hidden. The natural response would be to produce a phrase including the article, the name of the object, and the color. The question was whether people with WS would follow the correct rules, in other words matching the gender of the article, noun, and adjective.

Results showed that both people with WS and normally developing children showed better performance for real than nonce words and for concord than discord cases. Moreover, both groups showed very good performance (low error rates) for the known nouns (around 5% for the WS group and 2% for the normally developing 5-year-olds). But the people with WS performed worse than normal children overall, and especially in cases involving production of phrases for nonce nouns that represent discord (e.g., *un bicronne*). Karmiloff-Smith et al. concluded that WS children only "weakly extract the underlying system of morpho-phonological oppositions on word endings" consistent with the idea that they are "good at associative learning and poor at system and theory building" (1997, p. 256). The authors further suggested that system building could be especially difficult in French, where the system of gender agreement is based on a complex, multiple cue system and must be applied across several items, in other words, article/noun/adjective.[12] In sum, they argued that people with WS show very errorful performance on a complex morphology task, suggesting that they have not acquired the morphological system that is so easily and completely acquired by normally developing children by age 5.

A recent study by Boloh, Ibernon, Royer, Escudier, and Danillon (2009) challenges Karmiloff-Smith et al.'s conclusions, and suggests instead a subtly different interpretation of the data. In a nutshell, Boloh et al. show that people with WS indeed look much like normally developing 5-year-olds, and that their weakness corresponds to elements of the system that are not normally acquired until much later on—age 15 or later.

Boloh et al. point out three methodological problems in the Karmiloff-Smith study. First, there are two separate problems to be solved in Karmiloff-Smith et al.'s task: *attributing* the correct gender to the noun, and then using the morphosyntactic rule to generate gender *agreement* between the article and adjective. If the person does not correctly attribute gender to the noun, but does know the morphosyntactic rule, he or she would produce the wrong gender morphology (by attribution), but do so for both article and adjective. This pattern would suggest an intact morphological system that simply generates the wrong gender attribution to the noun. Second, the worst performance was in the discordant condition, where the noun's sound suggests one gender, but the article provided is for the other gender. Boloh et al. suggest that people with WS could perform poorly in this discordant condition because of inattention to the sound of the noun, or the article, not for lack of knowing the morphosyntactic rule. Finally, normally developing children between 4 and 10 typically default to masculine morphology

[12] They compare this kind of system to the English system of tense and number, which they suggest is much more predictable and applies to just a single element (i.e., the stem). They suggest that this difference may explain the difference between their findings of weakness in gender assignment vis-à-vis Bromberg et al.'s (1994) findings that people with WS perform better using morphosyntactic rules that apply to regular forms than they do in retrieving irregular forms (see also Clahsen & Almazan, 1998).

in a similar production task (Boloh & Ibernon, 2010). If people with WS do this too, then they would be expected to perform at random for some sets of items, with 100% "correct" on masculine items and 0% on feminine items. Because Karmiloff-Smith et al. did not separately analyze masculine and feminine endings, it is possible that poor performance in WS people reflects the normal default pattern (to masculine endings), which would yield a pattern of highly accurate performance for masculine nouns, and at best random performance for feminine nouns.

Boloh et al. carried out the same general task used by Karmiloff-Smith et al., but now looked separately at the issue of gender *attribution* for the noun and gender *agreement* for articles and adjectives. To examine gender attribution, they provided a noun phrase with a (neutral) number adjective (e.g., *Voici trois kibains*), and then examined the article that was produced in test (e.g., *Le kibain*). To examine gender agreement, they asked whether the article and adjective matched in gender, regardless of accuracy of the gender assignment (e.g., *Le kibain vert/La kibain verte*). They also systematically examined the effects of specific gender (comparing masculine and feminine nouns), to see whether the pattern of masculine default held for people with WS as well as normally developing children. Finally, they included a condition with discordant nouns (different genders suggested by noun itself versus its article).

They tested 24 people with WS (*M* age = 15.2, range = 9;10–21;6), 24 normally developing children matched to the WS people for mental age (*M* age = 7.9, range = 4.9–12.1), and 24 normally developing people matched to the WS people for chronological age (*M* age = 15.3, range = 9;8–21;2). For gender *attribution* (examining the gender of articles produced), all groups were at ceiling for words with masculine suffixes (89–94%), but ranged from 32% to 49% correct for words with feminine suffixes. This is consistent with the pattern of masculine default for gender assignment observed in normally developing children ages 4–10 (Boloh & Ibernon, 2010). These findings suggest that in normal development, the masculine default is close to ceiling by age 4 or 5, and that it remains through age 15 (and possibly longer). Across groups, performance of the WS group did not differ from the normally developing mental age matches on this measure, but was lower overall than the chronological age matches. The overall profile within groups, however, was the same, with better performance on masculine than feminine nouns.

On the measure of *agreement*, Boloh et al. found that people in all groups performed very well in the basic (i.e., not discordant) condition (82.8% for WS, 90% for MA matches, 94.3% for CA matches). Scores of children with WS were no different from those of mental-age-matched controls, but were lower than chronological age matches. This suggests that gender agreement emerges solidly by age 4 or 5 in normally developing children (the youngest MA matches), and reaches this level among people with WS (who are older than the 4–5-year-old normal children). Finally, Boloh et al. found that errors were most prominent in the discordant condition; here the group with WS performed no differently from children matched for mental age, and both showed more errors than chronological age matches. This suggests no improvement in the WS group past the level attained by mental age matches (range = 4;9–12;1). This suggests an area of developmental arrest for producing agreement in cases where the noun and article suggest different genders. The mature system requires using the article as the final arbiter for gender matching.

The findings of Boloh et al. are sobering. Contra Karmiloff-Smith et al.'s claim that people with WS only "weakly extract the underlying system of morpho-phonological oppositions on word endings" (1997, p. 256), Boloh et al. show that the agreement scores of people with WS are no different from mental age matches, and only slightly lower than chronological age matches. Importantly, Boloh et al. note that errors crossing gender categories (a masculine determiner with a feminine adjective) were "almost non-existent" (2009, p. 16) in WS or normally developing child controls. Although the WS group performed poorly in the discordant condition, this was no different from the performance of mental age matches.

At the same time, the results suggest a picture of slow development followed by developmental arrest among people with WS. The two places where Boloh et al. found substantial development between the younger and older normally developing children (average ages 7 and 15 years) were also the places where the WS people were found to be no different from the younger children. These were in correct production of articles for feminine-ending nouns and in performance in the discordant condition, where one must resist the influence of the noun suffix and stick to the article to determine gender assignment of the adjective. Control over some aspects of morphology appears to be a long developmental process. We speculate that if there is developmental arrest in WS at the functional level of a 4- or 5-year-old, then those aspects of morphology that are acquired late in normal development may never be fully acquired by people with WS.

6.5.4 Syntax

The integrity of syntactic and semantic properties of language has, from the start, provided the core test bed for claims that language is "spared" in people with WS. In some of the earliest published observations, Bellugi et al. (1994) reported that people with WS had excellent grammatical abilities, including ceiling performance in tasks requiring that they match pictures to passive sentences (e.g., "The horsed is chased by the man"), accurate processing of sentences containing negation and conditionals, and verbal completion of sentences using tag questions ("John and Mary like apples, *don't they*?"). This was true despite the fact that they were mentally retarded, on average, and could not pass the classic Piagetian conservation tasks that are normally mastered by age 7. One of the key comparison groups for Bellugi was individuals with Down syndrome, who performed worse in the language tasks than the group with Williams syndrome. These two aspects of the language profile in WS led to the inference that language was "spared" relative to overall intelligence, suggesting the independence of language from general cognition.

A fair amount of research over the past 20 years suggests that the empirical and logical basis for this inference is probably not valid. First, it turns out that language levels are rather well predicted by overall levels of intelligence (Mervis & Becerra, 2007). People with WS very often perform either at, or close to, the levels of mental-age-matched children in standardized measures of language. Second, it appears that the comparison between WS and DS is most accurately interpreted as significant weakness in language (relative to overall intelligence) among people with DS, rather than significant strength in language (relative to overall intelligence) among people with WS.

These facts have suggested to some that the original conclusion of spared language in people with WS has now been proven false (Mervis & Becerra, 2007; Thomas, Karaminis, & Knowland, 2010). Unfortunately, the new conclusion—that language in people with WS is *not* spared—has had the effect of throwing the baby out with the bathwater. We now review evidence from several careful and thorough studies showing that key properties of syntax do emerge in people with Williams syndrome. The studies also show that these key properties are acquired by normally developing children by around age 5, suggesting again that the WS language profile is surprisingly like that of a normal 5-year-old. Several studies further hint that some aspects of syntax that are normally acquired over a more lengthy time period may never be fully acquired by people with WS.

6.5.4.1 Subject- and Object-Relative Clauses

The control of embedded clauses—in which one must retrieve elements that are absent in the surface structure of the sentence—has long provided a test for a central property of syntax. For example, compare these two sentences:

(a) The horse that kicked the boy drank some water.
(b) The horse that the boy kicked drank some water.

Understanding both sentences requires that the listener know that each sentence actually has a main clause and an embedded clause, in other words, two separate subsentences. Each of these subsentences has its own subject and object, even though they do not explicitly appear. For example, in sentence (a), the horse is the subject of the main clause, and water is the object. The embedded sentence has the horse as its subject (though it doesn't appear again), and the boy as the object. In sentence (b), the horse and water are again the subject and object of the main clause; but now the boy is the subject and the horse is the object of the embedded sentence. The absence of the explicit subject of the embedded sentence in (a) and of the explicit object in (b) are called "gaps," with the former a "subject-gap" sentence, and the latter an "object gap" sentence. Understanding what belongs in these gaps leads hearers to the inference that the boy was kicked in sentence (a), but did the kicking in sentence (b).

Subject- and object-relative clauses have been widely tested as instances of complex syntax in normal children, in children who are impaired, and in normal adults. In studies of people with WS, the mastery of subject- and object-relative clauses has been used to test the claim of spared syntax, but with different investigators arriving at different conclusions.

A good starting point in understanding these different conclusions is Zukowski (2009), who makes a crucial distinction between *knowledge* of relative clauses and *processing* of these structures. She notes that measures of comprehension (i.e., accurate processing and interpretation) of relative clause structures have been offered as one key piece of evidence for the argument that syntax in people with WS is not "intact" (Karmiloff-Smith et al., 1997; Mervis, Morris, Bertrand, & Robinson, 1999). These studies have used the TROG (Bishop, 1983), in which people hear sentences with object or relative clauses and are asked to match the sentence to one of four pictures. Overall, performance in people with WS is at best the same as in mental-age-matched children, and sometimes worse—a pattern we have observed in other aspects of language as well.

But as Zukowski points out, the TROG makes it impossible to distinguish between failure on the relevant items due to lack of *knowledge* of relative clause structure, and failures due to impaired *processing* that affects these structures. She further notes that one pattern evident in performance on relative clauses in the TROG is also a hallmark for normal adult processing of these clauses: Object-relative clauses are harder to process than subject-relative clauses. For example, normal adults who clearly have mature and full knowledge of grammar still have difficulty comprehending object-gap relative clauses compared to very similar subject-gap relative clauses (see, e.g., Gibson, Desmet, Grodner, Watson, & Ko, 2005). The relative difficulty with object-gap relatives is accentuated among normal individuals who have low working memory (Just & Carpenter, 1992).

To determine whether people with WS have control over the grammatical structures involved in relative clauses with gaps, Zukowski designed an elicited production task that created felicitous conditions for producing subject-gap and object-gap relative clauses in three different types of syntactic contexts. The production task is a strong test of grammatical knowledge, since one cannot produce a novel complex sentence without having knowledge of the relevant structures; the production machinery must furthermore make use of the structure to produce a sequentially organized output—a sentence.

Zukowski tested 10 children and adolescents with WS (*M* age = 12;5, range 10;0–16;3), and 10 normally developing children (*M* age = 6;0, range 4;6–7;6) who were individually matched to the WS participants using the nonverbal portion of the KBIT (Kaufman & Kaufman, 1990). Although there were no differences in these scores or on the verbal portion of the KBIT, the normally developing children received higher scores on the TROG, suggesting that, overall, these children were more advanced in sentence comprehension than the participants with WS. All participants were tested on the relative clause trials from the TROG as well as a novel production task that created felicitous conditions for people to produce either object or subject-gap relative clauses.

In this novel production task, Zukowski presented computerized images of two identical characters or objects that the experimenter described with simple active declaratives (e.g., "Here is a girl standing on a truck and here is a girl jumping over a truck"; see Figure 6.13). The experimenter then pushed a spacebar, and an animated mouse appeared, looking at one of the characters. The experimenter then asked the participant to tell a third party (usually the parent, who is seated opposite the participant, and cannot see the display) which object/character the mouse is looking at. This request invites the participant to individuate one of the characters, which naturally can result in using a relative clause with either a subject or object gap. For example, if the experimenter says, "OK, tell your mom which truck Max (the mouse) is looking at," then the participant might respond, "The truck that the girl is standing on/jumping over," producing an object-gap relative. Or, in the case of one boy who is waving and another boy who is washing his hair, the experimenter asks, "OK, tell your mom which boy Max is looking at," and the participant can respond with a subject-gap relative clause (e.g., "Max is looking at the boy who is waving").

Zukowski first examined the TROG scores for the relative clause items among her WS participants; she found that these scores were

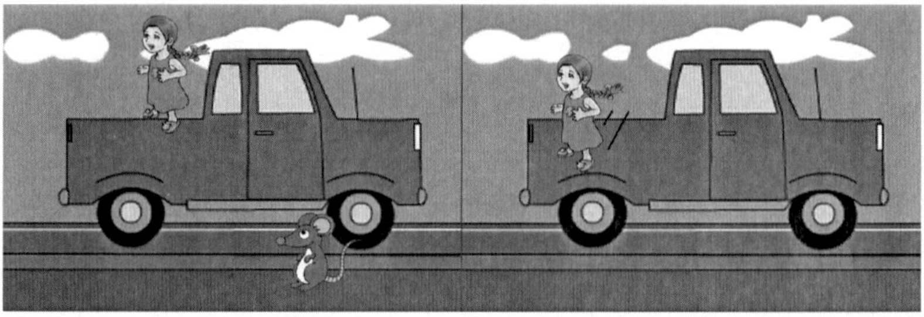

Figure 6.13. Types of test items used in Zukowski's (2009) study of production of sentences with object-relative and subject-relative clauses. In this example, each panel is described with simple active declaratives (e.g., "Here is a girl standing on a truck and here is a girl jumping over a truck"). Then an animated mouse appears, looking at one of the characters. The experimenter asks the participant to tell a third party which object/character the mouse is looking at. Here the mouse is in the left panel. So, the correct response would be: "Max (the mouse) is looking at the truck that the girl is standing on"—an example of a well-formed sentence with an object-gap relative clause. Zukowski's method proved to be effective in eliciting from WS participants complex grammatical productions such as these, even though the same participants performed poorly on a standardized test of their knowledge of relative clauses.

roughly in line with those reported by Karmiloff-Smith et al. (1997) and were lower than those of typically developing children. But the order of difficulty for the subject- and object-relative gaps was the same for both groups of WS participants and Zukowski's control group: All groups showed more difficulty with object gap than relative gap clauses. Indeed, the WS group showed roughly chance performance for object-gap items.

The crucial part of Zukowski's study, however, was the production task, which allowed her to determine much more clearly whether the scores in the TROG reflected lack of knowledge of the relevant grammatical structures or, alternatively, difficulty in mechanisms of processing. If people with WS can produce grammatical subject- and/or object-relative clauses, then they must have the grammatical knowledge required to generate these structures. Indeed, Zukowski found that almost every participant with WS successfully produced both structures in the appropriate inducing contexts. Not surprisingly, there was a strong asymmetry between subject-gap relatives and object-gap relatives, with the former produced much more frequently among all groups.[13] There were no group differences in production of the subject gaps; but in the object-gap condition, the people with WS produced fewer target sentences than either normal adults or normally developing children matched for mental age. This asymmetry is likely due to the relatively heavier dependence on working memory for object relatives, which is also reflected in the asymmetry in all groups in comprehension tasks such as the TROG. Although Zukowski did not test normally developing children who were even younger, we think it is quite possible that they would look comparable to the WS group. Notably, the error rates and patterns of the WS group were very similar to that of the normally developing children who were tested.

Three important points can be taken away from Zukowski's study. First, the data provide striking confirmation that people with WS are able to generate and produce grammatically well-formed relative clauses with both subject-relative and object-relative clauses. By the time they are about 10 years old, people with WS have the knowledge required to produce these complex linguistic structures. Second, this knowledge is normally acquired at least by the age of 5 or 6. Third, the poorer performance by WS people than by normally developing 6-year-olds on the TROG strongly suggests that factors other than the representation of linguistic knowledge per se adversely affect the performance of the WS group. Since the TROG requires that a person process a complex sentence, and then match it to one of four pictures, differences in working memory stand as an obvious possibility in explaining the difference. But the linguistic knowledge itself is present in both people with WS, at least

[13] Comparisons across groups (normal adults, people with WS, normally developing 6-year-olds matched to the WS group on mental age) showed that this subject-object gap asymmetry appeared for every group, although there were varying degrees of asymmetry. For example, normal adults produced subject-gap relatives 95.4% of the time in the appropriate inducing condition, whereas they produced object-gap relatives only 53.5% of the time in the appropriate inducing condition. Normally developing 6-year-olds produced subject-gap relatives 82.3% of the time in the appropriate inducing condition, and individuals with WS produced them 76.7% of the time. Object-gap relatives were produced 51% of the time among normally developing 6-year-olds in the appropriate inducing condition, and people with WS produced them 10% of the time.

by age 10, and by normally developing children, at least by age 6. This fact is consistent with the idea that people with WS undergo very slow development for this type of linguistic structure, but that they acquire it nonetheless.

6.5.4.2 Hierarchical Structure, C-Command, and the Interaction of "Not" and "Or"

Another case showing rich and complex linguistic knowledge in people with WS concerns several central properties of syntax and semantics. Musolino, Chunyo, and Landau (2010) examined the interaction of negation and disjunction ("or") as they are modulated by syntactic structure, in particular, hierarchical structure and the property of *c-command*, that is, the relationship between different nodes of the hierarchical tree. Their starting point was studies providing strong evidence for the existence of hierarchical structure and c-command in normally developing 5-year-olds (Lidz & Musolino, 2002). In these studies, children were given truth value judgment tasks, in which they were asked to judge the truth or falsity of complex sentences such as shown in (c) and (d) below. These sentences embody different hierarchical relationships between the elements of negation and disjunction, and therefore have quite different interpretations, as we now discuss.

In formal logic, one of De Morgan's laws of propositional logic states that when the logical relation of disjunction (*or*) is modified by negation, the result will be conjunction (for example, see Figure 6.14.) If we negate the disjunction "beer or wine," we get the reading "not beer" *and* "not wine." So if we say "John drank beer or wine," we mean he drank one or the other. But if we say "John didn't drink beer or wine," we mean that he drank *neither*—not beer and not wine.

Now it turns out that things are still more complex, since the effect of negation in the overall interpretation of a sentence depends on the position of the *negation* element in the hierarchical structure of the sentence. Specifically, each interpretation depends on the hierarchical position of the *negation* element relative to the element for disjunction, *or*. To illustrate, consider the following two sentences:

(c) The cat who meows will not be given a fish or milk.
(d) The cat who does not meow will be given a fish or milk.

$$\neg (P \vee Q) \Leftrightarrow (\neg P) \wedge (\neg Q)$$

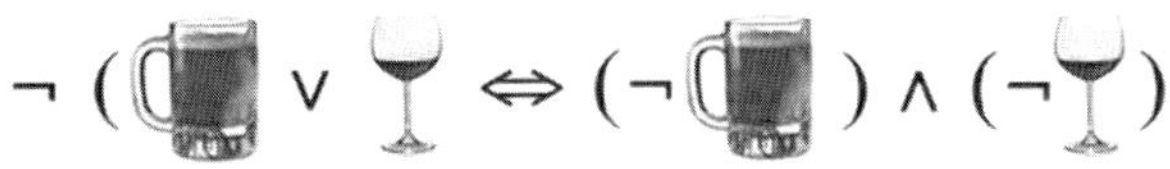

Figure 6.14. An illustration of one of De Morgan's laws of propositional logic: When the logical relation of disjunction is modified by negation, the result will be conjunction. For this image, the negation of the disjunction "beer or wine" yields the logical result "not beer" *and* "not wine."

In sentence (c), we understand that the cat did not get either item (i.e., he didn't get a fish AND he didn't get milk). In sentence (d), remarkably close to the other sentence in its individual elements, we understand something quite different—that the cat got either one or the other. The difference in meaning between these two sentences lies in the hierarchical location of the "negation" element (not) relative to the disjunction element (or). In sentence (c) but not (d), negation dominates (or c-commands) the disjunction element, allowing De Morgan's law to operate (see Figure 6.15).

Knowledge of De Morgan's laws, and it modulation by the hierarchical relation of the negation and disjunction element is a part of young children's knowledge, as shown by studies of Musolino and colleagues. Do people with WS also have such knowledge, and if so, what does this tell us about the nature and development of their linguistic knowledge more generally?

Musolino, Chunyo, and Landau (2010) carried out a series of studies in which they used the truth value judgment task to investigate this aspect of linguistic knowledge in 12 children and adults with WS (*M* age = 16;4, range = 11;10–21;11) and normally developing children. Two groups of normal children were included, 12 people in each group: The mental-age-matched group was around 6 years of age (*M* age = 6;1, range = 5;2–7;8) and was matched to the WS group using the KBIT matrices (nonverbal) scores (Kaufman & Kaufman, 1990). The second group was composed of normally developing children younger than the mental-age-matched group, averaging around age 4 (*M* age = 4;3, range = 4;0–4;11). Twelve normal adults were also tested.

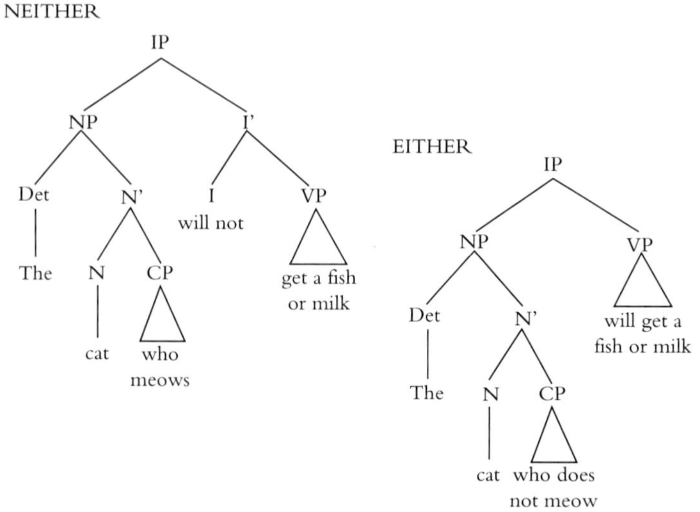

Figure 6.15. Two sentences whose lexical items are virtually identical have quite different meanings, caused by the different hierarchical relationships between the elements of negation (*not*) and disjunction (*or*). In the left panel, the relationship results in the meaning that the cat gets *neither* a fish nor milk; in the right panel, a different relationship results in a different meaning—this time, that the cat gets *either* one or the other. Musolino, Chunyo, and Landau (2010) tested children and adults with WS to determine whether they could represent complex grammatical facts such as these. The WS participants performed far above chance when asked to judge the meanings of such sentences, showing that they had knowledge of the relevant grammatical structures. Young normally developing children also master these structures by around age 4 or 5.

We asked two questions. The first concerned the nature of the linguistic knowledge possessed by children and adults with WS. Specifically, do they have knowledge of the semantics of negation and disjunction (*not*, *or*), and do they have knowledge of how the semantics of these terms interact under different hierarchical relations between the elements? If the WS group can determine the truth value of sentences that vary the hierarchical relation between *not* and *or*, and do so in a way that respects the relevant relationship of dominance (c-command), then we can conclude that their linguistic knowledge includes hierarchical structure, c-command, De Morgan's laws, and the relationship among these. The second question concerned the level of performance found among children and adults with WS, compared to normally developing children. If people with WS do have control over these linguistic structures and principles, how does this compare with that of normally developing individuals, and what does this tell us about language development—in both normal development and in Williams syndrome?

We included two experimental and four control conditions. The experimental conditions contrasted two different kinds of sentences. One type exhibited the proper hierarchical relations between negation (not) and disjunction (or) to yield the interpretation consistent with De Morgan's laws, as in sentence (c, above), and shown as (e) below. The second sentence had almost identical elements, but this time the negation and disjunction elements were in a hierarchical relation that violates De Morgan's law, as in sentence (f) below. Stimuli for these different conditions are shown in Figure 6.16.

(e) The cat who meows won't be given a fish or milk (i.e., the cat gets neither).

(f) The cat who doesn't meow will be given a fish or milk (i.e., the cat gets either).

The control conditions included four types of sentences that examined each of the components of these complex experimental sentences, in order to determine whether any aspect of the complex syntax and semantics relationships itself was especially difficult. These control conditions included sentences with relative clauses (e.g., "The man who has a red tie is walking the dog"), sentences with disjunction (e.g., "The policeman will get coffee or a doughnut"), sentences with negation (e.g., "The boy did not get a bicycle") and sentences with elements of negation and disjunction, which follow De Morgan's law (e.g., "The baseball player will not get the glove or the hat").

Experimental and control sentences were tested in contexts in which the participants viewed a simple set of animated vignettes that embodied either true or false situations corresponding to each sentence type (see Figure 6.16). The vignettes were accompanied by a prerecorded narration that introduced the characters, what he or she had, and so on.

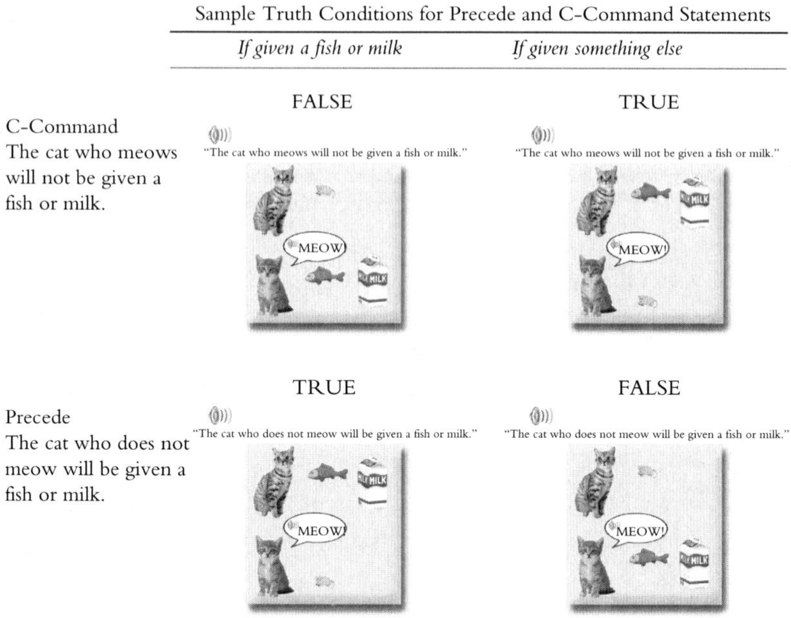

Figure 6.16. Sample scenes and true/false sentences accompanying each. The critical contrast is between the "C-command" sentences and the "Precede" sentences. Although both sentences have a *not* and an *or*, the hierarchical relationship between them is different in the two sentences, leading to two different truth value conditions. People watched animated vignettes and judged whether the sentence was true or false. For example, the sentence "The cat who meows will not be given a fish or milk" entails that the meowing cat gets neither, as shown in the upper right panel, where the cat gets a mouse, but neither a fish nor milk. Adapted from Musolino, Chunyo, and Landau (2010), with permission from Taylor & Francis.

Participants heard critical statements about what happened (i.e., the test sentences) at the beginning and end of each vignette. They were then asked to say whether the statement about the vignette was true or false. For example, in one vignette, two cats were portrayed, along with a fish, milk, and a mouse. One of the cats was shown meowing. Then that cat was given a mouse, and the other cat was given milk. The test sentence was "The cat that meows will not be given a fish or milk." For that particular vignette, the sentence was true. In other similar cases, it would be false (e.g., if the cat was given a fish).

In each of the six conditions (two experiments, four control), participants were tested on eight sentences, half true and half false, for a total of 48 test sentences. Analysis of the proportions correct for the four control conditions (negation, disjunction, relative clause, De Morgan) showed that the participants with WS and the normally developing children performed very well, achieving over 80% correct for each control, and with no reliable differences between the groups. In the experimental conditions, both groups again performed very well, with both groups achieving greater than 75% correct for each of the two experimental conditions. This result shows that people in both groups had control of the hierarchical relationships of *not* and *or*, and their interaction under the two different hierarchical relationships. Thus children and adults with WS do possess this linguistic knowledge.

At the same time, the WS participants performed reliably more poorly than the normally developing children (ages 5–7) who had been matched for mental age. Since the evidence points to knowledge of the complex structures in both groups, it seems likely that the difference in performance is linked to differences in the ability to process the complex sentences, which is likely to be strongly affected by differences in working memory, akin to the effects seen in the asymmetry between sentences with subject-relative and object-relative clauses (see Section 6.5.4.1). If so, then we might expect that normally developing younger children, who are likely to have weaker working memory, should perform worse than the 5–7-year-olds and might show comparable performance to the WS group.

A follow-up study of normally developing 4-year-old children showed that they did perform worse than the 5–7-year-olds on the experimental sentences (but not the control sentences), showing that there is some development on processing these complex structures between 4 and 7 years of age. More important, the WS group performed better than the 4-year-olds on the experimental sentences, although they had performed worse than the 5–7-year-olds. Figure 6.17 shows the performance of the WS group compared to the normally developing 5–7-year-olds (left panel) and 4-year-olds (right panel).

We can summarize the results of the Musolino et al. (2010) studies as follows. First, the absolute levels of performance by the people with WS provide compelling evidence that people with WS have control over

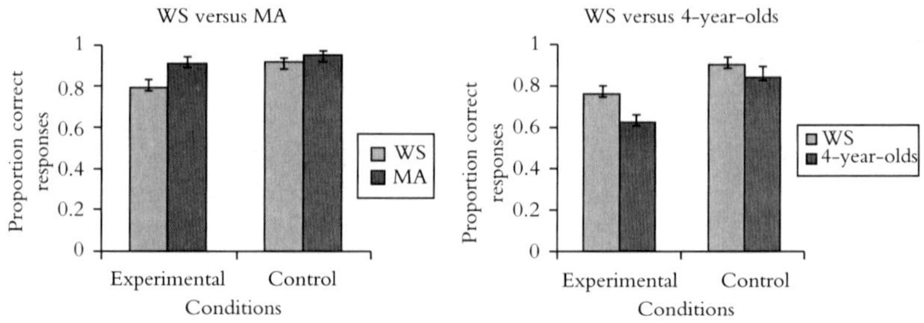

Figure 6.17. Proportion correct in the truth value judgment task testing hierarchical structure and its interaction with *not* and *or*. The left panel shows people with WS compared to normally developing children (*M* age = 6;1) matched for mental age to the WS participants. The right panel shows the same WS data plotted against normally developing 4-year-olds. In all cases, participants performed above chance. WS participants' level of performance was midway between the 4- and 6-year-olds. Adapted from Musolino, Chunyo, and Landau (2010), with permission from Taylor & Francis.

complex and rich aspects of linguistic structure—hierarchical structure, dominance relations, the relationship between *not* and *or*, and their modulation by different dominance relations. This is strong support for the idea that significant aspects of linguistic knowledge are, indeed, spared in WS. Second, the relative levels of performance, compared to normally developing children, show that the WS group (*M* age = 16) performs somewhat better than 4-year-olds, somewhat worse than children with an average age of 6 and roughly at the same level as 5-year-old normally developing children. This is precisely where we have seen this group fall on a number of other measures of language, and adds to our body of evidence that suggests that the WS individuals have undergone slow development, ending with arrest at the approximate level of a normally developing 5-year-old child. This slow development, however, includes the acquisition of rich linguistic knowledge—which is also acquired during the process of normal development by around age 5.

6.5.4.3 Binding, Raising, and Passives

The results from Zukowski and from Musolino et al. suggest that people with WS possess rich linguistic knowledge and control core aspects of grammatical structure. The results also suggest that these structures are acquired by normally developing young children at about 5 or 6 years of age. This pattern is consistent with the idea that people with WS develop a range of aspects of grammar but do so quite slowly—structures acquired by 5-year-old normally developing children are not acquired until adolescence or adulthood in people with WS. This raises the question of what happens with structures that are acquired at later developmental times by normally developing individuals.

One possibility is that language is severely *delayed* in people with WS; this is the hypothesis most widely offered by investigators, and would suggest that all structures are eventually acquired, but just on a very delayed timetable. For example, Wexler and colleagues (e.g., Perovic & Wexler, 2006, 2007) propose the specific grammatical delay hypothesis, which states that different aspects of grammar are differentially delayed in people with WS. A second possibility is that language in people with WS follows a pattern very similar to that of the spatial systems we have reviewed in previous chapters—it undergoes very slow development followed by arrest at an early functional level. This hypothesis has not been directly tested in the literature, but some recent data from Wexler and colleagues are remarkably consistent with it.

Wexler and colleagues (Perovic & Wexler, 2005, 2007, 2010) compared acquisition of three different kinds of structures whose acquisition in normal children ranges from early to quite late. They tested knowledge of three different kinds of grammatical processes: binding principles for reflexives and personal pronouns, passives, and raising. The patterns of performance across the three structure types were strikingly different: Performance on binding (linking pronouns with their anaphors) was strong in children and adults with WS, interpretation of passives was strong for action verbs but weak for psychological verbs, and knowledge of raising was uniformly poor.

Binding is acquired quite early in normally developing children, with good control of binding for reflexives by age 3, and binding options for personal pronouns acquired by around age 6 at least. Binding for reflexives allows a correct (reflexive) reading for the sentence "Mama bear washes herself" (meaning not another person), and binding options for personal pronouns allow a correct (nonreflexive) reading for the sentence "Mama bear washes her." Perovic and Wexler found that children and adolescents with WS (6–12 years old, 12–16 years old, respectively) performed at ceiling for binding of reflexives, and their performance was comparable to normally developing controls who were matched on vocabulary (using the PPVT); performance for the pronoun conditions was somewhat lower than the reflexive condition, but still very strong and no different from PPVT controls.

Passives, which were offered as a key example of sparing of language by Bellugi in early papers (Bellugi et al., 1988), resulted in a different story. Perovic and Wexler (2010) found that individuals with WS could accurately interpret passive action verbs (e.g., "Bart was pushed by Marge") and their performance was roughly in line with the normally developing children matched for scores on the PPVT. In contrast, the performance of people with WS for psychological verbs (e.g., "Bart was remembered by Marge") was poorer than for action verbs, and poorer than that of the normally developing PPVT controls, who performed quite well on both action and psychological verb passives. Perovic and Wexler note that there is a large literature showing that performance on passives for psychological verbs is at chance among normally developing 5-year-olds, and they argue that the action passives actually look strong early in normally developing children because these passive verbs are being represented as passive *adjectives*, which are often homophonous with the passive forms of the *verb* (e.g., "The toy is broken"). The fact that children and adolescents with WS also perform well on action verb passives, but poorly on psychological verb passives, suggests they are roughly equivalent to normally developing children around age 5.

Finally, Perovic and Wexler found that children and adolescents with WS (again, ages 6–16) performed poorly relative to normal controls on raising structures (e.g., "Marge seems to Homer to be driving a car"). Strikingly, their participants performed quite well on semantically equivalent sentences that did not involve raising (e.g., "It seems to Homer that Marge is driving a car"). Perovic and Wexler speculated that people with WS might never fully acquire raising structures.

The overall pattern shown in Perovic and Wexler's studies is consistent with the idea that people with WS develop slowly in their acquisition of binding and passives, that they may never develop control of raising structures, and, more generally, that they master what is acquired early in normal development, but may never fully normallly what normally develops later.

6.5.5 Summary of Pattern for Broad Aspects of Language

The pattern for nonspatial language looks remarkably similar to the pattern we observed for spatial language.

- Our studies of spatial language showed that people with WS have control over the semantic and syntactic organization of all key elements required to express the path component of motion events, the semantic organization of axial terms, and many more abstract uses of spatial terms.
- At the same time, we observed that each of these aspects of spatial language is also controlled by normally developing children between the ages of 4 and 5, and so appears quite early in the normal course of development. The normally later developments do not appear to be acquired by most people with WS, even into adulthood, suggesting developmental arrest.
- Our review of nonspatial language also suggests very slow development followed by arrest at an early functional level. People with WS show the same rich knowledge of syntax and semantics as is shown by young normally developing children. However, the WS mature performance falls on average at the level of a normally developing 5-year-old.

The pattern for spatial and nonspatial language has also been echoed in aspects of nonlinguistic spatial representation that we have reviewed in previous chapters. All of this raises the question of what kind of developmental model could account for this more general cognitive profile. In our final chapter, we turn to some possibilities.

7

Conclusions

Revisiting the Puzzle of Williams Syndrome

We began our book with the following puzzle: How could a small set of missing genes result in the unique cognitive profile of individuals with Williams syndrome? The original description of this profile centered on the severe impairment in spatial cognition, together with richly structured language. This unusual combination of strength and weakness across cognitive domains suggested to some a model in which specific genes have strong control over the development of specific cognitive systems. But in our first chapter, we cautioned that any simple model that attempts to explain the role of genes in the development of cognition would likely fail at present, and that detailed models await further understanding of the action of genes, as well as further understanding of the cognitive profile. Our goal in the book has been to understand, in detail, the nature of the spatial profile in people with Williams syndrome, in the hopes that it will ultimately contribute a theoretically driven and empirically rich body of knowledge that can be used to understand the complex path from genes to cognition.

In this final chapter, we put together the findings we have reported throughout the book and suggest a speculative hypothesis about the nature of the spatial profile in WS, how it emerges, and how it fits with the organization of normal spatial development. As a bonus, we also propose that this hypothesis can account for the WS profile in language. The hypotheses draw strongly on our original framework, in particular, on the three principles we articulated in Chapter 1: the importance of a detailed understanding of cognition, the importance of specialization of function in understanding the spatial profile in people with WS, and the importance of developmental timing—especially that of normal development—in understanding why the WS cognitive profile appears to be so unique. In a nutshell, we argue in support of the idea that people with WS do indeed have a cognitive profile that has both peaks and valleys within the domain of space and across the domains of space and language. But crucially, we also argue for *rethinking* the mechanisms underlying the profile. Specifically, we propose that the peaks and valleys in the WS spatial profile reflect the effects of at least two different developmental mechanisms, giving rise to two different—but mutually compatible—kinds of explanations for the spatial profile. We will propose that the same explanations can account for the WS profile for language.

We summarize in advance our interpretation of the data in the context of three principles. The first principle is the importance of cognition. A primary thesis of our book has been that understanding the link between genes and cognition requires hard work at each end of the causal chain. Citing Ramus (2006) again, this understanding "can only be as good as the characterization of the phenotype, and cognitive phenotyping is (or should be) in the hands of cognitive scientists" (p. 249). That is, regardless of what we know or come to know about the mechanisms underlying the genetic deletion in WS, or the structural and/or functional characteristics of the WS brain, we can fully understand the WS spatial profile only if we have a firm understanding at the level of *cognition*. An especially clear example comes from our analysis of the block construction task. There is no single region of the brain, or any single cognitive system, that is "the block construction system." This task—like many others—is complex, engaging a variety of mechanisms. Only by systematic task analysis can one dissect the range of cognitive components that are engaged when one re-creates a complex pattern. More generally, we have seen that the description of people with WS as having "severe spatial impairment" can be unfolded into a much more detailed profile across the several systems of human spatial representation. Our task has been to specify in as much detail as possible this *cognitive* end of the causal chain.

The second principle is *specialization of function*. We propose that the organization of spatial representation in people with WS—like that of normally developing individuals—is highly specialized. Specialization is evidenced in both normally developing children and in people with WS by the rich but structurally distinct nature of the representations underlying different spatial functions. It is also evidenced by our observations of different developmental trajectories in *normally developing* children across a broad range of spatial functions, with some functions reaching mature levels early in childhood, while others undergo prolonged developmental change, reaching maturity only in adolescence. Specialization is also reflected by evidence that in people with Williams syndrome, the spatial profile also shows relative strengths and weaknesses, with one key spatial system—reorientation—showing extreme fragility.

The third principle is *the importance of developmental timing*. We propose that for many (but not all) spatial functions, people with WS undergo very slow development, followed by developmental arrest at an early functional level. This results in a profile for many spatial functions that looks remarkably similar to that of a normally developing child between the ages of 4 and 6. Using the second and third principles, we will account for the range of cognitive findings we have reported.

The principles of specialization and developmental timing require that we embrace two ideas about the organization of human cognition in normal adults and children: One is that specialization of function plays a large role in the structure of the human mind and brain, and the second is that different spatial functions (and indeed, different aspects of cognition) undergo different developmental trajectories in normal and unusual development. This means that some aspects of spatial representation will develop early in life under normal circumstances, whereas other aspects will undergo a long developmental trajectory toward maturity. The same differences in developmental trajectory are likely to be true for spatial development in people with WS. Once we look through the lens of normal development, much of what appears to be unique in people with WS is actually remarkably like that of a much younger normally developing child. Equally important are those aspects of spatial representation that are *not* like that of a much younger child. Both sets of facts need to be explained.

In the next sections, we explore the two principles of specialization of function and developmental timing in the context of the cognitive evidence we have reported throughout the book. We begin with the hypothesis of specialization of function, returning to the two candidate divisions of labor that we discussed in Chapter 1—domain specificity within the visual system versus specificity over broader streams of the visual system (the dorsal and ventral streams). We then discuss the hypothesis of developmental timing, reviewing our findings on the spatial profile in people with WS relative to the normally developing groups we have tested. In this section, we also engage the issue of specialization, by asking about the character of the spatial acquisitions that are acquired early, and those that appear to undergo longer developmental trajectories.

The facts lead us to suggest that many of the early emerging spatial functions embody richly structured representations that are evidenced in people with WS as well as normally developing children who are much younger. We also argue that the same story holds for language. That is, early acquired aspects of representation in both space and language—richly structured as they are—show that specialization of function plays a strong role in guiding development in people with WS as well as those who are unaffected. But specialization of function is modulated by developmental trajectory—some functions are normally acquired early in development, some later. *We hypothesize that people with WS undergo very slow development followed by arrest at the functional level of a normally developing 4–6-year-old, resulting in a spatial (and language) profile for people with WS that embodies mature levels of acquisition for only those functions that are normally acquired early in development.*

Finally, we suggest a way of fitting what we know about space (and language) into the broader context of the WS cognitive profile. If, as we will argue, people with WS undergo slow development followed by arrest at the functional level of a 4–6-year old, then how can we account for the fact that they continue to grow and learn throughout their lifetime, showing systematic increases in vocabulary, becoming more skilled in the block construction task, and developing some skill in reading and mathematics? We conclude the book by speculating on how these additional skills and capacities coexist with the profile of severe limitations in many of the more basic cognitive functions, and we raise optimistic questions about possible effects of education and training in children and adults with WS.

7.1 Specialization of Function

In Chapter 1, we discussed two different divisions of labor in the visual-spatial systems that could be important in accounting for the WS spatial profile. One division posits a high degree of specialization in the mind and brain for different *domains*, including, for example, the representation of objects, places, faces, and navigation. The second division posits specialization across different *streams* of processing in the visual system, including functions primarily carried by the ventral stream (e.g., objects, faces, places), and those carried by the dorsal stream (e.g., visual-manual action, the representation of reference systems, attentive object tracking). Both of these hypotheses would be consistent with a profile of peaks and valleys in the spatial domain, which we have amply documented. In contrast, the profile of peaks and valleys within spatial representation would be *inconsistent* with the idea that all spatial systems develop using the same representational primitives, under the same general learning principles, at the same rate, and with the same developmental trajectories. The idea of such a "flat" profile can be ruled out, given the evidence.

7.1.1 Specialization of Function by Domain

Two kinds of evidence provide some support for this hypothesis. First, many aspects of spatial representations in people with WS embody rich, articulated structures that are also evident in normally developing individuals. Thus even in a genetic deficit that results in severe spatial impairment, the *qualitative* nature of spatial representations in people with WS are like those of normally developing individuals. Second, there is a stark contrast between two aspects of the WS profile: strength in the face domain and weakness in some aspects of reorientation.

7.1.1.1 Spatial Representation in People With WS Embodies Rich and Highly Differentiated Structure, as in Normal Development

One clear example concerns the representation of reference systems in people with WS. Reference systems—often conceived of as Cartesian coordinates centered on an object, an array, the body, and so on—are foundational to the representation of location. Without a system of axes and direction that is centered on an origin (i.e., the reference object), our ability to represent and remember the locations of objects would be radically deficient. In several studies, we showed that children and adults with WS possess representations of axes and direction within axes, and these mental structures are used in tasks as diverse as matching locations, copying locations, and naming locations. The existence of these basic representational systems among people with WS—as well as normally developing children—attests to the robust nature of this system in both normal and unusual development.

Specialization of function was also evident in the results of our language studies, which demonstrated the acquisition and control of complex linguistic structures among people with WS as well as normally developing children. The ability to understand the semantic difference between sentences such as "The cat who meowed will not be given a fish or milk" and "The cat who did not meow will be given a fish or milk" relies on the mental representation of hierarchical grammatical structures and relationships of dominance between elements such as "not" and "or." These representational elements and relationships are nowhere to be found in the spatial systems that we have studied, and the qualitative differences between the representations required for language and those required for representing and remembering locations attest to the high degree of specialization across different cognitive systems. Representations of both kinds are present in people with WS.

Specialization of function is also attested by our perceptual studies examining thresholds for motion coherence, biological motion, and form-from-motion. These different kinds of motion perception have somewhat different computational requirements, and have been linked to specific but different brain regions in adults (Oram & Perrett, 1994; Schenk & Zihl, 1997; Vaina et al., 1990). We reported that the three kinds of motion perception showed very different profiles among people with WS: Motion coherence thresholds were at the same level for WS children and adults as for normally developing 4–7-year-olds and normal adults. Biological motion thresholds for WS children and adults were lower (i.e., better) than the normally developing 4–7-year-olds, and no different from normal adults. And form-from-motion thresholds for WS children were higher (i.e., worse) than either normally developing 4–7-year-olds or normal adults, but thresholds for WS adults were no different from normally developing 4–7-year-olds, and higher (i.e., worse) than normal adults (Jordan et al., 2002; Reiss et al., 2005). These results suggest that the three different kinds of motion perception have distinct developmental signatures (with different developmental timetables), and that part of the WS profile may be linked to that signature—a topic we take up more extensively in the next section. More generally, however, the pattern of peaks and valleys within the several distinct systems of motion perception attests to the importance of considering specialization of function as a clear driving force in development.

7.1.1.2 Face Perception Versus Reorientation

The second kind of evidence for specialization of function by domain is the stark contrast between the abilities of people with WS when they engage in face perception tasks and their performance when they undergo disorientation and must reorient themselves in space. The evidence we reviewed on face perception strongly suggests that the representation of faces is quite similar to that of normally developing individuals of the same chronological age. Several studies of face perception have documented normal inversion effects among people with WS (Tager-Flusberg et al., 2003; see review in Chapter 3). Two independent studies using brain imaging techniques during passive viewing of faces showed similarity between people with WS and chronological age matches in both the location and size of the region that is activated during face processing (O'Hearn et al., 2010; Sarpal et al., 2008). The region in people with WS is the same as the one activated in normally developing children and adults (Kanwisher, 2010; Scherf et al., 2007).

In contrast, we found that at least some people with WS cannot use the geometric structure of the surrounding layout as the sole source of information in reorienting themselves after disorientation.[1] The task we used was one that has been very widely used in the field, with human toddlers, children, and adults, as well as a broad range of species, showing clear sensitivity to geometric properties of the surround (see Landau & Lakusta, 2009, for review). The signature geometric response after disorientation has been shown in all of these groups, and although there is debate on whether the reorientation system is modular (see, e.g., Cheng & Newcombe, 2005), there is no debate on whether the basic phenomenon of geometric responding exists and is privileged across many

[1] We should temper this with understanding that our experiment used just a single method of looking for sensitivity to geometric structure, so it is always possible that another method will reveal the ability to represent the geometry of scenes, and to use it in reorientation.

species. To our knowledge, the only evidence for a reliable failure to use geometric information comes from studies of rats, pigeons, and chicks with hippocampal lesions (Jones, Pearce, Davies, Good, & McGregor, 2007; Tommasi, Gagliardo, Andrew, & Vallortigara, 2003; Vargas, Petruso, & Bingman, 2004). The evidence we presented on reorientation in people with WS strongly suggests that this system of representation—underlying the capacity to reorient using the geometric structure of the environment—is severely compromised in some individuals. The contrast between the observed failures to reorient using geometric information and the strength in face processing reported for people with WS is clearly consistent with the theoretical idea that the spatial representational systems in humans are specialized, and that missing genes can ultimately have more significant impact on certain spatial systems while leaving others unimpaired in their basic structure.

In sum, two kinds of evidence are consistent with the hypothesis of specialization of function by domain. One is the set of rich structural differences across knowledge domains that are shown by people with WS as well as normally developing individuals. The second is the striking difference between the functionality of two distinct systems of representation in people with WS: face processing and the geometry-based system of reorientation.

7.1.2 Specialization of Function by Stream of Visual Processing: Dorsal Versus Ventral Streams

The differences between streams of processing in the visual system have long been useful to scientists in understanding the structure of the visual system as well as its breakdown under brain damage. Moreover, the idea has been appealing to developmental cognitive scientists, and has served as a handy organization by which to think about some puzzles in normal development. For example, decades of research have been dedicated to understanding the striking contrast between the failures shown by infants when they search manually for objects and their rich understanding of objects when measured by their looking time (see, e.g., Baillargeon, 2004). Several scientists have proposed that this discrepancy reflects a developmental lag in the dorsal stream (i.e., visual manual action) compared to the ventral stream (i.e., perceptual judgments measured by looking time) (see, e.g., Bertenthal, 1996; Johnson, Mareschal, & Csibra, 2008). Beyond the object concept in infants, a number of scientists have proposed that the dorsal stream generally lags behind the ventral stream in normal development (Johnson et al., 2008), and others have suggested that this lag may result in the dorsal stream being more sensitive to experience, as well as having greater susceptibility to neurological insult (Neville & Bavelier, 2000). Finally, several scientists have proposed that the cognitive profile in people with Williams syndrome is a dorsal stream deficit (Atkinson et al., 2003; Wang, Doherty, Rourke, & Bellugi, 1995).

However, evidence supporting an omnibus lag in the development of dorsal stream functions (relative to ventral stream) has not been forthcoming. Although there are selective cases where it appears that a particular dorsal stream function develops along a lengthier trajectory than a particular ventral stream function, there is no evidence that the dorsal stream in totality undergoes lengthier development, nor is there evidence that the ventral stream in totality undergoes rapid and early development. For example, Mareschal and Johnson (2003) found that 4-month-old infants were able to represent and detect changes of object identity but not object location, suggesting that identity (presumably a ventral stream function) matures earlier than object location (presumably a dorsal stream function). Similarly, Neville (reviewed in Neville & Bavelier, 2000) has shown that congenital deafness affects sensitivity to stimuli in the periphery of the visual field (which maps to the dorsal stream) more than sensitivity to stimuli in the central visual field (which maps to the ventral stream). At the same time, Street, James, Jones, & Smith (2011) found that 18-month-olds who could not insert an oriented object into a slot could nevertheless accurately orient their bare hand to the slot. The action of orienting the hand to a goal (the slot) would appear to be a clear case of engaging the sensorimotor areas of the brain, part of the dorsal stream, but it is acquired earlier than the more complex act of coordinating orientations of hand, object, and goal.

Part of the difficulty here is that we have limited understanding of the full complement of spatial functions that engage the dorsal versus the ventral stream. In addition, for the most part, studies of ventral stream functioning have not always been carried out with contrasts that allow comparisons to the development of dorsal stream functioning. Applying the dorsal versus ventral stream hypothesis to the case of Williams syndrome, we encounter the further difficulty that we need a rationale for deciding why the functions of one stream—but not the other—might be selectively impaired. Neville and Bavelier (2000) argued sensibly that dorsal stream functions will necessarily need to undergo longer postnatal development than ventral stream functions simply because experience is crucial to some functions that require tuning. Specifically, if a range of dorsal stream functions involve coordination between the world and one's growing body, then there will have to be developmental room to continually tune the system in accord with the changing body parameters. And a lengthier developmental trajectory will necessarily make the system more vulnerable to insult.

This idea by itself generates the interesting prediction that many (but not all) dorsal stream functions should undergo lengthier developmental trajectories than many (perhaps not all) ventral stream functions—an idea that we return to in the next section. But the case of Williams syndrome offers us a separate and additional rationale for making the prediction that this syndrome should be accompanied by selective impairment in dorsal stream functions. This is the evidence from studies of brain structure in people with WS. At least one part of the dorsal stream in people with WS—the area around the IPS—appears to have abnormal structure, possibly resulting in a variety of spatial-cognitive impairments in functions that normally engage the IPS and areas further upstream along the dorsal stream (Meyer-Lindenberg et al., 2004).

The hypothesis of dorsal stream abnormality in people with WS would predict that spatial functions engaging the IPS and parietal areas, as well as areas of the sensorimotor cortex, should be impaired, whereas functions engaging the ventral stream should be preserved. Because the area of the IPS is involved in many cognitive functions, including number (Hubbard, Piazza, Pinel, & Dehaene, 2005) and individuation (Xu & Chun, 2009), we might also expect deficits in these functions. Because the ventral stream supports functions such as object and face representation, the hypothesis would predict sparing of these functions, or at least distinct strength relative to dorsal stream functions.

On first glance, the evidence we have presented appears to fare well with respect to the hypothesis that Williams syndrome can be characterized as a dorsal stream deficit. We have shown that a wide variety of spatial functions normally engaging parts of the dorsal stream are severely impaired in children and adults with WS, with their performance systematically falling to the level of a normally developing 4- or 5-year-old child. The spatial functions we examined included the ability to track multiple moving objects, to represent and use axes and direction within axes, and to carry out visual-manual actions as apparently simple as posting a card into an oriented slot.

By contrast, we also showed that certain tasks involving object and face processing—domains that are known to involve the ventral stream—result in surprisingly strong performance. For example, children with WS could identify briefly presented objects under canonical viewpoints at high levels, close to the levels of normal adults. We described the findings of other labs that showed effects of face inversion in people with WS that were comparable to those in normal adults (Tager-Flusberg et al., 2003) as well as two sets of findings showing that the brain areas engaged during face processing in WS were similar in size and location to those of normal chronological age-matched controls. Finally, there were two distinct areas of difficulty within the general domain of object representation, and these, too, fit generally with the idea of dorsal stream impairment. For example, children with WS showed distinct weakness in recognizing objects under unusual views, with performance roughly like that of a normally developing 4–6-year-old child. Recognition under unusual views is often impaired in adults who sustain lesions to the parietal areas (Warrington, 1982), consistent with the idea that the weakness might reflect impairment in the dorsal stream. And children and adults with WS showed significant difficulties in object matching tasks that required perceiving and storing handedness (i.e., left-right relationships within the object), with performance roughly at the level of a normally developing 5-year-old. Like the case of unusual views, the representation of handedness has been tied to engagement of the parietal areas (Riddoch et al., 2004).

Although these findings do fit the idea of a dorsal stream deficit, there are a few crucial caveats. First is the case of motion coherence. Recall that children and adults with WS showed thresholds for perception of motion coherence that were no different from normal adults (Section 3.2.2.3). Motion coherence is considered to be a dorsal stream function, but here we have a pattern of performance that suggests that people with

WS acquire *this* spatial function at adult levels. Notably, we also saw that adult thresholds for motion coherence were attained in normally developing children by age 4. That is, the ability to detect motion coherence is early emerging (as measured by our task), and people with WS reach maturity on it. This clearly rules out the hypothesis of an omnibus dorsal stream deficit in people with WS.

Second, several studies have reported substantial weakness in areas of the ventral stream that are linked to the perception of houses and scenes (Meyer-Lindenberg et al., 2006; O'Hearn et al., 2010). These regions include the parahippocampal gyrus (parahippocampal place area, PPA), which has strong connections with the hippocampus and parietal areas, involved in navigation and reorientation. Thus, although aspects of object face perception are relatively strong in people with WS, other aspects of ventral stream processing are clearly impaired. The case of motion coherence shows strength in a dorsal stream task; the case of house perception shows weakness in a ventral stream task.

These cases suggest the need to reconsider the idea of a general dorsal stream deficit, with ventral stream sparing. Although the dorsal/ventral stream organization is useful, it appears to be limited in accounting for the detailed pattern of strengths and weaknesses in WS. As we will see in the next section, it is illuminating to think about overall patterns of strengths and weaknesses within the context of *normal* developmental trajectories. When we do this, we will see that much of the WS spatial profile may be driven by a factor that operates across spatial domains—and even includes language.

7.2 Developmental Timing

We have already hinted that examining the normal developmental trajectory of many different spatial functions might shed light on the pattern of strengths and weaknesses observed in people with WS. We now make this explicit by considering two questions: First, what is the nature of normal developmental trajectories across spatial functions? Second, how does the spatial profile of people with WS map onto that trajectory? We follow this discussion with a speculative hypothesis about a mechanism that would generate this mapping.

7.2.1 Two Examples

It should be obvious from the range of evidence we have presented that normally developing children show substantial changes in performance across the wide range of spatial tasks we have used. Let's start with two examples: object recognition and visual-manual action versus perception.

We showed that even 4-year-olds were very accurate at correctly identifying familiar objects when they were briefly presented (1/2-second exposure) as full-color, clear images in canonical viewpoints. The level of accuracy was above 80% for 4-year-olds, increasing to 90% for 6-year-olds and 95% for 12-year-olds, right around the level of normal adults. The levels were quite similar for black-and-white line drawings, even though all color and surface texture had been removed. The 4-year-olds' performance in this task suggests that object recognition from canonical viewpoints normally emerges quite early in development. We do not mean to suggest that this task, and only this task, should be used to evaluate "age of acquisition" of object recognition; we simply make the point that, for this particular task and set of stimuli, even 4-year-olds perform quite well, and there is not much change between their performance and that of normal adults.

By contrast, when the same objects were presented under unusual viewpoints, we observed substantial change over the same age range. The 4-year-olds now were correct only about 75% of the time, whereas 6-year-olds were correct about 78% of the time and 12-year-olds were correct about 88% of the time; normal adults were correct about 95% of the time. Thus there was more developmental change in recognition and accurate naming of unusual views objects between ages 4 and 12 than there was for canonical views. Recognition of objects from canonical views is acquired early in life, close to maturity by the age of 4; but recognition from unusual viewpoints requires considerably more developmental time, not reaching mature levels until adolescence. Moreover, comparing the normal 4- and 6-year-olds suggests that much development in recognition of objects presented in unusual views takes place between the ages of 6 and 12. The idea that object perception undergoes development is consistent with findings from Scherf et al. (2007) showing significant changes in the size and location of brain areas engaged during passive viewing of objects between the ages of 6 and 12. Although Scherf et al. focused on ventral stream activation, they did not use objects that explicitly varied in viewpoint, and their participants did not identify the objects they saw. Based on our evidence and the evidence for parietal involvement in the recognition of objects presented in unusual views (e.g., Warrington, 1982; see Chapter 3), we suspect that the developmental changes we observed in unusual view recognition may be correlated with changes in the parietal areas over development.

Taking this developmental trajectory as the lens through which to examine performance by people with WS, we observe that WS children and adolescents (7–15 years, *M* age = 11) were slightly better than normal 4-year-olds in the canonical views condition, but no different from them in the unusual views condition. The WS group was also no different from normally developing 6-year-olds, perhaps not surprising as there was little developmental change between 4 and 6 among the normally developing children.

This pattern suggests the following: Children and adolescents with WS recognize briefly presented objects in canonical orientations at roughly the level of normally developing 4–6-year-olds. They do so when objects are presented in full color and with textural information, and when the objects are presented as line drawings, which requires that identification be done on the basis of overall shape without color or texture. This achievement is considerable: The task of recognizing objects at far better than chance levels under the demanding conditions of our experiment, suggests an object recognition system that has a great deal of structure. But importantly, this considerable achievement is also reached by normally developing 4-year-olds.

The case of visual-manual action and perception makes a similar point. In our tasks, we asked people to either "post" a card into an oriented slot (like a letter being inserted into a mailbox slot) or tell us when the card had been rotated (by someone else) to a position that would allow insertion. The results showed that normally developing 4-year-olds were considerably less accurate when they were asked to post than when they were asked to judge the orientation; by the time children were 6 years of age, they were quite accurate in both tasks, with no difference between perception and action. There was substantial developmental change from ages 4 to 6 in accuracy for the posting task, but less in the perceptual match task, showing that the visual-manual action task was still undergoing development at a time when the "comparable" perceptual matching task was close to ceiling. Thus, there were substantial differences in the developmental trajectories of the two tasks, with visual-manual action normally undergoing a longer trajectory than perceptual matching. This is similar to what we observed in the case of object recognition, with little development in normal children beyond age 4 in the recognition of objects under canonical views, but substantial development between 4 and 12 in the recognition of unusual views.

In the posting task, the performance of children and adults with WS was no different from normally developing 4-year-olds, suggesting that the WS group had reached this level of accuracy and essentially remained there.[2] The WS group also showed more accurate performance on the perceptual match task than the posting task, as was also true of the normally developing 4-year-olds. This case again reveals a pattern in which different spatial functions—even those that have much in common on the surface—normally undergo different trajectories: In this case, a type of visual-manual action lags behind perceptual matching. The WS pattern of worse performance in the action task than the perception task suggests that the WS individuals, as a group, were quite similar to normally developing 4-year-olds.

Both of these cases suggest the possibility that spatial functions that normally reach maturity early in development are likely to be those that develop fully in people with WS; by contrast, functions that normally undergo a longer developmental trajectory may never reach maturity. In people with WS, many spatial functions appear to reach the level of a normally developing 4- or 5-year-old child and remain there through adulthood.

7.2.2 Extension to Other Spatial Functions

The WS pattern of achievement for spatial functions that normally emerge early in development—by roughly age 4 or 5—is echoed across

[2] It is quite possible that training would have a beneficial effect on performance in this task, improving the accuracy of adolescents and adults with WS. Here, we simply make the point that without any training, the pattern for adults is very much like that of normal 4-year-olds.

a number of different cases we have reported in previous chapters. For example, the pattern is consistent with our review of perceptual functions that we described as part of "mid-level" vision (see Chapter 3). Consider the perception of illusions. The mechanisms by which we perceive illusions require that visual information be integrated over space. From that perspective, one might assume that people with WS would be faulty, or perform poorly in judging, say, which of two displays shows the "longer" arrow. Yet we found that, for three of four illusions we tested, people with WS showed the same thresholds and magnitude of perceived illusions as normal adults; crucially, these adult-like thresholds also reached maturity in normally developing children around age 4 (Palomares, Ogbonna, Landau, & Egeth, 2009).

Similarly, when we examined the ability to integrate oriented elements to generate the percept of a line, we found that people with WS had thresholds that were like those of normal adults; and these thresholds were attained by normally developing children by around age 5 (Palomares, Landau, & Egeth, 2009). By contrast, thresholds for orientation *discrimination* among people with WS were far from adult-like, and were more like those of normally developing 4-year-olds, who had not reached maturity. Unlike orientation *integration*, the task of explicitly *discriminating* orientation appears to undergo a lengthy developmental trajectory, with mature (adult-like) normal performance not appearing until age 9 or older. In these cases, people with WS—older children, adolescents, and adults—performed like normal adults when the function itself reached maturity early in normal development. But when the function was one that undergoes a lengthy developmental trajectory toward maturity—like explicit judgment of orientation—people with WS again performed like normally developing 4- or 5-year-olds. In this case, we have two critical facts. The first is the age equivalence—the person with WS is performing like a normal 4–5-year-old. The second is that the spatial function in question normally undergoes considerably more growth, with maturity only reached years later. Under this combination of facts, the person with WS has a "severe deficit" because he or she is like a person who is much younger, *and* has apparently never undergone the continued development needed for mature performance. The issue, thus, is *where* in the developmental curve the WS system finds itself: If the spatial function normally reaches maturity by age 4, people with WS will have reached this point by adolescence or adulthood, and will therefore show mature performance. If the spatial function normally continues to develop past age 4, 5, or 6, it seems likely that people with WS will still show a 4- or 5-year-old pattern, and hence—as adults—will never have reached maturity, and will be severely impaired.

Other examples that fit this pattern come from our review of the variety of spatial functions generally required to represent objects in places (Chapter 4). There, we saw that children and adults with WS were qualitatively similar to normal 6-year-olds in their representation of two sets of orthogonal axes, but that their use of direction within each axis was weaker than children of this age. This difficulty with direction had serious consequences for the use of spatial terms indicating locations *above/below/right/left*, and we observed errors of direction in language comprehension (e.g., *left* for *right*) even among adults with WS. Although we did not have evidence from normally developing children younger than about age 5 on the axes tasks, the literature tells us that such directional errors in language are common among 4- and 5-year-olds. Again, this is consistent with the idea that people with WS reach the level of 4–5-year-olds in their use of directional language, but that they have difficulty moving past this point to systematically sort out *left* and *right*. In copying tasks, we saw that people with WS could make a reasonable copy of a dot relative to a square, but that the level of accuracy in angular disparity and distance was no different from that of normally developing 4-year-olds, and worse than 6-year-olds. The same was true of tracking multiple objects, where we repeatedly saw equivalence between older children and adults with WS and normally developing 4-year-olds, all of whom could track fewer objects than normally developing children who were age 6 and beyond.

7.2.3 Extension to Language

Perhaps most surprising, the same pattern appears to hold for language. Our review of the literature as well as our own data showed that for many aspects of language, people with WS possess rich representations that can be used to both produce and comprehend complex aspects of language. They can produce complex relative clauses, and can understand sentences that exhibit varying relationships between logical operators such as *not* and *or*, and interpret these appropriately, depending on the hierarchical structure between the operators. They can produce spatial prepositions that aptly describe exemplars of spatial relationships holding between concrete entities such as cups and tables and much more abstract entities such as classrooms and buildings. But the performance of people in our WS group tends to lie below that of normally developing mental age matches; on average, it is more likely to match the level of normally developing 5-year-olds. These aspects of language are largely formed during normal development by the time children are 5 years old. People with WS acquire these same aspects of language, but clearly not on the same timetable as the normally developing child.

What kind of developmental mechanism accounts for these findings? We now turn to a speculative hypothesis.

7.3 A Developmental Mechanism: Slow Development and Arrest at an Early Functional Level

The patterns of performance we have just summarized suggest that for a wide range of spatial tasks, older children (e.g., 10-year-olds), adolescents, and adults with WS show a profile that patterns most closely with a normally developing child between the ages of 4 and 6. There may be some variation within this age range. Some of the tasks (e.g., posting a card into a slot, multiple object tracking, copying locations) show a clear equivalence with normal 4-year-olds, whereas other tasks (e.g., perceptual matching of a card to a slot, recognizing objects from unusual viewpoints) may be better approximated with a 5- or 6-year-old age equivalent. The fact remains, however, that in these tasks, adolescents and adults with WS appear to reach the level of a normally developing 4–6-year-old and go no further. Equally important, these levels of performance—although comparable to much younger normally developing children—still embody the same qualitative signatures. That is, the normal 4-year-old equivalent in a WS adult is characterized not only by *quantitative* similarity in overall performance, but also by *qualitative* similarity in the fine-grained nature of errors that occur. Remarkably, patterns of performance shown in language tasks—whether spatial language or not—also fit this pattern. The question is why.

We have already argued that the straightforward hypothesis of a dorsal stream deficit does not perfectly fit the facts. Exceptions to the pattern of dorsal stream deficit include adult-like performance on motion coherence (a function of MT, a dorsal stream structure), and performance on house processing tasks (engaging the parahippocampal areas, ventral stream structures) that is worse than mental age matches. Still, there is something significant in the fact that there is strength in aspects of object recognition typically engaging the ventral stream (i.e., canonical recognition), face processing, and biological motion; and the fact that there is real weakness in aspects of spatial representation that tend to engage parts of the dorsal stream, such as visual-manual action, use of reference systems in copying tasks, and representation of handedness in objects.

A different hypothesis builds on the idea that developmental trajectories themselves are key. Let's first assume that normal developmental trajectories for spatial representation vary substantially. Some spatial functions—such as recognizing objects from their canonical perspectives—develop early, whereas other spatial functions—such as accurate copying of figures or mental rotation—undergo a long developmental trajectory. This hypothetical scenario for normal development is shown in Figure 7.1. The two curves represent two different sets of spatial functions, one early emerging (i.e., normally mature by age 4) and one emerging over a much longer developmental timetable, maturing possibly in adolescence (normally mature by age 12).

Now let's assume that the WS growth curves for these functions are fundamentally the same as in normally developing individuals, but much slower. Then, for any given spatial function, people with WS should show a growth curve that moves along the same developmental path, but at, say, half the normal rate of growth. We indicate this in Figure 7.1 by simply posting chronological ages for the WS group that are more than double the chronological ages for the normally developing group. This much seems consistent with the overall delay shown in cognitive functions among children with WS; for example, using standardized measures, children with WS show initial delay in language functions (Mervis & Becerra, 2007).

So far, the model proposes that there is slow development in people with WS. But this model leaves aside an important fact: Adults with WS do not seem to catch up, at least for the spatial (and language) functions

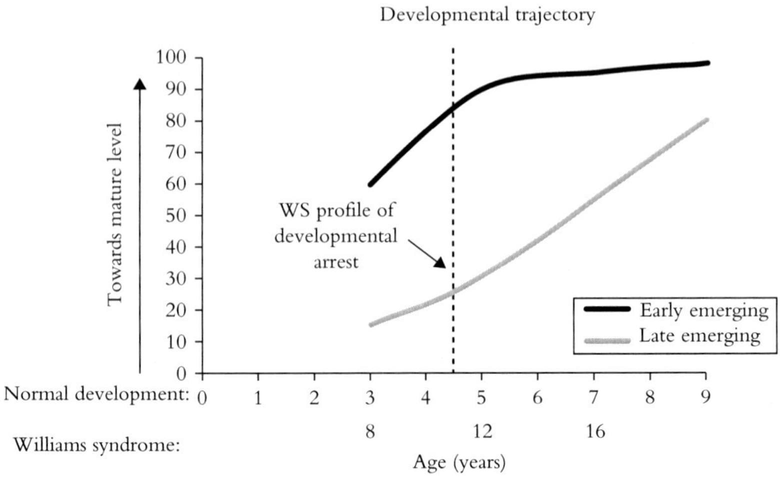

Figure 7.1. Model of hypothesized mechanisms underlying WS profile for spatial representations. The model shows a hypothetical developmental curve for early emerging spatial functions (black) contrasted with late emerging spatial functions (gray). The ages for development of the two kinds of spatial functions are shown on the x-axis. For normally developing children, we show development of the two sets of functions from age 3 to 9, to illustrate that some functions are close to maturity by around age 4 or 5, whereas others do not reach maturity until much later. For people with WS, we hypothesize very slow developmental trajectories, illustrated by more than doubling the age at which different functions are achieved. We also hypothesize that there is, around chronological age 10 or 12, developmental arrest. If this is true, then the 10–12-year-old WS person would reach the same developmental points as the normally developing 4- or 5-year-old, but would go no further, resulting in arrest at this functional level. See text for further discussion.

we have described. This means that spatial development for the functions we are considering must come to a halt at some point, resulting in arrest. If this is true, then we would have a combination of very slow growth coupled with *arrest* at an early functional level, consistent with what we have observed.

To model this point, we simply drop a vertical line across both types of spatial functions—those normally reaching maturity early and those emerging on a longer developmental trajectory. In our model, we have drawn the line at the chronological ages of 4–5 for normally developing children, and the "equivalent" of around age 10–12 for the WS group.

For this particular time point, we can observe that for both normally developing children and people with WS, there is a heavy imbalance in the "maturity" of different spatial functions. Early emerging functions are close to maturity, while late emerging functions have proceeded only part of the way along the full developmental trajectory to maturity. This means that the typical 4–5-year-old child will show an imbalance across spatial functions, consistent with what we have seen—some functions undergo very little development between 4 and adulthood, whereas others show a great deal of development. But the model also suggests that the person with WS, who has developed through age 10–12, will exhibit a similar imbalance across spatial functions. If this pattern were to persist, caused by developmental arrest during this time, then we would have a persisting pattern of spatial imbalance, with early emerging functions fully developed, but later emerging functions showing very little if any growth.

Why would we posit a "stopping point" at the chronological age of 10–12 years in people with WS? Admittedly, this age range is just a guess, but it is an educated guess based on several points. The first is based on the cognitive profile that we have observed, suggesting that from early adolescence onward in WS, there is not much development across the spatial functions we have examined.

The second is based on the fact that the WS pattern for language mirrors the WS pattern for spatial functions we have studied: mastery of early emerging structures, but more severe difficulties and lack of full mastery for later emerging structures. It has long been assumed that language learning is subject to some kind of sensitive period, originally thought to coincide with puberty (Lenneberg, 1967) but more recently acknowledged to reflect a complex set of factors including age of onset as well as trajectory (Newport, Bavelier, & Neville, 2001). The sensitive period is a time of development during which the organism is maximally susceptible to experience. In the case of language, people who learn a language before the age of 8–10 years tend to show native-like proficiency as adults, whereas people who learn a language (usually a second language) after this time period tend to show poorer proficiency in both morphology and syntax (Johnson & Newport, 1991; Newport, 1990). Spatial language—the basic words that encode spatial relationships—is subject to similar limitations, with performance in adulthood declining as the age of learning onset increases (Munnich & Landau, 2010). Having observed that the pattern for language in people with WS is remarkably similar to that for a range of spatial functions, we speculate that development across this quite wide range of cognitive functions may slow or even stop around the time of puberty. Because people with WS undergo quite early puberty (with a recent estimate 1 year before non-WS children, P. Kaplan, pers. comm.), this would suggest that a range of cognitive functions might undergo developmental arrest at this point.[3]

Our hypothesis is clearly quite speculative and raises many questions. One question is whether the developmental curves we have assumed—for example, a rate of slowed development, and a point of arrest—are correct. A second question is whether puberty does indeed have the assumed slowing or halting effect on development. A third question is whether the assumed sensitive period for language is likely to be the same as a possible sensitive period for the spatial functions we have considered. Evidence on the role of sensitive periods in visual development suggests that different visual functions are subject to differently timed sensitive periods (see Lewis & Maurer, 2005). To our knowledge, evidence on the role of sensitive periods in higher-level spatial cognitive tasks is currently limited (but see Bavelier, Levi, Li, Dan, & Hensch, 2010, for recent discussion). However, some studies have addressed the role of early visual experience in navigation (Loomis et al., 1993); these suggest that early visual experience is helpful but not necessary for constructing mental representation of spatial layouts. Further studies (especially longitudinal ones) would allow us to determine whether the assumed point

[3] The idea of slow growth is consistent with at least one domain that is quite unrelated to cognition—physical growth. People with WS have short stature, falling on average in the 3rd percentile for height. Longitudinal growth charts show slowing of physical growth after around age 10–12, and somewhat later for males (Martin, Smith, Cole & Preece, 2007). Early puberty is suggested as one possible factor in growth retardation. Recent studies show that mice that have had deletions on chromosome 5 in the WBS region also show growth retardation, with lower weight than normal mice at all times of measurements, from 1 to 5 weeks through 32 weeks postnatal. Physical growth is, of course, not likely to be the perfect model for cognitive growth but we suggest it as an analogy.

of halted development is correct, whether there is some other age range that better fits the point of arrest, or whether we are altogether incorrect in our characterization.

Finally, a fourth and crucial question is, what kind of theory explains why certain spatial-cognitive systems normally develop early and why others undergo a longer developmental trajectory? There are several possibilities. One is that, consistent with views we have discussed, many ventral stream functions develop early, whereas many dorsal stream functions—requiring, as they do, calibration for the growing body—develop along a much lengthier trajectory simply because they must continue to adapt along with physical growth. Although we have ruled out an omnibus hypothesis of early development for all ventral stream functions and lengthier development for all dorsal stream functions, it is still possible that there is a relative imbalance across the streams in terms of developmental trajectory. This is clearly an empirical question. A second possibility is that knowledge systems considered "core" to human cognition develop early in some form (Spelke & Kinzler, 2007). This would include systems such as objects, space, number, time, and language. This has a certain appeal, but given the great range of spatial systems that we have observed, it seems hard to characterize "space" as a single core system that emerges early. A better prospect is to dissect a range of candidate systems, and to determine empirically which aspects of representation emerge early and which undergo more lengthy development. This is what we have tried to do for the domain of space. Our results suggest that tracking developmental profiles within a domain can lead to new insights about normal development, as well as shed light on our understanding of WS.

7.4 Is That All There Is? What Slow Development and Early Arrest Cannot Account For

Although our account fits much of the data on spatial development, and although we have argued that it also fits aspects of the data on language development, there are a number of cases where the account does not fit. We believe that these fall into two very different classes. One is a set of clear violations of the hypothesis of slow development followed by arrest. These include biological motion processing, face processing, and reorientation. The second is a range of cognitive capacities that show continued growth over the lifetime, and may require special support from the environment to flourish. These include the continued acquisition of vocabulary, the acquisition of reading and mathematical skills, and improvements in copying. The two kinds of violation shed further light on why people with WS show such an unusual profile and, perhaps more important, what avenues exist for promoting continued growth throughout adolescence and adulthood.

7.4.1 Spatial Systems That Flourish and Spatial Systems That Fail

For both biological motion and face processing, people with WS perform as well or better than 4- or 6-year-olds, and sometimes substantially better (biological motion). Where we have measures of brain activation—for face processing—the patterns for people with WS appear most similar to chronological age matches, and more mature than mental age matches who are around 6 years of age (O'Hearn et al., 2010). These data suggest that biological motion perception and face processing flourish in the context of the severe impairments in other spatial systems.

For the case of reorientation, we have quite a different situation: Here, at least some people with WS fail to use the geometric structure of the environment in contexts where even 18-month-old normally developing toddlers succeed. These data do not fit the profile of navigation tasks more generally; as we saw in Chapter 5, people with WS can keep track of their own movements through the environment, can use allocentric frames of reference to locate objects, and can use landmarks to locate objects after they have been disoriented and must regain their orientation.

How can we account for these two very different cases, one in which spatial functions thrive, and the other in which a completely different kind of spatial function fails? At present, we are far from a full explanation. One important set of findings is that the brain systems that support these cognitive functions are relatively normal in the case of biological motion and face processing, but show abnormalities in the case of reorientation. A number of studies have shown that the region supporting face processing (FFA) has normal size for chronological age in people with WS, and is activated to the same extent (O'Hearn et al., 2010; Sarpal et al., 2008). Other studies have reported that abnormal structure and functioning in both the hippocampal formation and parietal regions, especially the intraparietal sulcus, in people with WS (Meyer-Lindenberg et al., 2004, 2005). The strong connectivity between these regions, and their importance in a range of navigation functions, is consistent with the severe difficulties that some people with WS have in the reorientation task.

But the existence of correlated brain function abnormalities takes us only a part of the way to understanding why these spatial systems show abnormal functioning. Do the brain regions start out with severely abnormal structure and functioning, leading to immediate and persistent strength and/or weakness in these spatial functions? Or do the brain regions start out with small differences in structure and functioning, leading the person with WS to engage in kinds of activities that might lead to increasing strength in one function and weakness in another? The latter kind of explanation is consistent with the idea of developmental cascades in which cognitive patterns and behavioral tendencies can cascade as development proceeds (Elman et al., 1996; Karmiloff-Smith, 1998). For example, it has been noted that toddlers with WS are "fixated" on other people's eyes, although they also show abnormalities in early communicative gestures including pointing and gaze following (John & Mervis, 2010). It is possible that the fascination with eyes may be part of an early complex that drives attention to the face more generally, resulting in a kind of early emerging "expertise" with faces that puts children with WS on a par with normally developing children in the development of face recognition. Reorientation difficulties could emerge through a similar process, if, for example, children with WS are severely constrained in their independent locomotion. This could be a natural outcome of early locomotor difficulties, and perhaps even the consequence of parents protecting their children by limiting independent exploration of space.

All this is speculative, of course. What we do know, however, is that the patterns of expertise in biological motion, face processing, and reorientation form a most unusual part of the spatial profile of people with WS. They are unusual in that they violate the pattern observed in many other aspects of spatial representation we have described. And they are unusual because they present us with a clear pattern of peaks and valleys relative to the rest of the spatial profile: peaks for biological motion and face processing; a valley for reorientation.

7.4.2 Cognitive Systems That Continue to Grow

Our hypothesis of slow development followed by arrest at an early functional level encounters another important set of violations. These include vocabulary growth, the acquisition of reading and mathematical skills, and copying ability—an admittedly complex skill that draws on many more basic spatial capacities. These violations provide compelling evidence that people with WS do not show *exactly* the same cognitive profile of a 4- or 5-year-old. People with WS obviously mature physically and emotionally, and they also mature cognitively. If we are right that there is a large range of spatial (and language) capacities that are similar to the level of a 4- or 5-year-old, we cannot argue that the *entire cognitive profile* is limited in this way. Importantly, each of the violations in this category, in its own way, tells a slightly different story about the nature of overall cognitive development in people with WS. This in turn sheds additional light on the relative weakness in the spatial domain.

7.4.2.1 Vocabulary Growth

In Chapter 6, we described a number of studies showing that people with WS undergo a slow start to language learning, and that their development then continues, but that, when tested as older children or adults, they seem to have reached the level of performance of normally developing 5-year-olds. This pattern spanned a range of different functions, including complex syntax, morphology, and spatial language. Particularly surprising were some of the latter findings: Even for many uses of the basic spatial prepositions such as *in*, *on*, *above*, and *over*, people with WS fit the profile of normally developing 5-year-old children, with good performance on some items that are quite abstract (e.g., Naples is *on* the coast) but poor performance on other similarly abstract items (e.g., "bird *in* the tree"). We used these data to argue that language learning might actually fit the same profile as much of spatial representation—slow development, followed by arrest at an early functional level. This conclusion is clearly subject to further empirical testing; in particular, the hypothesis predicts that people with WS should show poor performance on any structures that are normally acquired after about age 6.

But one large fact looms as a clear violation to this hypothesis: the continued acquisition of vocabulary. When people with WS are tested on vocabulary tests such as the KBIT-verbal (KBIT 2; Kaufman & Kaufman, 2004) or the PPVT (Dunn & Dunn, 1997), their scores continue to climb over time. They climb slowly, and so their normal age equivalences are not likely to be comparable to chronological age matches. But the fact that they continue to climb over developmental time, through adulthood, shows that this is an aspect of language learning that is not subject to developmental arrest in the same sense as shown for aspects of grammar.

This difference may be explained by appeal to the idea of a sensitive period, suggested earlier in this chapter. We know that the acquisition of morphology, syntax, and some aspects of semantics (e.g., spatial prepositions) are subject to sensitive period effects—the earlier that one learns a language, the better the language is learned. But this does not hold for "open-class" words that constitute a large part of our vocabulary. These words are largely nouns and verbs, said to be part of the "open" class because new members of the class enter into the vocabulary of a community quite easily and with little resistance. For example, we all have learned words such as "Bluetooth" and "iPod," just as past generations learned words such as "Kleenex" and "refrigerator." These words often start as brand names, but the last two examples show that over generations, they come to represent classes of items, not just the original branded item. Learners of all ages are susceptible to acquisition of new nouns and verbs on a regular basis: We are happy to accept new nouns representing categories of newly discovered artifacts, animals, foods, and so on. We also readily accept new verbs, often derived from new nouns; for example, we now "e-mail" each other and "download" documents. Such new words are acquired throughout the lifetime, and as far as we know, with equal facility over age, consistent with the idea that learning new words engages mechanisms that are not subject to fixed time frames or cut off due to the end of biological maturation.

Although we do not have clear empirical data, we think it is highly likely that people with WS also continually grow their open-class vocabularies in the same ways that people without WS do. But the hypothesized normalcy of this process suggests another unusual aspect of the WS profile: Adults with WS may have the vocabulary of a 16-year-old (or better), but only the grammatical or morphological system of a 5-year-old. Does this mean that each word in the active vocabulary of a WS adult will have the same complex and rich semantic representation of a normally developing person with the same vocabulary? We do not know the answer to this question. But studies of biological knowledge in people with WS indicate limits in their understanding of terms such as "person," "animal," and "living thing," which remain at the level of much younger normally developing 4–6-year-olds. By contrast, normally developing children go on to develop qualitatively different concepts by age 10, for example, coalescing concepts of "animal" and "plant" into a larger category of "living things" (Johnson & Carey, 1996).

The combination of a large vocabulary and more shallow meaning representations for late acquired words would suggest a possible split between the acquisition of the word per se (e.g., the ability to use it in basic sentences) and the more prolonged developmental process of enriching the semantic representations for these words. With few limits on the former, but more severe limits on the latter, a person would be expected to produce sentences filled with a range of words, both frequent and infrequent, but to reveal, upon further questioning, little depth of knowledge of the meanings of those words. This profile seems to fit the original observations made by Bellugi et al. (1994): The verbal description of an elephant by an adolescent with WS showed extensive vocabulary, but the description more generally had little depth.

7.4.2.2 Reading and Mathematical Skills

The idea that people with WS show slow development followed by arrest at an early functional level would predict that both reading and mathematical skills should also be limited to the level of a normally developing 4- or 5-year-old child. Although we know little about these skills in people with WS, the evidence is not consistent with this prediction. Many (if not all) people with WS learn to read, and many of the people who never learned to read are now adults, perhaps from a cohort where there was little support for their special educational needs. The few existing studies on reading in people with WS indicate that there can be difficulties in the area of phonological coding (Laing et al., 2001; Menghini et al., 2004) as well as problems stemming from the visual-spatial disorder (Dessalegn, Landau, & Rapp, 2012). But reading levels in some people with WS can reach seventh- or eighth-grade equivalents, as we have seen in our lab; anecdotally, there are some adults with WS who enjoy reading. In addition, people with WS learn basic mathematical skills. Our study of a small sample of children and adolescents with WS showed that, on average, they performed at the third-grade level on a standardized measure, the Test of Early Mathematical Abilities (Ginsburg & Baroody, 1990; O'Hearn & Landau, 2007).

How can we square these results with our hypothesis that many basic aspects of space and language are arrested at the level of a 4- or 5-year-old child? It turns out that these two sets of results are not necessarily inconsistent with each other. Let's consider mathematical skills first. There is evidence that basic numerical representations in people with WS are impaired, which would also predict impairment in the learning of basic mathematical skills such as addition and subtraction. One of the most compelling cases concerns the representation of numbers in the approximate number system (ANS)—our remarkable ability to estimate both large and small numerosities from briefly presented displays that prevent explicit counting. A large literature shows that this system is present in nonhuman animals as well as human infants, children, and adults (Dehaene, 1999; Feigenson, Dehaene, & Spelke, 2004; Xu & Spelke, 2000); recent evidence shows that the resolution of the ANS (as specified by the Weber fraction) increases between ages 3 and 6, and does not become adult-like until even later in development (Halberda & Feigenson, 2008). Research using single-cell recording and brain imaging techniques tells us that the ANS engages an area of the parietal lobe in animals and in humans (specifically, the intraparietal sulcus, IPS; Dehaene et al., 2003). We have discussed a wide range of evidence showing that people with WS have severe difficulty with tasks that engage this area of the brain, and that there appear to be structural and functional abnormalities that are correlated with these difficulties (Meyer-Lindenberg et al., 2004, 2006).

Given our hypothesis of slow development followed by arrest at an early functional level, and given the fact that similar regions of the brain are engaged in a wide range of spatial tasks as well as tasks of judging approximate number, we would predict that people with WS should show severe impairments in the latter tasks. Indeed, recent work in our lab shows that this is the case, with performance among adolescents and adults with WS showing the same profile as normally developing 4–6-year-old children (Libertus, Halberda, Feigenson, & Landau, in preparation). Our results are consistent with data from other labs (Ansari, Donlan, & Karmiloff-Smith, 2007; Krajcsi et al., 2009) and suggest that the ANS is severely impaired in people with WS, falling to the same level as many of the spatial tasks we have discussed in the book. However, people with WS perform on average like normally developing 6–8-year-olds on at least one standardized math achievement test (the TEMA-2, Ginsburg & Baroody, 1990; see O'Hearn & Landau, 2007).

Recent evidence on normally developing children shows large individual differences in the resolution of the ANS at age 14, and this variation across children is a strong predictor of their performance on standardized math achievement tests measured in first through sixth grades (Halberda, Mazzocco, & Feigenson, 2008). From this, we should predict that ANS resolution in people with WS should predict their level of mathematical skill. In other words, the math skills of people with WS should be overall like those of a 4–6-year-old. But based on O'Hearn and Landau's findings, people with WS appear to move beyond this level, and although there are admittedly serious constraints on the ultimate levels of math skill achieved by this group, they clearly learn more about numerical computations than would be predicted only by the level of resolution in their ANS. It seems likely that the same variation in the ANS observed by Halberda et al. (2008) is present in people with WS, and if so, an important question would be whether this variation also predicts variation in the level achieved in math skills, as measured by standardized math tests.

These findings suggest that formal education plays a strong role in moving people with WS beyond the severe constraints imposed by the naturally developing approximate number system. They learn to add and subtract and to multiply, and several of our WS participants have even moved on to basic algebra in their late teens. The variation in achievement here is likely correlated with more general cognitive capacities such as working memory and general intelligence. But the level of mathematical skill is not rendered immutable by a severely immature basic sensitivity to numerosity. Rather, people with WS can move beyond this constraint. This fact holds promise for assistive technology in learning math, and for promoting life skills that involve number—things as basic as understanding how to deal with money.

The same kind of story may apply to reading. Although we have argued that many spatial and language functions in people with WS fit with the profile of a normally developing 4- or 5-year-old, people with WS do learn to read at levels that are higher than the average 4–5-year-old child. There have been only a handful of systematic studies of reading in people with WS, and these confirm development of some skill, with a number of reports showing acquisition at a second- or third-grade level. Although people with WS rarely reach a level commensurate with their chronological age, we have seen cases of individuals who read at the high school level, often close to their chronological age level. The overall profile of spatial and language abilities as we have described it would not predict reading levels of around second or third grade—estimated by many parents to be the endpoint—and certainly would not predict levels beyond that. How do we explain the ability to read in the context of the spatial and linguistic profile we have described?

There are two answers to this question. The first is that learning to read, like schooled mathematics, requires explicit training. Given appropriate techniques, people with WS can clearly build on their existing phonological and visual-spatial skills and learn some of the mappings between sound and form. These initial mappings can lead to reading levels of a second or third grader, but often this is final level attained by individuals with WS. Beyond this, we simply do not know what pushes some people with WS to continue developing their reading skills, although we suspect that, among other things, environment and motivation make a difference. Perhaps more important, the degree of strength in reading may be linked to a clear diagnosis of the root problem in reading, the development of compensatory mechanisms on the part of the individual, and the tailoring of appropriate interventions.

For example, we have evidence suggesting that the limits on reading in some people with WS may be more linked to the visual-spatial disorder than to phonological disorders, as has been assumed in several studies (Laing et al., 2001; Menghini et al., 2004). Tests for phonological skill include, for example, the ability to rhyme, to pronounce a word "minus" the starting or ending sound, and to read nonwords (which could never have been learned, and so must be pronounced by mapping the sequences of letters onto sounds). Results have shown that phonological awareness among adolescents with WS is poorer than normally developing mental-age-matched controls (Laing et al., 2001; Menghini et al., 2004). If poor phonological awareness is the root cause of poor reading in people with WS, then it would stand to reason that tutoring in phonological awareness should improve reading level.

We know of no systematic studies testing this hypothesis. But we do know that there are cases of people with WS for whom the crucial stumbling block is the visual-spatial component of reading, not phonological awareness. We carried out an in-depth study of two 16-year-olds with WS who had been longtime research participants in our program (Dessalegn, Landau, & Rapp, 2012). The two individuals, one male and one female (MWS, FWS), were both in ninth-grade public schools, and both had IQs in the high 80's when tested for reading abilities. The female had undergone extensive reading tutoring over a period of several years before being tested in our reading research. The tutoring focused on phonological awareness. Indeed, both FWS and MWS performed similarly on tests from an extensive phonological battery (CTOPP; Wagner, Torgesen, Rashotte, & Pro-Ed., 1999). However, their overall levels of word reading were strikingly different: FWS achieved a word reading grade of 2.6 (word reading age = 7;9 years) and MWS achieved a grade of 7.8 (word reading age = 13;1 years). Tests of nonword reading showed the same profile, with FWS achieving a reading grade of 2.5 (reading age = 7;10 years) and MWS achieving a grade of 16.9 (nonword reading age = 18;6 years). Their word spelling was at the level of first and sixth grades, respectively.

When tested for visual-spatial skills that were deemed especially relevant for reading letters and words, we found very large differences between the two. FWS performed more poorly than MWS on tests requiring detection and discrimination of mirror image letters, and on tests requiring the detection of visual features of words such as *bow/dow* or *dad/bad* that also involve mirror image reversals. FWS also performed more poorly than MWS on tests requiring representation in memory of the orientation of objects, and her errors in both reading and spelling were consistent with the idea that she had a severe deficit in the representation and retention of orientation. Despite these deficits, FWS learned to read, and was also able to use compensatory strategies to read texts that exceeded her estimated reading grade of 2.5. Even people with extreme deficits in visual-spatial representation can learn to compensate by using "top-down" contextual information to better predict words as they read text (for a particularly striking example, see the case of A.H., studied by McCloskey, 2009).

The two case studies of people with WS remind us that reading is comprised of many basic processes, which are cobbled together to create a new system that requires exposure to explicit instruction, motivation, and systematic practice to develop. In the process of assembling this complex system, the learner may fail to grow and thrive for many different reasons.

7.4.2.3 Copying

We conclude this section with an example that we offered in the earliest sections of our book: copying—the hallmark deficit for people with WS. Throughout the book, we have offered evidence that the copying task involves many basic mechanisms of spatial representation, and we have argued that people with WS—even in adulthood—tend to show deficits in these mechanisms that pattern after a very early time in normal development. Given this, it makes sense that our WS participants have tremendous difficulty carrying out copying tasks, whether by drawing or by assembling blocks.

Surprisingly, however, people with WS do show growth and change in their ability to copy figures. Bertrand and Mervis (1996) found growth in copying by children with WS over a period of 3 to 4 years. At age 9–10, the children had a mean age equivalent of 5;9 on a standardized copying task (VMI; Beery & Buktenica, 1967), but the same children had a mean age equivalent of 7;3 three to four years later, at age 13–14. Of course, this growth is quite slow, with development of only about 18 months over a chronological age period of 3 to 4 years. Like Mervis, we too have observed improvement in copying among our WS participants.

As they come into our lab over the years, their scores on the DAS block task do change, albeit very slowly. Tutoring in writing skills may well enhance the ability to produce good figure copies, even if the growth is limited.

How can we account for this improvement, if we have hypothesized that many basic functions remain at the level of a 4- or 5-year-old child? The answer is that copying—like reading and math—can be improved by providing strategic guidance to the user. Such guidance can be provided by verbal instruction (e.g., "Start by drawing a straight line. Now go to the end of the line, place a point where you want to end up, and draw another straight line"). This kind of strategic copying is not what most of us use to produce copies, but for the spatially impaired individual, it might be very useful. Indeed, instruction (and practice) is clearly used to improve handwriting—a skill that most people with WS find very challenging. Another kind of guidance might be provided by mechanical means. In a pilot experiment, we employed a haptic robot to guide the pen held by a person with WS over a straight line, moving from point to point using force fields that "push" the user into the channel required for a straight line (Lee, Okamura, & Landau, 2009; see Figure 7.2).

Although this was only a pilot study with three individuals, we found that brief practice using the haptic robot led to substantial improvement in copying simple triangles. The practice might have helped by actually training specific routes, or it might have helped by encouraging the user to look ahead to the goal point, as he or she moved the pen. In either case, we suspect that strategies such as these might do much to promote improvement. Like reading and formal math, copying is a skill that can be nurtured, even if the basic mechanisms required for the skill are not—and perhaps will never be—fully mature.

7.5 Remaining Puzzles

In closing, we sense that our book has raised more questions than it has answered. Our goal has been to thoroughly document the nature of the spatial systems in people with WS, and to relate it to the normal development of these systems. Our larger goal was to add to our scientific understanding of the relationship between genes, brains, and spatial

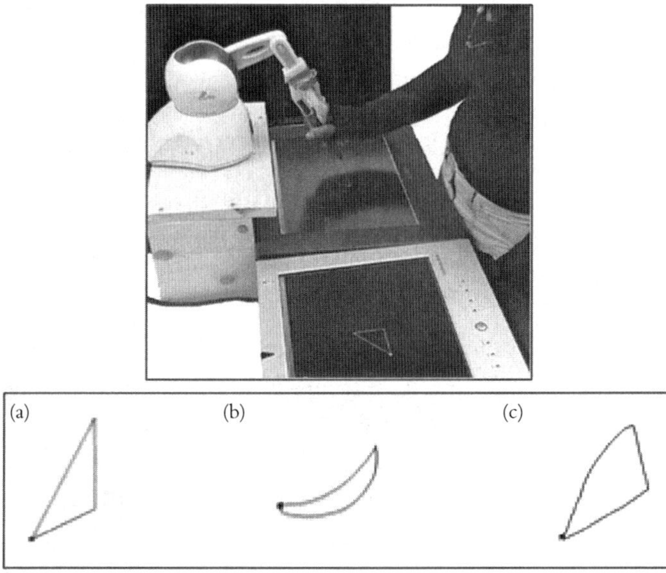

Figure 7.2. Upper panel: A haptic robot holding a stylus is held by a participant, who attempts to trace the triangle on the screen. Force fields are applied as the person moves along the lines of the triangle, keeping the stylus within channels when the user veers outside of these. The screen to the person's left displays the target triangle, which she is trying to copy. Lower panel: Sample results. Prior to training, people with WS and normally developing children were shown target triangles (a) and copied them with no assistance (b). They were then trained to copy triangles using the haptic robot, which guided their action over the three legs of a set of triangles. After this training, people were tested without the robot on their ability to copy new triangles—never part of the training (c). There was clear improvement in the copies of both WS participants and normally developing children. Adapted from Lee, Okamura, and Landau (2009), Copyright © 2009 IEEE. Reprinted with permission.

cognition, specifically asking how a small group of missing genes could result in the development of such an unusual cognitive profile.

We believe we have gone some way toward these goals. We have documented the striking peaks and valleys across the broad range of spatial functions, and we have argued that the overall profile of people with WS can be fully understood only in the context of normal development. Our hypothesis, admittedly speculative, is that people with WS develop a range of spatial functions that appear to be quite similar to those of early developing functions in normal children: What normally reaches maturity early will also reach maturity in people with WS. We have further suggested, however, that the timetable for arriving at these developmental milestones is quite different in people with WS than normal children—with a slow-moving developmental trajectory that is "stretched out" in time. At some point, for many spatial functions, this developmental trajectory simply stops, resulting in arrested development for individuals with WS. This has been the story for a range of spatial functions, including object representation, multiple object tracking, representation of location for the purposes of copying and language, and visual-manual action, among others.

Along with the hypothesis of slow development and arrest at an early functional level, we also documented two sets of systems that do not fit this profile: one was an example of extreme weakness, and one of clear strength. For the weakness, reorientation using geometry is a challenge for at least some people with WS. The evidence also suggests real strength in face perception and biological motion perception—possibly both linked to the social profile of people with WS. Finally, we suggested that some kinds of knowledge continue to emerge over the lifetime, allowing people with WS to move beyond the restrictions imposed by their most severe deficits.

There are many remaining puzzles. At the molar level, we wonder why some of the spatial and linguistic functions seem to halt in their development, while other kinds of learning continue. We wonder whether our concept of the sensitive period and its role in normal and abnormal development really align properly with the various spatial systems we have studied: Are there actually sensitive periods for their development, similar to those observed in language learning, or is this just entirely the wrong idea? We wonder why is it so easy to build a vocabulary of nouns and verbs over one's lifetime, but so hard to learn grammatical facts as an older learner. All these are empirical questions; and we hope that our book will have stimulated research to address them.

Finally, we wonder what the answer is to the biggest puzzle of our story: How does the absence of 25 genes eventually result in the complex cognitive profile we have observed? We believe that we have offered the details of a cognitive phenotype, in the hopes that eventually these will be useful in understanding the long and complex causal chain connecting genes, brains, and cognition.

Appendix A

Percent Production of All Path Terms Over All 80 Events

Simple Path Terms	Normal Adults	Normal Children	Children with WS
across	22.2	5.3	2.9
against	0.1	0.2	—
along	0.8	0.2	—
around	3.1	2.5	2.5
at	0.3	0.7	—
away	—	3.6	2.7
back	0.2	0.7	1.7
backwards	2.7	3.3	1.5
behind	0.7	0.7	0.2
beside	—	0.2	—
by	1.3	0.5	0.6
down	5.2	8.3	10.1
downhill	0.3	—	—
downward	0.1	—	—
forwards	—	0.4	—
from	1.2	0.8	0.4
in	1.6	5.1	4.8
inside	0.2	—	—
into	3	1	3.4

Simple Path Terms	Normal Adults	Normal Children	Children with WS
near	—	0.5	—
off	13.7	18	15.2
on	3.8	9.4	5.3
onto	1.2	1.3	0.8
out	3.9	3.8	1.7
over	9	10.6	26.9
past	1.7	3	0.8
through	6.7	6.3	2.3
to	3.1	2.6	5
toward(s)	1.7	—	—
under	0.1	0.2	—
up	2.5	3.6	2.5
uphill	0.3	—	—
Other	—	—	0.4
Compound Path Terms			
around and around	—	0.7	0.8
away from	2.3	1.2	0.8
back of/back to	—	0.3	0.2
close to	—	0.2	—
down from/down off	0.1	0.2	0.4
from x to y	1.2	0.7	—
in back of/in front of	0.2	0.4	0.2
in front of	—	0.2	—
in and out	—	0.2	0.8
in his way	—	0.5	—
in the middle	—	—	0.2
in through	—	—	0.2
left to right	0.1	—	—
next to	—	0.2	0.2
on left side of	0.1	—	—
on over	—	—	0.2

Compound Path Terms	Normal Adults	Normal Children	Children with WS
on top of	2	0.2	0.4
out around	—	—	0.2
over and over	—	—	1.3
over to	0.6	0.2	1.5
over towards	0.1	—	—
perpendicular to	0.1	—	—
right in front	—	—	0.2
up and down	0.1	2.8	1.1
up to	2	0.2	0.2

Adapted from Landau and Zukowski (2003), with permission from Taylor & Francis.

Appendix B

Spatial Stimuli in Munnich and Landau's (2010) Study

Stimuli Contrasting *In* and *On*

	Base Items	Contrast Items
1a.	***There are pretzels IN the bag***	***There are pretzels ON the bag***
1b.	***There is a blue ball IN the container***	*There is a blue ball ON the container*
2a.	There are grapes IN the bowl (grapes heaping beyond rim)	**There are grapes ON the plate**
2b.	**There are passengers IN the seats**	**There is a person ON the sofa**
3a.	There are pretzel sticks IN the napkin (napkin folded around pretzels)	***There are pretzel sticks ON the napkin***
3b.	**There is a flower IN the book**	***There is a flower ON the book***
4a.	**There is an owl IN the tree**	**There are birds ON the branch**
4b.	**There is a classroom IN the building**	**There is a classroom ON the second floor**
5a.	**There is a square IN the circle**	**There is a square ON the chalkboard**
5b.	**There are blue circles IN the orange box**	**There are blue circles ON the page**
6a.	**There is a crack IN the pavement**	**There is yellow paint ON the pavement**
6b.	**There is a dent IN the can**	**There is writing ON the can**

Stimuli Contrasting *In* and *On*

	Base Items	Contrast Items
7a.	There is chocolate IN the ice cream (chocolate ice cream)	**There is chocolate ON the ice cream (chocolate topping)**
7b.	**There are nuts IN the cookie**	There are nuts ON the roll (nuts are spread over top of roll)
8a.	**There is a woman IN the car**	There are people ON the flight (people are in their seats on airplane)
8b.	**There are two women IN the canoe**	There are passengers ON the ferry
9a.	**There is a city called Naples IN Florida**	**There is a city called Naples ON the coast**
9b.	**There is an airport IN Paytonville**	**There is an airport ON the island**
10a.	**There is a red book IN the stack**	There is a red book ON the stack
10b.	**There is a blue shirt IN the stack**	There is a blue shirt ON the stack

Note. **Bold** = very good items; *Ital* = prototypical items

Stimuli Contrasting *On*, *Over*, and *Under*

	Base Items	Contrast Items
1a.	***There is a lizard ON the table***	**There is a lizard OVER the table**
1b.	**There is an apple sticker *ON* the table**	**There is an apple sticker *OVER* the table (hanging from string)**
2a.	**There is a lizard UNDER the table (crawling on bottom side)**	***There is a lizard UNDER the table (on floor beneath table)***
2b.	**There is an apple sticker UNDER the table (stuck to bottom side)**	**There is an apple sticker UNDER the table (hanging from table by string)**
3a.	**There is peanut butter ON the ball (top side)**	**There is peanut butter OVER the ball (on spoon above ball)**
3b.	**There is chocolate pudding ON the orange (top side)**	**There is chocolate pudding OVER the orange (on spoon above orange)**
4a.	**There is peanut butter ON the ball (bottom side)**	**There is peanut butter UNDER the ball (on surface beneath ball)**
4b.	There is chocolate pudding ON the orange (bottom side)	**There is chocolate pudding UNDER the orange (on surface beneath orange)**

Stimuli Contrasting *On*, *Over*, and *Under*

	Base Items	Contrast Items
5a.	There is peanut butter ON the ceiling	**There is an apple sticker ON the ceiling**
5b.	**There is chocolate pudding ON the ceiling**	There is a lizard ON the ceiling
6a.	***There is a blanket ON the man (blanket folded up)***	**There is a blanket OVER/ON the man (blanket covers man)**
6b.	There is aluminum foil ON the bowl (foil folded, on rim of bowl)	There is aluminum foil OVER/ON the bowl (foil covers bowl)
7a.	**There is a blanket UNDER the man (blanket folded up)**	***There is a blanket UNDER the man (blanket spread out)***
7b.	**There is aluminum foil UNDER the bowl (foil folded up)**	***There is aluminum foil UNDER the bowl (foil spread out)***
8a.	**There is a sweater ON the woman (wearing sweater over her shirt)**	**There is a sweater OVER the shirt (wearing sweater over her shirt)**
8b.	**There is an apron ON the man (wearing apron)**	**There is an apron OVER the man's clothing (wearing apron)**
9a.	There is a white pin ON the man (pin is on man's shirt)	**There is a white pin ON the shirt (pin is on man's shirt)**
9b.	*There is a lizard ON the person's leg*	**There is a lizard ON the jeans (man is wearing jeans)**
10a.	***There is a watch ON the table***	**There is a watch ON the man's wrist**
10b.	***There is a label ON the floor***	**There is a label ON the bottle (label goes all the way around bottle)**

Note: **Bold** = very good items; *Ital* = prototypical items.
Reprinted from Munnich and Landau (2010), with permission from Taylor & Francis.

References

Acredolo, L. P. (1978). Development of spatial orientation in infancy. *Developmental Psychology, 14*(3), 224–234.

Acredolo, L. P., & Evans, D. (1980). Developmental changes in the effects of landmarks on infant spatial behavior. *Developmental Psychology, 16*(4), 312–318.

Aguirre, G. K., & D'Esposito, M. (1999). Topographical disorientation: A synthesis and taxonomy. *Brain, 122*(9), 1613.

Aguirre, G. K., Zarahn, E., & D'Esposito, M. (1998). Neural components of topographical representation. *Proceedings of the National Academy of Sciences of the United States of America, 95*(3), 839.

Allison, T., Puce, A., & McCarthy, G. (2000). Social perception from visual cues: Role of the STS region. *Trends in Cognitive Sciences, 4*, 267–278.

Alvarez, G. A., & Franconeri, S. L. (2007). How many objects can you track? Evidence for a resource-limited attentive tracking mechanism. *Journal of Vision, 7*(13), 1–10.

Ansari, D., Donlan, C., & Karmiloff-Smith, A. (2007). Typical and atypical development of visual estimation abilities. *Cortex, 43*, 758–768.

Atkinson, J., Anker, S., Braddick, O., Nokes, L., Mason, A., & Braddick, F. (2002). Visual and visuospatial development in young children with Williams syndrome. *Developmental Medicine & Child Neurology, 43*, 330–337.

Atkinson, J., Braddick, O., Anker, S., Curran, W., Andrew, R., Wattam-Bell, J., & Braddick, F. (2003). Neurobiological models of visuospatial cognition in children with Williams syndrome: Measures of dorsal-stream and frontal function. *Developmental Neuropsychology, 23*(1&2), 139–172.

Atkinson, J., Braddick, O., Rose, F. E., Searcy, Y. M., Wattam-Bell, J., & Bellugi, U. (2006). Dorsal-stream motion processing deficits persist into adulthood in Williams syndrome. *Neuropsychologia, 44*(5), 828–833.

Atkinson, J., King, J., Braddick, O., Nokes, L., Anker, S., & Braddick, F. (1997). A specific deficit of dorsal stream function in Williams' syndrome. *Neuroreport, 8*(8), 1919–1922.

Bae, G.Y., & Flombaum, J. (2012). Close encounters of the distracting kind: Identifying the cause of visual tracking errors. *Attention, Perception, & Psychophysics, 74*, 703–715.

Baillargeon, R. (2004). Infants' physical world. *Current Directions in Psychological Science, 13*, 89–94.

Ballard, D. H., Hayhoe, M. M., Pook, P. K., & Rao, P. N. (1997). Deictic codes for the embodiment of cognition. *Behavioral and Brain Sciences, 20*, 723–742.

Banks, W. P., & Prinzmetal, W. (1976). Configurational effects in visual information-processing. *Perception & Psychophysics, 19*(4), 361–367.

Bavelier, D., Levi, D. M., Li, R. W., Dan, Y., & Hensch, T. K. (2010). Removing brakes on adult brain plasticity: From molecular to behavioral interventions. *The Journal of Neuroscience, 30*(45), 14964–14971.

Beery, K. E., & Buktenica, N. A. (1967). *Developmental Test of Visual-Motor Integration.* Cleveland, OH: Modern Curriculum Press.

Bellugi, U., Bihrle, A., Jernigan, T., Trauner, D., & Doherty, S. (1990). Neuropsychological, neurological, and neuroanatomical profile of Williams syndrome. *American Journal of Medical Genetics, 37*(S6), 115–125.

Bellugi, U., Korenberg, J. R., & Klima, E. S. (2001). Williams syndrome: An exploration of neurocognitive and genetic features. *Clinical Neuroscience Research, 1*(3), 217–229.

Bellugi, U., Lichtenberger, L., Mills, D., Galaburda, A., & Korenberg, J. R. (1999). Bridging cognition, the brain and molecular genetics: Evidence from Williams syndrome. *Trends in Neurosciences, 22*(5), 197–207.

Bellugi, U., Marks, S., Bihrle, A., & Sabo, H. (1993). Dissociation between language and cognitive functions in Williams syndrome. In D. Bishop & K. Mogford (Eds.), *Language development in exceptional circumstances* (pp. 177–189). Hillsdale, NJ: Lawrence Erlbaum Associates, 177–189.

Bellugi, U., Marks, S., Bihrle, A., & Sabo, H. (1988). Dissociation between language and cognitive functions in Williams syndrome. In D. Bishop & K. Mogford (Eds.), *Language development in exceptional circumstances* (pp. 177–189). Edinburgh: Churchill Livingstone.

Bellugi, U., Sabo, H., & Vaid, J. (1988). Spatial deficits in children with Williams syndrome. In J. Stiles-Davis, M. Kritchevsky, & U. Bellugi (Eds.), *Spatial cognition brain bases and development* (pp. 273–297). Hillsdale, NJ: Lawrence Erlbaum Associates.

Bellugi, U., Wang, P. P., & Jernigan, T. L. (1994). Williams syndrome: An unusual neuropsychological profile. In S. Broman & J. Grafman (Eds.), *Atypical cognitive deficits in developmental disorders: Implications for brain function* (pp. 23–56). Hillsdale, NJ: Lawrence Erlbaum Associates.

Bertenthal, B. (1996). Origins and early development of perception, action, and representation. *Annual Review of Psychology, 47*, 431–459.

Bertrand, J., & Mervis, C. B. (1996). Longitudinal analysis of drawings by children with Williams syndrome: Preliminary results. *Visual Arts Research, 22*(2), 19–34.

Beuren, A., Apitz, J., & Harmjanz, D. (1962). Supravalvular aortic stenosis in association with mental retardation and a certain facial appearance. *Stroke, 26*(6), 1235–1240.

Biederman, I. (1987). Recognition-by-components: A theory of human image understanding. *Psychological Review, 94*, 115–147.

Bihrle, A. M., Bellugi, U., Dean, D., & Marks, S. (1989). Seeing either the forest or the trees: Dissociation in visuospatial processing. *Brain and Cognition, 11*(1), 37–49.

Bishop, D. V. M. (1983). *Test for the Reception of Grammar (TROG)*. Oxford, UK: Medical Research Council.

Blanke, O., Brooks, A., Mercier, M., Spinelli, L., Adriani, M., Lavanchy, L., et al. (2007). Distinct mechanisms of form-from-motion perception in human extrastriate cortex. *Neuropsychologia, 45*(4), 644–653.

Boddaert, N., Mochel, F., Meresse, I., Seidenwurm, D., Cachia, A., Brunelle, F., Lyonnet, S., & Zilbovicius, M. (2006). Parieto-occipital grey matter abnormalities in children with Williams syndrome. *NeuroImage, 30*(3), 721–725.

Boloh, Y., & Ibernon, L. (2010). Gender attribution and gender agreement in 4- to 10-year-old French children. *Cognitive Development, 25*(1), 1–25.

Boloh, Y., Ibernon, L., Royer, S., Escudier, F., & Danillon, A. (2009). Gender attribution and gender agreement in French Williams syndrome. *Research in Developmental Disabilities, 30*(6), 1523–1540.

Bouchard, T. J., Lykken, D. T., McGue, M., Segal, N. L., & Tellegen, A. (1990). Sources of human psychological differences: The Minnesota study of twins reared apart. *Science, 250*(4978), 223–228.

Brady, T. F., Konkle, T., Alvarez, G. A., & Oliva, A. (2008). Visual long-term memory has a massive storage capacity for object details. *Proceedings of the National Academy of Sciences, 105*(38), 14325–14329.

Bridgeman, B., Peery, S., & Anand, S. (1997). Interaction of cognitive and sensorimotor maps of visual space. *Perception & Psychophysics, 59*(3), 456–469.

Bromberg, H., Ullman, M., Marcus, G., & Kelly, K. (1994). *A dissociation of memory and grammar: Evidence from Williams syndrome.* Paper presented at the Eighteenth Annual Boston University Conference on Language Development, Boston, MA.

Bullens, J., Nardini, M., Doeller, C. F., Braddick, O., Postma, A., & Burgess, N. (2010). The role of landmarks and boundaries in the development of spatial memory. *Developmental Science, 13*(1), 170–180.

Burgess, N. (2008). Spatial cognition and the brain. *Annals of the New York Academy of Sciences, 1124*, 77–97.

Burgess, N., Jeffery, K. J., & O'Keefe, J. (1999). Integrating hippocampal and parietal functions: A spatial point of view. In N. Burgess, K. J. Jeffery, & J. O'Keefe (Eds.), *The hippocampal and parietal foundations of spatial cognition* (pp. 3–29). New York: Oxford University Press.

Carey, S. (2009). *The origin of concepts.* New York: Oxford University Press.

Carey, S., & Diamond, R. (1994). Are faces perceived as configurations more by adults than by children? *Visual Cognition, 1*, 253–274.

Carlson-Radvansky, L., & Irwin, D. E. (1993). Frames of reference in vision and language: Where is "above"? *Cognition, 46*(3), 223–244.

Casey, B. J., Tottenham, N., Liston, C., & Durston, S. (2005). Imaging the developing brain: What have we learned about cognitive development? *Trends in Cognitive Sciences, 9*(3), 104–110.

Chafee, M. V., Crowe, D. A., Averbeck, B. B., & Georgopoulos, A. P. (2005). Neural correlates of spatial judgement during object construction in parietal cortex. *Cerebral Cortex, 15*(9), 1393.

Cheng, K. (1986). A purely geometric module in the rat's spatial representation. *Cognition, 23*(2), 149–178.

Cheng, K. (2008). Whither geometry? Troubles of the geometric module. *Trends in Cognitive Science, 12*(9), 355–361.

Cheng, K., & Newcombe, N. (2005). Is there a geometric module for spatial orientation? Squaring theory and evidence. *Psychonomic Bulletin & Review, 12*(1), 1–23.

Chianetti, C., & Vallortigara, G. (2008). Is there an innate geometric module? Effects of experience with angular geometric cues on spatial reorientation based on the shape of the environment. *Animal Cognition, 11*, 139–146.

Clahsen, H., & Almazan, M. (1998). Syntax and morphology in Williams syndrome. *Cognition, 68*(3), 167–198.

Clamp, M., Fry, B., Kamal, M., Xia, X., Cuff, J., Lin, M. F., Kellis, M., Lindblad-Toh, K., & Lander, E. S. (2007). Distinguishing protein-coding and noncoding genes in the human genome. *Proceeding of the National Academy of Science, 104*(49), 19428–19433.

Clark, E. V. (1971). On the acquisition of the meaning of before and after. *Journal of Verbal Learning and Verbal Behavior, 10*(3), 266–275.

Clark, E. V. (1980). Here's the top: Nonlinguistic strategies in the acquisition of orientational terms. *Child Development, 51*(2), 329–338.

Colby, C. L., & Goldberg, M. E. (1999). Space and attention in parietal cortex. *Annual Review of Neuroscience, 22*, 319–349.

Cowan, N. (2000). The magical number 4 in short-term memory: A reconsideration of mental storage capacity. *Behavioral and Brain Sciences, 24*, 87–185.

Culham, J. C., Brandt, S. A., Cavanagh, P., Kanwisher, N. G., Dale, A. M., & Tootell, R. B. H. (1998). Cortical fMRI activation produced by attentive tracking of moving targets. *Journal of Neurophysiology, 80*(5), 2657.

Culham, J. C., & Kanwisher, N. G. (2001). Neuroimaging of cognitive functions in human parietal cortex. *Current Opinion in Neurobiology, 11*(2), 157–163.

Dehaene, S. (1999). *The number sense: How the mind creates mathematics.* New York: Oxford University Press.

Dehaene, S., Piazza, M., Pinel, P., & Cohen, L. (2003). Three parietal circuits for number processing. *Cognitive Neuropsychology, 20*(3), 487–506.

Deruelle, C., Mancini, J., Livet, M., Casse-Perrot, C., & De Schonen, S. (1999). Configural and local processing of faces in children with Williams syndrome. *Brain and Cognition, 41*(3), 276–298.

Deruelle, C., Rondan, C., Livet, M. O., Mancini, J. (2003). Exploring face processing in Williams syndrome. *Cognition, Brain, Behavior, 7*, 157–172.

Dessalegn, B., & Landau, B. (2008). More than meets the eye—The role of language in binding and maintaining feature conjunctions. *Psychological Science, 19*(2), 189–195.

Dessalegn, B., Landau, B., & Rapp, B. (2012). The impact of a visual-spatial deficit on reading acquisition: Evidence from Williams syndrome. *Neurocase*, iFirst, 1–20.

Dilks, D., Hoffman, J. E., & Landau, B. (2008). Vision for perception and vision for action: Normal and unusual development. *Developmental Science, 11*(4), 474–486.

Dittrich, W. H., Troscianko, T., Lea, S., & Morgan, D. (1996). Perception of emotion from dynamic point-light displays represented in dance. *Perception, 25*, 727–738.

Doeller, C. F., & Burgess, N. (2008). Distinct error-correcting and incidental learning of location relative to landmarks and boundaries. *Proceedings of the National Academy of Sciences, 105*(15), 5909.

Doeller, C. F., King, J. A., & Burgess, N. (2008). Parallel striatal and hippocampal systems for landmarks and boundaries in spatial memory. *Proceedings of the National Academy of Sciences, 105*(15), 5915.

Duchaine, B., & Nakayama, K. (2005). Dissociations of face and object recognition in developmental prosopagnosia. *Journal of Cognitive Neuroscience, 17*(2), 249–261.

Dunn, L. M., & Dunn, L. M. (1997). *Peabody Picture Vocabulary Test–Third Edition.* Circle Pines, MN: American Guidance Service.

Eckert, M. A., Hu, D., Eliez, S., Bellugi, U., Galaburda, A., Korenberg, J., Mills, D., & Reiss, A. L. (2005). Evidence for superior parietal impairment in Williams syndrome. *Neurology, 64*(1), 152.

Edmonston, N. K., & Litchfield Thane, N. (1988). *TRC: Test of Relational Concepts.* Austin, TX: Pro-Ed.

Eichenbaum, H. (2000). A cortical-hippocampal system for declarative memory. *Nature Reviews Neuroscience, 1*(1), 41–50.

Elliott, C. D. (1990). *Differential Abilities Scales.* San Antonio, TX: Psychological Corporation.

Elman, J. L., Bates, E., Johnson, M. H., Karmiloff-Smith, A., Parisi, D., Plunkett, K. (1996). *Rethinking innateness: Connectionism in a developmental framework.* Cambridge, MA: MIT Press.

Epstein, R. A. (2008). Parahippocampal and retrosplenial contributions to human spatial navigation. *Trends in Cognitive Sciences, 12*(10), 388–396.

Epstein, R., Harris, A., Stanley, D., & Kanwisher, N. (1999). The parahippocampal place area: Recognition, navigation, or encoding? *Neuron, 23*(1), 115–125.

Epstein, R., & Kanwisher, N. (1998). A cortical representation of the local visual environment. *Nature, 392*(6676), 598–601.

Ewart, A. K., Morris, C. A., Atkinson, D., Jin, W., Sternes, K., Spallone, P., Stock, A. D., Leppert, M., & Keating, M. T. (1993). Hemizygosity at the elastin locus in a developmental disorder, Williams syndrome. *Nature Genetics, 5*(1), 11–16.

Farah, M. J. (2004). *Visual agnosia.* Cambridge, MA: MIT Press.

Farah, M. J., Rabinowitz, C., Quinn, G. E., & Liu, G. T. (2000). Early commitment of neural substrates for face recognition. *Cognitive Neuropsychology, 17*(1), 117–123.

Farah, M. J., Wilson, K. D., Drain, M., & Tanaka, J. N. (1998). What is "special" about face perception? *Psychological Review, 105*(3), 482–498.

Faria, A. F., Landau, B., O'Hearn, K., Li, X., Jiang, H., Zhang, J., Oishi, K., Zhang, J., & Susumu, M. (2012). Quantitative analysis of gray and white matter in Williams syndrome, *Neuroreport, 23*(5), 283–289.

Farran, E. K. (2005). Perceptual grouping ability in Williams syndrome: Evidence for deviant patterns of performance. *Neuropsychologia, 43*(5), 815–822.

Farran, E. K. (2006). Orientation coding: A specific deficit in Williams syndrome? *Developmental Neuropsychology, 29*(3), 397–414.

Farran, E. K., Blades, M., Boucher, J., & Tranter, L. J. (2010). How do individuals with Williams syndrome learn a route in a real-world environment? *Developmental Science, 13*(3), 454–468.

Farran, E. K., Jarrold, C., & Gathercole, S. E. (2003). Divided attention, selective attention and drawing: Processing preferences in Williams syndrome are dependent on the task administered. *Neuropsychologia, 41*(6), 676–687.

Feigenson, L., Dehaene, S., & Spelke, E. (2004). Core systems of number. *Trends in Cognitive Sciences, 8*(7), 307–314.

Feist, M. I., & Gentner, D. (1998). On plates, bowls, and dishes: Factors in the use of English IN and ON. *Proceedings of the Twentieth Annual Conference of the Cognitive Science Society: August 1–4, 1998, University of Wisconsin-Madison*, 345.

Ferrara, K., & Landau, B. (2012). Reorientation in people with Williams syndrome: A second look. Manuscript in preparation.

Fisher, S. E. (2006). Tangled webs: Tracing the connections between genes and cognition. *Cognition, 101*(2), 270–297.

Fodor, J. A. (1983). *The modularity of mind.* Cambridge, MA: MIT Press.

Franconeri, S., Jonathan, S. V., & Scimeca, J. M. (2010). Tracking Multiple Objects Is Limited Only by Object Spacing, Not by Speed, Time, or Capacity. *Psychological Science, 21*(7), 920–925.

Frangiskakis, J. M., Ewart, A. K., Morris, C. A., Mervis, C. B., Bertrand, J., Robinson, B. F., Klein, B. P., Ensing, G. J., Everett, L. A., & Green, E. D. (1996). LIM-kinase 1 hemizygosity implicated in impaired visuospatial constructive cognition. *Cell, 86*(1), 59–70.

Franz, V., Hesse, C., & Kollath, S. (2009). Visual illusions, delayed grasping, and memory: No shift from dorsal to ventral control. *Neuropsychologia, 47*(6), 1518–1531.

Freire, A., Lewis, T. L., Maurer, D., & Blake, R. (2006). The development of sensitivity to biological motion in noise. *Perception, 35*(5), 647–657.

Frisby, J. P., & Stone, J. V. (2010). *Seeing: The computational approach to biological vision.* Cambridge, MA: MIT Press.

Galaburda, A. M., & Bellugi, U. (2000). Multi-level analysis of cortical neuroanatomy in Williams syndrome. *Journal of Cognitive Neuroscience, 12*(Suppl. 1), 74–88.

Galaburda, A. M., Holinger, D. P., Bellugi, U., & Sherman, G. F. (2002). Williams syndrome—Neuronal size and neuronal-packing density in primary visual cortex. *Archives of Neurology, 59*(9), 1461–1467.

Gallistel, C. R. (1990). *The organization of learning.* Cambridge, MA: MIT Press.

Gaser, C., Luders, E., Thompson, P. M., Lee, A. D., Dutton, R. A., Geaga, J. A., Hayashi, K. M., Bellugi, U., Galaburda, A. M., & Korenberg, J. R. (2006). Increased local gyrification mapped in Williams syndrome. *NeuroImage, 33*(1), 46–54.

Gathercole, S. E. (1998). The development of memory. *The Journal of Child Psychology and Psychiatry and Allied Disciplines, 39*(01), 3–27.

Gazzaniga, M., Ivry, R. B., & Mangun, G. R. (2008). *Cognitive neuroscience: The biology of the mind* (3rd ed.). New York: Norton.

Georgopoulos, M. A., Georgopoulos, A. P., Kurz, N., and Landau, B. (2004). Figure copying in Williams syndrome and normal subjects. *Experimental Brain Research, 157*, 137–146.

Gibson, E., Desmet, T., Grodner, D., Watson, D., & Ko, K. (2005). Reading relative clauses in English. *Cognitive Linguistics, 16*(2), 313–353.

Ginsburg, H., & Baroody, A. (1990). *Test of early mathematics ability.* Austin, TX: ProEd.

Glessner, J. T., Wang, K., et al. (2009). Autism genome-wide copy number variation reveals ubiquitin and neuronal genes. *Nature, 459*(7246), 569–573.

Gogtay, N., Giedd, J. N., Lusk, L., Hayashi, K. M., Greenstein, D., Vaituzis, A. C., Nugent, T. F., Herman, D. H., Clasen, L. S., & Toga, A. W. (2004). Dynamic mapping of human cortical development during childhood through early adulthood. *Proceedings of the National Academy of Sciences, 101*(21), 8174–8179.

Golarai, G., Ghahremani, D. G., Whitfield-Gabrieli, S., Reiss, A., Eberhardt, J. L., Gabrieli, J. D. E., & Grill-Spector, K. (2007). Differential development of high-level visual cortex correlates with category-specific recognition memory. *Nature Reviews Neuroscience, 10*(4), 512–522.

Golarai, G., Hon, S., Haas, B. W., Galaburda, A. M., Mills, D. L., Bellugi, U., Grill-Spector, K., & Reiss, A. L. (2010). The fusiform face area is enlarged in Williams syndrome. *The Journal of Neuroscience, 30*(19), 6700–6712.

Gopnik, M. (1990). Feature-blind grammar and dysphasia. *Nature, 344*, 715.

Gopnik, M., & Crago, M. (1991). Familial aggregation of a developmental language disorder. *Cognition, 39*(1), 1–50.

Gouteux, S., Thinus-Blanc, C., & Vauclair, J. (2001). Rhesus monkeys use geometric and non-geometric information during a reorientation task. *Journal of Experimental Psychology: General, 130*, 505–519.

Gouteux, S., Vauclair, J., & Thinus-Blanc, C. (2001). Reorientation in a small-scale environment by 3-, 4-, and 5-year-old children. *Cognitive Development, 16*, 853–869.

Gray, V., Karmiloff-Smith, A., Funnell, E., & Tassabehji, M. (2006). In-depth analysis of spatial cognition in Williams syndrome: A critical assessment of the role of the LIMK1 gene. *Neuropsychologia, 44*(5), 679–685.

Grefkes, C., & Fink, G. R. (2005). The functional organization of the intraparietal sulcus in humans and monkeys. *Journal of Anatomy, 207*(1), 3.

Gregory, E., Trzcinski, N., Hoffman, J. E., & Landau, B. (2009). The representation of action in memory: A developmental study. Poster presented at the Annual Meeting of the Vision Sciences Society, Naples, Florida.

Gregory, R. L. (1974). *The intelligent eye.* New York: McGraw-Hill.

Grill-Spector, K., Golarai, G., & Gabrieli, J. (2008). Developmental neuroimaging of the human ventral visual cortex. *Trends in Cognitive Sciences, 12*(4), 152–162.

Grill-Spector, K., & Kanwisher, N. (2005). Visual recognition. *Psychological Science, 16*, 152–160.

Grossberg, S., Kuhlmann, L., & Mingolla, E. (2007). A neural model of 3D shape-from-texture: Multiple-scale filtering, boundary grouping, and surface filling-in. *Vision Research, 47*(5), 634–672.

Gunn, A., Cory, E., Atkinson, J., Braddick, O., Wattam-Bell, J., Guzzetta, A., et al. (2002). Dorsal and ventral stream sensitivity in normal development and hemiplegia. *Neuroreport, 13*(6), 843–847.

Haaxma, R., & Kuypers, H. (1975). Intrahemispheric cortical connexions and visual guidance of hand and finger movements in the rhesus monkey. *Brain, 98*(2), 239.

Hafting, T., Fyhn, M., Molden, S., Moser, M. B., & Moser, E. I. (2005). Microstructure of a spatial map in the entorhinal cortex. *Nature, 436*, 801–806.

Halberda, J., & Feigenson, L. (2008). Developmental change in the acuity of the "number sense": The approximate number system in 3-, 4-, 5-, and 6-year-olds and adults. *Developmental Psychology, 44*(5), 1457–1465.

Halberda, J., Mazzocco, M. M. M., & Feigenson, L. (2008). Individual differences in non-verbal number acuity correlate with maths achievement. *Nature, 455*(7213), 665–668.

Hartley, T., Bird, C. M., Chan, D., Cipolotti, L., Husain, M., Vargha-Khadem, F., & Burgess, N. (2007). The hippocampus is required for short-term topographical memory in humans. *Hippocampus, 17*(1), 34–48.

Hayward, W. G., & Tarr, M. J. (1995). Spatial language and spatial representation. *Cognition, 55*, 39–84.

Hermer, L., & Spelke, E. (1996). Modularity and development: The case of spatial reorientation. *Cognition, 61*(3), 195–232.

Hermer-Vazquez, L., Moffet, A., & Munkholm, P. (2001). Language, space, and the development of cognitive flexibility in humans: The case of two spatial memory tasks. *Cognition, 79*, 263–299.

Hermer-Vazquez, L., Spelke, E., & Katsnelson, A. S. (1999). Sources of flexibility in human cognition: Dual-task studies of space and language. *Cognitive Psychology, 39*, 3–36.

Herskovits, A. (1986). *Language and spatial cognition: An interdisciplinary study of the prepositions in English*. Cambridge: Cambridge University Press.

Himmelbach, M., Nau, M., Zundorf, I., Erb, M., Perenin, M-T., & Karnath, H.-O. (2009). Brain activation during immediate and delayed reaching in optic ataxia. *Neuropsychologia, 47*, 1508–1517.

Hoeft, F., Barnea-Goraly, N., Haas, B. W., Golarai, G., Ng, D., Mills, D., Korenberg, J., Bellugi, U., Galaburda, A., & Reiss, A. L. (2007). More is not always better: Increased fractional anisotropy of superior longitudinal fasciculus associated with poor visuospatial abilities in Williams syndrome. *Journal of Neuroscience, 27*(44), 11960.

Hoffman, J. E., Landau, B., & Pagani, B. (2003). Spatial breakdown in spatial construction: Evidence from eye fixations in children with Williams syndrome. *Cognitive Psychology, 46*(3), 260–301.

Hubbard, E. M., Piazza, M., Pinel, P., & Dehaene, S. (2005). Interactions between number and space in parietal cortex. *Nature Reviews Neuroscience, 6*(6), 435–448.

Hubel, D. H., & Wiesel, T. N. (1962). Receptive fields, binocular interaction and functional architecture in the cat's visual cortex. *Journal of Physiology, 1*, 106–154.

Hulleman, J. (2005). The mathematics of multiple object tracking: From proportions correct to number of objects tracked. *Vision Research, 45*, 2298–2309.

Hupbach, A., & Nadel, L. (2005). Reorientation in a rhombic environment: No evidence for an encapsulated geometric module. *Cognitive Development, 20*, 279–302.

Huttenlocher, J., & Presson, C. C. (1973). Mental rotation and the perspective problem. *Cognitive Psychology, 4*(2), 277–299.

Huttenlocher, P. R. (2002). *Neural plasticity: The effects of environment on the development of the cerebral cortex*. Cambridge, MA: Harvard University Press.

Ihara, H., & Fujita, I. (2000). A cognitive approach to errors in case marking in Japanese agrammatism: The priority of the goal -ni over the source -kara. In A. Foolen & F. Van der Leek (Eds.), *Constructions in cognitive linguistics: Selected papers from the fifth international cognitive linguistics conference* (pp. 124–140). Amsterdam: John Benjamins.

Jackendoff, R. (1983). *Semantics and cognition*. Cambridge, MA: MIT Press.

Jackendoff, R. (1994). *Patterns in the mind: Language and human nature*. New York: Basic Books.

Jackowski, A. P., & Schultz, R. T. (2005). Foreshortened dorsal extension of the central sulcus in Williams syndrome. *Cortex, 41*(3), 282–290.

Jacobs, J., Kahana, M. J., Ekstrom, A. D., Mollison, M.V., & Fried, I. (2010). A sense of direction in human entorhinal cortex. *Proceedings of the National Academy of Sciences, 107*(14), 6487.

Jarrold C., Baddeley, A. D., & Hewes, A. K. (1999). Genetically dissociated components of working memory: Evidence from Down's and Williams syndrome. *Neuropsychologia, 37*, 647–651.

Johansson, G. (1973). Visual perception of biological motion and a model for its analysis. *Perception and Psychophysics, 14*, 201–211.

John, A., & Mervis, C. B. (2010). Comprehension of the communicative intent behind pointing and gazing gestures by young children with Williams syndrome or Down syndrome. *Journal of Speech Language and Hearing Research*, 53, 950–960

Johnson, J. S., & Newport, E.L. (1991). Critical period effects in second language learning: The influence of maturational state on the acquisition of a second language. *Cognition, 39*, 215–258.

Johnson, M. H., Mareschal, D., & Csibra, G. (2008). The development and integration of dorsal and ventral visual pathways in object processing. In C. A. Nelson & M. Luciana (Eds.), *Handbook of developmental cognitive neuroscience* (pp. 467–478). Cambridge, MA: MIT Press.

Johnson, S. C., & Carey, S. (1996). Knowledge enrichment and conceptual change in folkbiology: Evidence from Williams syndrome. *Cognitive Psychology, 37*, 156–200.

Jones, P. M., Pearce, J. M., Davies, V. J., Good, M. A., & McGregor, A. (2007). Impaired processing of local geometric features during navigation in a water maze following hippocampal lesions in rats. *Behavioral Neuroscience, 121*, 1258–1271.

Jones, W., Hesselink, J., Courchesne, E., Duncan, T., Matsuda, K., & Bellugi, U. (2002). Cerebellar abnormalities in infants and toddlers with Williams syndrome. *Developmental Medicine and Child Neurology, 44*(10), 688–694.

Jordan, H., Reiss, J. E., Hoffman, J. E., & Landau, B. (2002). Intact perception of biological motion in the face of profound spatial deficits: Williams syndrome. *Psychological Science, 13*(2), 162–167.

Jovicich, J., Peters, R. J., Koch, C., Braun, J., Chang, L., & Ernst, T. (2001). Brain areas specific for attentional load in a motion-tracking task. *Journal of Cognitive Neuroscience, 13*(8), 1048–1058.

Just, M. A., & Carpenter, P. A. (1992). A capacity theory of comprehension: Individual differences in working memory. *Psychological Review, 98*, 122–149.

Kanwisher, N. (2010). Functional specificity in the human brain: A window into the functional architecture of the mind. *Proceedings of the National Academy of Sciences, 107*(25), 11163–11170.

Karmiloff-Smith, A. (1997). Crucial differences between developmental cognitive neuroscience and adult neuropsychology. *Developmental Neuropsychology, 13*(4), 513–524.

Karmiloff-Smith, A. (1998). Development itself is the key to understanding developmental disorders. *Trends in Cognitive Sciences, 2*, 389–398.

Karmiloff-Smith, A. (2007). Atypical epigenesis. *Developmental Science, 10*(1), 84.

Karmiloff-Smith, A., Grant, J., Berthoud, I., Davies, M., Howlin, P., & Udwin, O. (1997). Language and Williams syndrome: How intact is intact? *Child Development, 68*(2), 246–262.

Karmiloff-Smith, A., Thomas, M., Annaz, D., Humphreys, K., Ewing, S., Brace, N., Van Duuren, M., Pike, G., Grice, S., & Campbell, R. (2004). Exploring the Williams syndrome face-processing debate: The importance of building developmental trajectories. *Journal of Child Psychology and Psychiatry, 45*(7), 1258–1274.

Kaufman, A. S., & Kaufman, N. L. (1990). *Kaufman Brief Intelligence Test.* Circle Pines, MN: American Guidance Service.

Kaufman, A. S., & Kaufman, N. L. (2004). *Kaufman Brief Intelligence Test* (2nd ed.). Circle Pines, MN: American Guidance Service.

Kelly, D. M., Spetch, M. L., & Heth, C. D. (1998). Pigeons' encoding of geometric and featural properties of a spatial environment. *Journal of Comparative Psychology, 112*, 259–269.

Kesler, S. R., Haberecht, M. F., Menon, V., Warsofsky, I. S., Dyer-Friedman, J., Neely, E. K., et al. (2004). Functional neuroanatomy of spatial orientation processing in Turner syndrome. *Cerebral Cortex, 14*(2), 174–180.

Key, A. F., Pani, J. R., & Mervis, C. B. (1998). *Visuospatial constructive ability of people with Williams Syndrome.* Paper presented at the Sixth Annual Workshop on Object Perception and Memory, Dallas, TX.

Kippenhan, J. S., Olsen, R. K., Mervis, C. B., Morris, C. A., Kohn, P., Meyer-Lindenberg, A., & Berman, K. F. (2005). Genetic contributions to human gyrification: Sulcal morphometry in Williams syndrome. *Journal of Neuroscience, 25*(34), 7840.

Klatzky, R. L., Clark, E. V., & Macken, M. (1973). Asymmetries in the acquisition of polar adjectives: Linguistic or conceptual? *Journal of Experimental Child Psychology, 16*(1), 32–46.

Klatzky, R. L., Loomis, J. M., Beall, A. C., Chance, S. S., & Golledge, R. G. (1998). Spatial updating of self-position and orientation during real, imagined, and virtual locomotion. *Psychological Science, 9*(4), 293–298.

Knierim, J. J., & Hamilton, D. A. (2011). Framing spatial cognition: Neural representations of proximal and distal frames of reference and their roles in navigation. *Physiological Reviews, 91*(4), 1245–1279.

Kourtzi, Z., & Kanwisher, N. (2001). Representation of perceived object shape by the human lateral occipital complex. *Science, 293*(5534), 1506–1509.

Krajcsi, A., Lukács, Á., Igacs, J., Racsmany, M., & Pleh, C. (2009). Numerical abilities in Williams syndrome: Dissociating the analogue magnitude system and verbal retrieval. *Journal of Clinical and Experimental Neuropsychology, 31*(4), 439–446.

Kravitz, D. J., Saleem, K. S., Baker, C. I., & Mishkin, M. (2011). A new neural framework for visuospatial processing. *Nature Reviews Neuroscience, 12*, 217–230.

Laing, E., Hulme, C., Grant, J., & Karmiloff-Smith, A. (2001). Learning to read in Williams syndrome: Looking beneath the surface of atypical reading development. *The Journal of Child Psychology and Psychiatry and Allied Disciplines, 42*(06), 729–739.

Lakusta, L., Dessalegn, B., & Landau, B. (2010). Impaired geometric reorientation caused by genetic defect. *Proceedings of the National Academy of Sciences, 107*(7), 2813.

Lakusta, L., & Landau, B. (2005). Starting at the end: The importance of goals in spatial language. *Cognition, 96*(1), 1–33.

Lakusta, L., & Landau, B. (2012). Language and memory for motion events: Origins of the asymmetry between source and goal paths. *Cognitive Science, 36*(3), 517–544.

Lakusta, L., Wagner, L., O'Hearn, K., & Landau, B. (2007). Conceptual foundations of spatial languages: Evidence for a goal bias in infants. *Language Learning and Development, 3*(3), 179–197.

Lakusta, L., Yoshida, H., Landau, B., & Smith, L. (2006). *Cross-linguistic evidence for a goal/source asymmetry: The case of Japanese.* Poster presented at the International Conference on Infant Studies, Kyoto, Japan.

Landau, B., Gleitman, H., & Spelke, E. (1981). Spatial knowledge and geometric representation in a child blind from birth. *Science, 213*(4513), 1275–1278.

Landau, B., & Hoffman, J. E. (2005). Parallels between spatial cognition and spatial language: Evidence from Williams syndrome. *Journal of Memory & Language, 53*(2), 163–185.

Landau, B., & Hoffman, J. E. (2007). Explaining selective spatial breakdown in Williams syndrome: Four principles of normal spatial development and why they matter. In J. M. Plumert & J. P. Spencer (Eds.), *The emerging spatial mind* (pp. 290–319). New York: Oxford University Press.

Landau, B., Hoffman, J., & Kurz, N. (2006). Object recognition with severe spatial deficits in Williams syndrome: Sparing and breakdown. *Cognition, 100*(3), 483–510.

Landau, B., & Jackendoff, R. (1993). "What" and "where" in spatial language and spatial cognition. *Behavioral and Brain Sciences, 16*(2), 217–265.

Landau, B., & Lakusta, L. (2009). Spatial representation across species: Geometry, language, and maps. *Current Opinion in Neurobiology, 19*(1), 12–19.

Landau, B., Smith, L., & Jones, S. (1998). Object perception and object naming in early development. *Trends in Cognitive Sciences, 2*(1), 19–24.

Landau, B., & Spelke, E. (1988). Geometric complexity and object search in infancy. *Developmental Psychology, 24*(4), 512–521.

Landau, B., Spelke, E., & Gleitman, H. (1984). Spatial knowledge in a young blind child. *Cognition, 16*(3), 225–260.

Landau, B., & Zukowski, A. (2003). Objects, motions, and paths: Spatial language in children with Williams syndrome. *Developmental Neuropsychology, 23*(1), 107–139.

Learmonth, A. E., Newcombe, N. S., & Huttenlocher, J. (2001). Toddlers' use of metric information and landmarks to reorient. *Journal of Experimental Child Psychology, 80*(3), 225–244.

Lee, J., Okamura, A., & Landau, B. (2009). Haptics as an aid to copying for people with Williams Syndrome. *Third Joint EuroHaptics Conference and Symposium on*

Haptic Interfaces for Virtual Environment and Teleoperator Systems, Salt Lake City, UT, March 18–20, 356–361.

Lee, S. A., & Spelke, E. S. (2008). Children's use of geometry for reorientation. *Developmental Science, 11*, 743–749.

Lenneberg, E. H. (1967). *Biological foundations of language*. New York: Wiley.

Lever, C., Wills, T., Cacucci, F., Burgess, N., & O'Keefe, J. (2002). Long-term plasticity in hippocampal place-cell representation of environmental geometry. *Nature, 416*, 90–94.

Lewis, T. L., & Maurer, D. (2005). Multiple sensitive periods in human visual development: Evidence from visually deprived children. *Developmental Psychobiology, 46*(3), 163–183.

Libertus, M., Halberda, J., Feigenson, L, & Landau, B. (in preparation). Representation of approximate number in people with Williams syndrome.

Li, H., Roy, M., Kuscuoglu, U., Spencer, C. & Francke, U. (2009). Induced chromosome deletions cause hypersociability and other features of Williams-Beuren syndrome in mice. *EMBO Molecular Medicine, 1*, 50–65.

Lidz, J., & Musolino, J. (2002). Children's command of quantification. *Cognition, 84*, 113–154.

Loomis, J., Klatzky, R. L., Golledge, R. G., Cicinelli, J. G., Pellegrino, J. W., & Fry, P. A. (1993). Nonvisual navigation by blind and sighted: Assessment of path integration ability. *Journal of Experimental Psychology: General, 122*(1), 73–91.

Lowery, M. C., Morris, C. A., Ewart, A., Brothman, L. J., Zhu, X. L., Leonard, C. O., Carey, J. C., Keating, M., & Brothman, A. R. (1995). Strong correlation of elastin deletions, detected by FISH, with Williams syndrome: Evaluation of 235 patients. *American Journal of Human Genetics, 57*(1), 49.

Macmillan, N. A., & Creelman, C. D. (1991). *Detection theory: A user's guide*. New York: Cambridge University Press.

Maguire, E. A., Gadian, D. G., Johnsrude, I. S., Good, C. D., Ashburner, J., Frackowiak, R. S. J., & Frith, C. D. (2000). Navigation-related structural change in the hippocampi of taxi drivers. *Proceedings of the National Academy of Sciences, 97*(8), 4398.

Marcus, G. F. (2004). *The birth of the mind*. New York: Basic Books.

Marenco, S., Siuta, M. A., Kippenhan, J. S., Grodofsky, S., Chang, W., Kohn, P., Mervis, C. B., Morris, C. A., Weinberger, D. R., & Meyer-Lindenberg, A. (2007). Genetic contributions to white matter architecture revealed by diffusion tensor imaging in Williams syndrome. *Proceedings of the National Academy of Sciences, 104*(38), 15117.

Mareschal, D., & Johnson, M. H. (2003). The "what" and "where" of object representations in infancy. *Cognition, 88*(3), 259–276.

Marr, D. (1982). *Vision*. San Francisco: W. H. Freeman.

Marr, D., & Nishihara, H. K. (1978). Representation and recognition of the spatial organization of three-dimensional structure. *Proceedings of the Royal Society of London, Series B: Biological Sciences, 200*, 269–294.

Martin, N. D.T., Smith, W. R., Cole, T. J., & Preece, M. A. (2007). New height, weight, and head circumference charts for British children with Williams syndrome. *Archives of Disease in Childhood, 92*, 598–601.

Mather, G., & Murdoch, L. (1994). Gender discrimination in biological motion display based on dynamic cues. *Proceedings of the Royal Society of London, Series B: Biological Sciences, 258*, 273–279.

Mathers, P. H., Grinbeg, A., Mahon, K. A., & Jamrich, M (1997). The *Rx* homeobox gene is essential for vertebrate eye development. *Nature, 387*, 604–607.

Maurer, D., Le Grand, R., & Mondloch, C. J. (2002). The many faces of configural processing. *Trends in Cognitive Science, 6*, 255–260.

Mazard, A., Schiltz, C., & Rossion, B. (2006). Recovery from adaptation to facial identity is larger for upright than inverted faces in the human occipito-temporal cortex. *Neuropsychologia, 44*(6), 912–922.

McCloskey, M. (2009). *Visual reflections: A perceptual deficit and its implications*. New York: Oxford.

McGregor, A., Hayward, A. J., Pearce, J. M., & Good, M. A. (2004). Hippocampal lesions disrupt navigation based on the shape of the environment. *Behavioral Neuroscience, 118*, 1011–1021.

McKone, E., & Boyer, B. L. (2006). Sensitivity of 4-year-olds to featural and second-order relational changes in face distinctiveness. *Journal of Experimental Child Psychology, 94*(2), 134–162.

McKone, E., Crookes, K., & Kanwisher, N. (2009). The cognitive and neural development of face recognition in humans. In Gazzaniga, M. (Ed.), *The Cognitive Neurosciences* (pp. 467–482). Cambridge, MA: MIT Press.

McKone, E., Kanwisher, N., & Duchaine, B. (2007). Can generic expertise explain special processing for faces? *Trends in Cognitive Sciences, 11*(1), 8–15.

Meng, Y., Zhang, Y., Tregoubov, V., Janus, C., Cruz, L., Jackson, M., Lu, W., MacDonald, J. F., Wang, J. Y., Falls, D. L., & Jia, Z. (2002). Abnormal spine morphology and enhanced LTP in LIMK-1 knockout mice. *Neuron, 35*(1), 121–133.

Menghini, D., Verucci, L., & Vicari, S. (2004). Reading and phonological awareness in Williams syndrome. *Neuropsychology, 18*(1), 29–37.

Mervis, C. B. (2004). Cross-etiology comparisons of cognitive and language development. In M. L. Rice & S. F. Warren (Eds.), *Developmental language disorders: From phenotypes to etiologies* (pp. 153–186). Mahwah, NJ: Erlbaum Associates.

Mervis, C. B., & Becerra, A. M. (2007). Language and communicative development in Williams syndrome. *Mental Retardation and Developmental Disabilities Research Reviews, 13*(1), 3–15.

Mervis, C. B., & John, A. E. (2008). Vocabulary abilities of children with Williams syndrome: Strengths, weaknesses, and relation to visuospatial construction ability. *Journal of Speech, Language, and Hearing Research, 51*(4), 967.

Mervis, C. B., & Klein-Tasman, B. P. (2004). Methodological issues in group-matching designs: α levels for control variable comparisons and measurement characteristics of control and target variables. *Journal of Autism and Developmental Disorders, 34*(1), 7–17.

Mervis, C. B., Morris, C. A., Bertrand, J., & Robinson, B. (1999). Williams syndrome: Findings from an integrated program of research. In H. Tager-Flusberg (Ed.), *Neurodevelopmental disorders: Contributions to a new framework from the cognitive neurosciences* (pp. 65–110). Cambridge, MA: MIT Press.

Mervis, C. B., Robinson, B. F., Bertrand, J., Morris, C. A., Klein-Tasman, B. P., & Armstrong, S. C. (2000). The Williams syndrome cognitive profile. *Brain and Cognition, 44*(3), 604–628.

Meyer-Lindenberg, A., Kohn, P., Mervis, C. B., Kippenhan, J. S., Olsen, R. K., Morris, C. A., & Berman, K. F. (2004). Neural basis of genetically determined visuospatial construction deficit in Williams syndrome. *Neuron, 43*(5), 623–631.

Meyer-Lindenberg, A., Mervis, C. B., & Berman, K. F. (2006). Neural mechanisms in Williams syndrome: A unique window to genetic influences on cognition and behaviour. *Nature Reviews Neuroscience, 7*(5), 380–393.

Meyer-Lindenberg, A., Mervis, C. B., Sarpal, D., Koch, P., Steele, S., Kohn, P., Marenco, S., Morris, C. A., Das, S., & Kippenhan, S. (2005). Functional, structural, and metabolic abnormalities of the hippocampal formation in Williams syndrome. *Journal of Clinical Investigation, 115*(7), 1888–1895.

Milner, A. D., & Goodale, M. A. (1995). *The visual brain in action*. Oxford: Oxford University Press.

Milner, A. D., & Goodale, M. A. (2008). Two visual systems re-viewed. *Neuropsychologia, 46*(3), 774–785.

Mondloch, C. J., Le Grand, R., & Maurer, D. (2002). Configural face processing develops more slowly than featural face processing. *Perception, 31*(5), 553–566.

Morris, C. A. (2006a). The dysmorphology, genetics, and natural history of Williams-Beuren syndrome. In C. A. Morris, H. Lenhoff, & P. Wang (Eds.), *Williams-Beuren syndrome: Research, evaluation, and treatment* (pp. 3–17). Baltimore, MD: Johns Hopkins University Press.

Morris, C. A. (2006b). Genotype-phenotype correlations in Williams-Beuren syndrome. In C. A. Morris, H. Lenhoff, & P. Wang (Eds.), *Williams-Beuren syndrome: Research, evaluation, and treatment* (pp. 59–82). Baltimore, MD: Johns Hopkins University Press.

Morris, C. A., Mervis, C. B., Hobart, H. H., Gregg, R. G., Bertrand, J., Ensing, G. J., Sommer, A., Moore, C. A., Hopkin, R. J., & Spallone, P. A. (2003). GTF2I hemizygosity implicated in mental retardation in Williams syndrome: Genotype-phenotype analysis of five families with deletions in the Williams syndrome region. *American Journal of Medical Genetics Part A, 123*(1), 45–59.

Morton, J. (2004). *Understanding developmental disorders: A causal modeling approach.* Malden, MA: Wiley-Blackwell.

Moscovitch, M., Winocur, G., & Behrmann, M. (1997). What is special about face recognition? Nineteen experiments on a person with visual object agnosia and dyslexia but normal face recognition. *Journal of Cognitive Neuroscience, 9*(5), 555–604.

Muller, M., & Wehner, R. (1988). Path integration in desert ants, *Cataglyphis fortis. Proceedings of the National Academy of Sciences, 85*, 5287–5290.

Munnich, E., & Landau, B. (2010). Developmental decline in the acquisition of spatial language. *Language Learning and Development, 6*(1), 32–59.

Munnich, E., Landau, B., & Dosher, B. A. (2001). Spatial language and spatial representation: A cross-linguistic comparison. *Cognition, 81*(3), 171–207.

Musolino, J., Chunyo, G., & Landau, B. (2010). Uncovering knowledge of core syntactic and semantic principles in individuals with Williams syndrome. *Language Learning and Development, 6*(2), 126–161.

Musolino, J., & Landau, B. (2010). When theories don't compete: Response to Thomas, Karaminis, and Knowland's commentary on Musolino, Chunyo, and Landau. *Language Learning and Development, 6*(2), 170–178.

Nakayama, K., & Silverman, G. H. (1988). The aperture problem. I: Perception of nonrigidity and motion direction in translating sinusoidal lines. *Vision Research, 28*, 739–746.

Nardini, M., Atkinson, J., Braddick, O., & Burgess, N. (2008). Developmental trajectories for spatial frames of reference in Williams syndrome. *Developmental Science, 11*(4), 583–595.

Nardini, M., Burgess, N., Breckenridge, K., & Atkinson, J. (2006). Differential developmental trajectories for egocentric, environmental and intrinsic frames of reference in spatial memory. *Cognition, 101*(1), 153–172.

Navon, D. (1977). Forest before trees—precedence of global features in visual-perception. *Cognitive Psychology, 9*(3), 353–383.

Neville, H. J., & Bavelier, D. (2000). Specificity and plasticity in neurocognitive development in humans. In M. Gazzaniga (Ed.), *The new cognitive neurosciences* (pp. 83–98). Cambridge, MA: MIT Press.

Newcombe, N. S., & Huttenlocher, J. (1992). Children's early ability to solve perspective-taking problems. *Developmental Psychology, 28*(4), 635–643.

Newcombe, N. S., & Huttenlocher, J. (2000). *Making space: The development of spatial representation and reasoning*. Cambridge, MA: MIT Press.

Newcombe, N., Huttenlocher, J., Drummey, A. B., & Wiley, J. G. (1998). The development of spatial location coding: Place learning and dead reckoning in the second and third years. *Cognitive Development, 13*, 185–201.

Newcombe, N., & Ratliff, K. R. (2007). Explaining the development of spatial reorientation: Modularity-plus-language versus the emergence of adaptive combination. In J. M. Plumert & J. P. Spencer (Eds.), *The emerging spatial mind* (pp. 53–76). New York: Oxford University Press.

Newport, E. L. (1990). Maturational constraints on language learning. *Cognitive Science, 14*(1), 11–28.

Newport, E. L., Bavelier, D., & Neville, H. J. (2001). Critical thinking about critical periods: Perspectives on a critical period for language acquisition. In E. Dupoux

(Ed.), *Language, Brain and Cognitive Development* (pp. 481–502). Cambridge, MA: MIT Press.

Newsome, W. T., Britten, K. H., & Movshon, J. A. (1989). Neuronal correlates of a perceptual decision. *Nature, 341*(6237), 52–54.

Newsome, W. T., & Pare, E. B. (1988). A selective impairment of motion perception following lesions of the middle temporal visual area (MT). *Journal of Neuroscience, 8*(6), 2201–2211.

Ogawa, K., & Inui, T. (2009). The role of the posterior parietal cortex in drawing by copying. *Neuropsychologia, 47*(4), 1013–1022.

O'Hearn, K., Courtney, S., Street, W., & Landau, B. (2009). Working memory impairment in people with Williams syndrome: Effects of delay, task and stimuli. *Brain and Cognition, 69*, 495–503.

O'Hearn, K., Hoffman, J. E., & Landau, B. (2010). Developmental profiles for multiple object tracking and spatial memory: Typically developing preschoolers and people with Williams syndrome. *Developmental Science, 13*(3), 430–440.

O'Hearn, K., & Landau, B. (2007). Mathematical skill in individuals with Williams syndrome: Evidence from a standardized mathematics battery. *Brain and Cognition, 64*(3), 238–246.

O'Hearn, K., Landau, B., & Hoffman, J. E. (2005). Multiple object tracking in people with Williams syndrome and in normally developing children. *Psychological Science, 16*(11), 905.

O'Hearn, K., Roth, J. K., Courtney, S. M., Luna, B., Street, W., Terwillinger, R., & Landau, B. (2011). Object recognition in Williams syndrome: Uneven ventral stream activation. *Developmental Science, 14*(3), 549–565.

O'Keefe, J., & Burgess, N. (1996). Geometric determinants of the place fields of hippocampal neurons. *Nature, 381*(6581), 425–428.

O'Keefe, J., & Nadel, L. (1978). *The hippocampus as a cognitive map.* Oxford: Clarendon Press.

Olsen, R. K., Kippenhan, J. S., Japee, S., Kohn, P., Mervis, C. B., Saad, Z. S., Morris, C. A., Meyer-Lindenberg, A., & Berman, K. F. (2009). Retinotopically defined primary visual cortex in Williams syndrome. *Brain, 132*(3), 635.

Oram, M. W., & Perrett, D. I. (1994). Responses of anterior superior temporal polysensory (STPa) neurons to "biological motion" stimuli. *Journal of Cognitive Neuroscience, 6*, 99–116.

Osborne, L. R. (2006). The molecular basis of a multisystem disorder. In C. A. Morris, H. M. Lenhoff, and P. P. Wang (Eds.), *Williams-Beuren syndrome: Research, evaluation, and treatment* (pp. 18–58). Baltimore, MD: Johns Hopkins University Press.

Osborne, L. R., & Mervis, C. B. (2007). Rearrangements of the Williams–Beuren syndrome locus: Molecular basis and implications for speech and language development. *Expert Reviews in Molecular Medicine, 9*(15), 1–16.

Palmeri, T. J., & Gauthier, I. (2004). Visual object understanding. *Nature Reviews Neuroscience, 5*(4), 291–303.

Palomares, M., Landau, B., & Egeth, H. (2008). Visuospatial interpolation in typically developing children and in people with Williams syndrome. *Vision Research, 48*(23–24), 2439–2450.

Palomares, M., Landau, B., & Egeth, H. (2009). Orientation perception in Williams syndrome: Discrimination and integration. *Brain and Cognition, 70*(1), 21–30.

Palomares, M., Ogbonna, C., Landau, B., & Egeth, H. (2009). Normal susceptibility to visual illusions in abnormal development: Evidence from Williams syndrome. *Perception, 38*(2), 186.

Pani, J. R., Mervis, C. B., & Robinson, B. F. (1999). Global spatial organization by individuals with Williams syndrome. *Psychological Science, 10*(5), 453–458.

Parrish, E. E., Giaschi, D. E., Boden, C., & Dougherty, R. (2005). The maturation of form and motion perception in school age children. *Vision Research, 45*(7), 827–837.

Pavlova, M., Krägeloh-Mann, I., Sokolov, A., & Birbaumer, N. (2000). Simultaneous masking of a point-light walker in children. In C. Bonnet (Ed.), *Fechner Day 2000* (pp. 279–284). Strasbourg, France: ISP.

Perenin, M. T., & Vighetto, A. (1988). Optic ataxia: Specific disruption in visuomotor mechanisms. *Brain, 111*, 643–674.

Perovic, A., & Wexler, K. (2005). *New data on passives in Williams syndrome: Evidence for a grammatical delay.* Paper presented at the Thirtieth Annual Boston University Conference on Language Development, Boston, MA.

Perovic, A., & Wexler, K. (2006). Knowledge of binding, raising and passives in Williams syndrome. *The Proceedings of the Inaugural Conference on Generative Approaches to Language Acquisition–North America (GALANA)*, (4), 273–284.

Perovic, A., & Wexler, K. (2007). Complex grammar in Williams syndrome. *Clinical Linguistics & Phonetics, 21*(9), 729–745.

Perovic, A., & Wexler, K. (2010). Development of verbal passive in Williams syndrome. *Journal of Speech, Language, and Hearing Research, 53*(5), 1294–1306.

Piaget, J. (1954). *The construction of reality in the child.* Oxford, UK: Basic Books.

Piaget, J., & Inhelder, B. (1967). The child's conception of space. *The Coordination of Perspectives, 8*, 209–246.

Pinker, S. (1994). *The language instinct: The new science of language and mind.* New York: Harper Perennial.

Pinker, S. (1999). *Words and rules.* New York: Basic Books.

Pylyshyn, Z. W. (2000). Situating vision in the world. *Trends in Cognitive Sciences, 4*(5), 197–207.

Pylyshyn, Z. W. (2006). *Seeing and visualizing: It's not what you think.* Cambridge, MA: MIT Press.

Pylyshyn, Z. W., & Storm, R. W. (1988). Tracking multiple independent targets: Evidence for a parallel tracking mechanism. *Spatial Vision, 3*(3), 179–197.

Ramus, F. (2006). Genes, brain, and cognition: A roadmap for the cognitive scientist. *Cognition, 101*(2), 247–269.

Reddy, L., & Kanwisher, N. (2006). Coding of visual objects in the ventral stream. *Current Opinion in Neurobiology, 16*(4), 408–414.

Regier, T., & Carlson, L. A. (2001). Grounding spatial language in perception: An empirical and computational investigation. *Journal of Experimental Psychology General, 130*(2), 273–298.

Regier, T., & Zheng, M. (2007). Attention to endpoints: A cross-linguistic constraint on spatial meaning. *Cognitive Science, 31*, 705–719.

Reiss, A. L., Eckert, M. A., Rose, F. E., Karchemskiy, A., Kesler, S., Chang, M., Reynolds, M. F., Kwon, H., & Galaburda, A. (2004). An experiment of nature: Brain anatomy parallels cognition and behavior in Williams syndrome. *Journal of Neuroscience, 24*(21), 5009–5015.

Reiss J. E., Hoffman, J. E., & Landau, B. (2005). Motion processing specialization in Williams syndrome. *Vision Research, 45*(27), 3379–3390.

Riddoch, M. J., Humphreys, G., Jacobson, S., Pluck, G., Bateman, A., & Edwards, M. (2004). Impaired orientation discrimination and localisation following parietal damage: On the interplay between dorsal and ventral processes in visual perception. *Cognitive Neuropsychology, 21*(6), 597–623.

Rizzolatti, G., & Matelli, M. (2003). Two different streams form the dorsal visual system: Anatomy and functions. *Experimental Brain Research, 153*(2), 146–157.

Rondan, C., Santos, A., Mancini, J., Livet, M. O., & Deruelle, C. (2008). Global and local processing in Williams syndrome: drawing versus perceiving. *Child Neuropsychology, 14*(3), 237–248.

Rose, F. E., Lincoln, A. J., Lai, Z., Ene, M., Searcy, Y. M., & Bellugi, U. (2007). Orientation and affective expression effects on face recognition in Williams syndrome and autism. *Journal of Autism and Developmental Disorders, 37*(3), 513–522.

Sack, A. T. (2009). Parietal cortex and spatial cognition. *Behavioural Brain Research, 202*(2), 153–161.

Sarpal, D., Buchsbaum, B. R., Kohn, P. D., Kippenhan, J. S., Mervis, C. B., Morris, C. A., Meyer-Lindenberg, A., & Berman, K. F. (2008). A genetic model for understanding higher order visual processing: Functional interactions of the ventral visual stream in Williams syndrome. *Cerebral Cortex, 18*(10), 2402.

Schendan, H. E., & Stern, C. E. (2007). Where vision meets memory: Prefrontal-posterior networks for visual object constancy during categorization and recognition. *Cerebral Cortex, 18*(7), 1695–1711.

Schenk, T., & Zihl, J. (1997). Visual motion perception after brain damage: II. Deficits in form-from-motion perception. *Neuropsychologia, 35*, 1299–1310.

Scherer, S.W., & Osborne, L. R. (2007). Williams-Beuren syndrome. In P. Stankiewicz & J. R. Lupski (Eds.), *Genomic disorders: The genomic basis of disease* (pp. 221–236). Totowa, NJ: Humana Press.

Scherf, K. S., Behrmann, M., Humphreys, K., & Luna, B. (2007). Visual category-selectivity for faces, places and objects emerges along different developmental trajectories. *Developmental Science, 10*(4), F15–F30.

Scherf, K. S., Behrmann, M., Kimchi, R., & Luna, B. (2009). Emergence of global shape processing continues through adolescence. *Child Development, 80*(1), 162–177.

Schiltz, C., & Rossion, B. (2006). Faces are represented holistically in the human occipito-temporal cortex. *NeuroImage, 32*(3), 1385–1394.

Schmitt, J. E., Eliez, S., Warsofsky, I. S., Bellugi, U., & Reiss, A. L. (2001). Corpus callosum morphology of Williams syndrome: Relation to genetics and behavior. *Developmental Medicine and Child Neurology, 43*(03), 155–159.

Scholl, B. J. (2009). What have we learned about attention from multiple object tracking (and vice versa)? In D. Dedrick & L. Trick (Eds.), *Computation, cognition, and Pylyshyn* (pp. 49–78). Cambridge, MA: MIT Press.

Shusterman, A., & Spelke, E. S. (2005). Language and the development of spatial reasoning. In P. Curruthers, S. Laurence, & S. Stitch (Eds.), *The innate mind: Structure and content* (pp. 89–108). New York: Oxford University Press.

Simon, T. J. (2007). Cognitive characteristics of children with genetic syndromes. *Child and Adolescent Psychiatric Clinics of North America, 16*(3), 599–616.

Skoczenski, A. M., & Norcia, A. M. (2002). Late maturation of visual hyperacuity. *Psychological Science, 13*(6), 537–541.

Sovrano, V. A., Bisazza, A., & Vallortigara, G. (2007). How fish do geometry in large and in small spaces. *Animal Cognition, 10*, 47–54.

Soechting, J. F., & Flanders, M. (1992). Moving in three-dimensional space: Frames of reference, vectors, and coordinate systems. *Annual Review of Neuroscience, 15*, 167–191.

Spelke, E. S. (1990). Principles of object perception. *Cognitive Science, 14*(1), 29–56.

Spelke, E. S. (2000). Core knowledge. *American Psychologist, 55*(11), 1233–1243.

Spelke, E. S., & Kinzler, K. D. (2007). Core knowledge. *Developmental Science, 10*(1), 89–96.

Street, S. Y., James, K. H., Jones, S. S., & Smith, L. B. (2011). Vision for action in toddlers: The posting task. *Child Development, 82*(6), 2083–2094.

Stromme, P., Bjomstad, P. G., & Ramstad, K. (2002). Prevalence estimation of Williams syndrome. *Journal of Child Neurology, 17*(4), 269.

Supalla, T. R. (1982). *Structure and acquisition of verbs of motion and location in American Sign Language*. Cambridge, MA: Bradford Books/MIT Press.

Suzuki, W. A., & Amaral, D. G. (1994). Perirhinal and parahippocampal cortices of the macaque monkey: Cortical afferents. *Journal of Comparative Neurology, 350*(4), 497–533.

Tager-Flusberg, H., Plesa-Skwerer, D., Faja, S., & Joseph, R. M. (2003). People with Williams syndrome process faces holistically. *Cognition, 89*(1), 11–24.

Talmy, L. (1978). The relation of grammar to cognition: A synopsis. *Proceedings of the 1978 Workshop on Theoretical Issues in Natural Language Processing*, 14–24.

Talmy, L. (1983). How language structures space. In H. Pick (Ed.), *Spatial orientations: Theory, research, and application* (pp. 225–282). New York: Plenum Press.

Tanaka, J. W., & Farah, M. J. (1993). Parts and wholes in face recognition. *Quarterly Journal of Experimental Psychology, 46A*, 225–245.

Tarr, M. J., & Pinker, S. (1989). Mental rotation and orientation-dependence in shape-recognition. *Cognitive Psychology, 21*(2), 233–282.

Tassabehji, M., Hammond, P., Karmiloff-Smith, A., Thompson, P., Thorgeirsson, S. S., Durkin, M. E., Popescu, N. C., Hutton, T., Metcalfe, K., Rucka, A., Stewart, H., Read, A. P., Maconochie, M., & Donnai, D. (2005). GTF2IRD1 in craniofacial development of humans and mice. *Science, 310*(5351), 1184–1187.

Tassabehji, M., Metcalfe, K., Karmiloff-Smith, A., Carette, M. J., Grant, J., Dennis, N., Reardon, W., Splitt, M., Read, A. P., & Donnai, D. (1999). Williams syndrome: Use of chromosomal microdeletions as a tool to dissect cognitive and physical phenotypes. *The American Journal of Human Genetics, 64*(1), 118–125.

Thomas, M. S. C., Karaminis, T. N., & Knowland, V. C. P. (2010). What is typical language development? *Language Learning and Development, 6*(2), 162–169.

Thomas, M., & Karmiloff-Smith, A. (2005). Can developmental disorders reveal the component parts of the human language faculty? *Language Learning and Development, 1*(1), 65–92.

Thomas, M. S. C., & Richardson, F. (2006). Atypical representational change: conditions for the emergence of atypical modularity. In Y. Munakata & M. H. Johnson (Eds.), *Processes of change in brain and cognitive development: Attention and performance XXI* (pp. 315–347). Oxford: Oxford University Press.

Tomaiuolo, F., Di Paola, M., Caravale, B., Vicari, S., Petrides, M., & Caltagirone, C. (2002). Morphology and morphometry of the corpus callosum in Williams syndrome: A T1-weighted MRI study. *Neuroreport, 13*(17), 2281–2284.

Tommasi, L., Gagliardo, A., Andrew, R. J., & Vallortigara, G. (2003). Separate processing mechanisms for encoding of geometric and landmark information in the avian hippocampus. *European Journal of Neuroscience, 17*, 1695–1702.

Trick, L. M., Jaspers-Fayer, F., & Sethi, N. (2005). Multiple-object tracking in children: The "catch the spies" task. *Cognitive Development, 20*(3), 373–387.

Turati, C., Bulf, H., & Simion, F. (2008). Newborns' face recognition over changes in viewpoint. *Cognition, 106*(3), 1300–1321.

Udwin, O., & Yule, W. (1991). A cognitive and behavioural phenotype in Williams syndrome. *Journal of Clinical and Experimental Neuropsychology, 13*, 232–244.

Ungerleider, L. G., & Mishkin, M. (1982). Two cortical visual systems. In D. J. Ingle, M. A. Goodale, & R. J. W. Mansfield (Eds.), *Analysis of visual behavior* (pp. 549–586). Cambridge, MA: MIT Press.

Vachon, P., Voss, P., Lassonde, M., Leroux, J. M., Mensour, B., Beaudoin, G., et al. (2009). Global motion stimuli and form-from-motion stimuli: Common characteristics and differential activation patterns. *International Journal of Neuroscience, 119*(10), 1584–1601.

Vaina, L. M., LeMay, M., Bienfang, D. C., Choi, A. Y., & Nakayama, K. (1990). Intact "biological motion" and "structure from motion" perception in a patient with impaired motion mechanisms: A case study. *Visual Neuroscience, 5*, 353–369.

Vaina, L. M., Solomon, J., Chowdhury, S., Sinha, P., & Belliveau, J. W. (2001). Functional neuroanatomy of biological motion perception in humans. *Proceedings of the National Academy of Sciences, 98*(20), 11656–11661.

Vallortigara, G., Zanforlin, M., & Pasti, G. (1990). Geometric modules in animals' spatial representations: A test with chicks (*Gallus gallus domesticus*). *Journal of Comparative Psychology, 104*, 248–254.

Van Essen, D. C., Dierker, D., Snyder, A. Z., Raichle, M. E., Reiss, A. L., & Korenberg, J. (2006). Symmetry of cortical folding abnormalities in Williams syndrome revealed by surface-based analyses. *Journal of Neuroscience, 26*(20), 5470.

Van Marle, K., & Scholl, B. J. (2003). Attentive tracking of objects versus substances. *Psychological Science, 14*(5), 498.

Vargas, J. P., Petruso, E. J., & Bingman, V. P. (2004). Hippocampal formation is required for geometric navigation in pigeons. *European Journal of Neuroscience, 20*, 1937–1944.

Vargha-Khadem, F., Gadian, D. G., Copp, A., & Mishkin, M. (2005). FOXP2 and the neuroanatomy of speech and language. *Nature Reviews Neuroscience, 6*, 131–138.

Vicari, S., Brizzolara, D., Carlesimo, G., Pezzini, G., & Volterra, V. (1996). Memory abilities in children with Williams syndrome. *Cortex, 32*, 503–514.

Wagner, R. K., Torgesen, J. K., Rashotte, C. A., & Pro-Ed. (1999). *Comprehensive test of phonological processing: CTOPP.* Austin, TX: Pro-Ed.

Wang, P. P., Doherty, S., Rourke, S. B., & Bellugi, U. (1995). Unique profile of visuo-perceptual skills in a genetic syndrome. *Brain and Cognition, 29*(1), 54–65.

Wang, R., & Spelke, E. (2002). Human spatial representation: Insights from animals. *Trends in Cognitive Science, 6*, 376–382.

Warrington, E. K. (1982). Neuropsychological studies of object recognition. *Philosophical Transactions of the Royal Society of London Series B: Biological Sciences, 298*(1089), 15–33.

Williams, J. C. P., Barratt-Boyes, B. G., & Lowe, J. B. (1961). Supravalvular aortic stenosis. *Stroke, 24*(6), 1311–1318.

Wills, T. J., Cacucci, F., Burgess, N., & O'Keefe, J. (2010). Development of the hippocampal cognitive map in preweanling rats. *Science, 328*(5985), 1573.

Wolfe, J. M., Place, S. S., & Horowitz, T. S. (2007). Multiple object juggling: Changing what is tracked during extended multiple object tracking. *Psychonomic Bulletin & Review, 14*(2), 344–349.

Xu, Y. D., & Chun, M. M. (2006). Dissociable neural mechanisms supporting visual short-term memory for objects. *Nature, 440*(7080), 91–95.

Xu, Y. D., & Chun, M. M. (2009). Selecting and perceiving multiple visual objects. *Trends in Cognitive Sciences, 13*(4), 167–174.

Xu, F., & Spelke, E. S. (2000). Large number discrimination in 6-month-old infants. *Cognition, 74*, B1–B11.

Yin, R. K. (1969). Looking at upside-down faces. *Journal of Experimental Psychology, 81*, 141–145.

Yovel, G., & Kanwisher, N. (2005). The neural basis of the behavioral face-inversion effect. *Current Biology, 15*(24), 2256–2262.

Zigler, E. (1967). Cultural/familial mental retardation: A continuing dilemma. *Science, 155*, 292–298.

Zilbovicius, M., Meresse, I., Chabane, N., Brunelle, F., Samson, Y., & Boddaert, N. (2006). Autism, the superior temporal sulcus and social perception. *Trends in Neurosciences, 29*(7), 359–366.

Zukowski, A. (2009). Elicited production of relative clauses in children with Williams syndrome. *Language and Cognitive Processes, 24*(1), 1–43.

Author Index

Note: Page numbers followed by "*f*" and "*t*" denote figures, and tables, respectively

Subject Index

Note: Page numbers followed by "*f*" and "*t*" denote figures, and tables, respectively